# Learning and Teaching
# NURSING

(A Book on Nursing Education and Educational Technology)

*As per the Revised INC Syllabus for BSc Nursing, 2021 (Also Covering the Old Syllabus)*

**FIFTH EDITION**

**B Sankaranarayanan** MSc N (Edn and Admn)
Principal
National Hospital College of Nursing
Calicut, Kerala, India

**Sindhu Gopinathan** BSc N
Principal
Baby Memorial School of Nursing
Calicut, Kerala, India

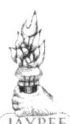

**JAYPEE BROTHERS MEDICAL PUBLISHERS**
*The Health Sciences Publisher*
New Delhi | London

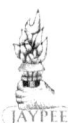 **Jaypee Brothers Medical Publishers (P) Ltd**

**Headquarters**
Jaypee Brothers Medical Publishers (P) Ltd.
EMCA House
23/23-B, Ansari Road, Daryaganj
New Delhi 110 002, India
Landline: +91-11-23272143, +91-11-23272703
+91-11-23282021, +91-11-23245672
E-mail: jaypee@jaypeebrothers.com

**Corporate Office**
Jaypee Brothers Medical Publishers (P) Ltd.
4838/24, Ansari Road, Daryaganj
New Delhi 110 002, India
Phone: +91-11-43574357
Fax: +91-11-43574314
E-mail: jaypee@jaypeebrothers.com

**Overseas Office**
JP Medical Ltd.
83, Victoria Street, London
SW1H 0HW (UK)
Phone: +44-20 3170 8910
E-mail: info@jpmedpub.com

**EU GPSR** Authorised Representative
Logos Europe, 9 rue Nicolas Poussin
17000, La Rochelle, France
Phone: +33 (0) 6 67 93 73 78
E-mail: Contact@logoseurope.eu

Website: www.jaypeebrothers.com
Website: www.jaypeedigital.com

© 2022, Jaypee Brothers Medical Publishers

The views and opinions expressed in this book are solely those of the original contributor(s)/author(s) and do not necessarily represent those of editor(s) of the book.

All rights reserved by the author. No part of this publication may be reproduced, stored or transmitted in any form or by any means, electronic, mechanical, photocopying, recording or otherwise, without the prior permission in writing of the publishers.

All brand names and product names used in this book are trade names, service marks, trademarks or registered trademarks of their respective owners. The publisher is not associated with any product or vendor mentioned in this book.

Medical knowledge and practice change constantly. This book is designed to provide accurate, authoritative information about the subject matter in question. However, readers are advised to check the most current information available on procedures included and check information from the manufacturer of each product to be administered, to verify the recommended dose, formula, method and duration of administration, adverse effects and contraindications. It is the responsibility of the practitioner to take all appropriate safety precautions. Neither the publisher nor the author(s)/editor(s) assume any liability for any injury and/or damage to persons or property arising from or related to use of material in this book.

This book is sold on the understanding that the publisher is not engaged in providing professional medical services. If such advice or services are required, the services of a competent medical professional should be sought.

Every effort has been made where necessary to contact holders of copyright to obtain permission to reproduce copyright material. If any have been inadvertently overlooked, the publisher will be pleased to make the necessary arrangements at the first opportunity.

Inquiries for bulk sales may be solicited at: jaypee@jaypeebrothers.com

*Learning and Teaching Nursing*

*Fourth Edition:* 2012
*Fifth Edition:* **2022**

ISBN: 978-93-5465-724-5

# Dedicated to

*Her holiness Shri Mata Amritanandamayi Devi*
for enabling the members of
Amrita Institute of Medical Sciences and Research Centre,
especially Dr SG Rao, Dr R Krishnakumar, Dr Suresh, Mrs Remani RN
and their team to rekindle the light of our life in
an exceptionally miraculous manner

# PREFACE TO THE FIFTH EDITION

A profession is a dynamic integration of various faculties of knowledge. Moreover, knowledge is the quickest and safest path to success in any area of life. Since nursing is a caring profession, lack of knowledge from the part of nurses may give rise to unforgiving mistakes. Thus, it is the duty of all nursing professionals to acquire knowledge and transfer it to the future generations. This will in turn contribute to the development of our profession. This text serves its very purpose by equipping you to attain the nursing expertise in a commendable manner and thereafter transferring it in a comprehensible way. Considering the transnational acceptance of our profession, this book prepares men and women for the rewarding career of nursing in an international environment.

## Who will Benefit from this Book?

All categories of nursing professionals and nursing students will benefit from knowing how to acquire knowledge and transferring it to others in a fruitful manner. As such, this book is prepared as a lifelong companion to all nursing professionals who wish to share their nursing expertise to future generations. The content of this book meticulously satisfies the requirements of graduate as well as postgraduate students. Unlike other healthcare professions, in nursing the knowledge of its members working in the clinical area is neither preserved nor transferred properly. Perhaps, this may be the main obstacle in our journey towards a more independent practice. This book will help the nurses working in the clinical area to transfer their knowledge in a comprehensible manner. Since nurses working in the clinical area represent the cream of our profession, this will contribute to the development of our profession. The aim behind this work is not to redefine the concept of nursing education but to refine it in a student friendly manner. It is earnestly hoped that the simple yet authentic explanation followed throughout this book with the help of suitable examples will make the subject of nursing education more palatable and interesting to the nursing community.

## Organization of the Book

Essentials of nursing education is explained by way of 14 well organized chapters, which are especially designed to serve the very purpose of this book. Depending on your need, you can select the type and volume of information. *Chapter 1* deals with the basis of general education and nursing education. *Chapter 2* explains the philosophy of nursing education in the simplest way. *Chapter 3* brilliantly narrates the various aspects of educational objectives. *Chapter 4* is concerned with nursing curriculum. Under nursing curriculum all practical aspects of nursing education like course planning, unit planning and lesson planning are discussed properly. *Chapter 5* on learning will guide you in acquiring nursing skills in a commendable manner. *Chapter 6* deals with the various aspects of teaching–learning process and teaching–learning methods. *Chapter 7* deals with teaching and learning in the digital age. *Chapter 8* deals with communication and human relations. *Chapter 9* will assist you in the judicious use of audiovisual aids. *Chapter 10* explains all about evaluation in a down-to-earth manner. *Chapter 11* is devoted to the vital component of present day education system namely guidance and counseling. *Chapter 12* describes discipline in a very concise manner. *Chapter 13* describes ethics and evidence-based nursing education. *Chapter 14* deals with communication and human relations.

## Revision Work for this Edition

This fifth edition is the result of the feedback and encouragement we received from the stakeholders of nursing education. While contents that are relevant has been retained many new content areas have been added and many others updated and expanded. Four new chapters namely "Teaching and learning nursing in digital age", classroom management, ethics and evidence-based nursing education and Communication and Human Relations is added for **complying with new Indian Nursing Council Syllabus.**

## Chapter by chapter content changes are as follows:

*Chapter 1: Basis of Nursing Education*
- New description of meaning of education.
- New description of concept of education.
- New description of principles of education.
- Update on aims of education.
- New description of transformational education.
- New description of relationship-based education.
- New description of competency-based education.
- New description of value education.
- New description of education and life.
- New description of factors influencing trends in education.
- Update on trends in education.
- Update on aims of nursing education.
- Update on trends in nursing education.
- New description of issues in nursing education.
- New description of challenges before nursing education.

*Chapter 2: Philosophy and Education*
- Update on meaning of philosophy.
- Update on educational philosophy.
- New description of functions of educational philosophy.
- New description of importance of educational philosophy.
- New description of philosophy and teacher.
- New description of eclecticism as philosophy of nursing education.

*Chapter 3: Educational Objectives*
- Update on definition of educational objectives.
- New description of purpose of educational objectives.
- New description of revised Bloom's taxonomy.
- New description of Bloom's taxonomy and nursing education.
- New description of criteria of behavioral objectives.
- New description of writing good objectives.
- New description of setting learner friendly objectives for teaching nursing.

*Chapter 4: Curriculum*
- New description of components of curriculum.
- Update on criteria for a desirable curriculum.
- Update on types of curriculum.
- New description of nature of twenty first century curriculum.
- New description of steps in developing official curriculum.
- New description of aspects of curriculum development.
- New description of constraints in the selection of learning experience.

❖ New description of curriculum for excellence in nursing education.
❖ New description of concept of happiness curriculum and nursing education.
❖ New description of principles of unit planning.
❖ New description of steps in unit planning.
❖ New description of criteria of lesson planning.

Chapter 5: Learning
❖ New description of definition of learning.
❖ New description of modern concepts of learning.
❖ New description of characteristics of learning.
❖ New description of factors influencing learning.
❖ New description of principles of learning.
❖ New description of nature of learning.
❖ New description of barriers to learning.
❖ New description of first principles thinking and learning.
❖ New description of approaches to learning.
❖ New description of determinants of learning.
❖ New description of types of learners.
❖ New description of characteristics of present day learners.
❖ New description of emotional intelligence and learning.
❖ New description of environment and learning.
❖ New description of definition of learning nursing.
❖ New description of principles of learning nursing.
❖ New description of active learning strategies.

Chapter 6: Teaching–Learning Methods
❖ New description of learner-centered principles of teaching.
❖ New description of Hay Mcber model of teacher effectiveness.
❖ New description of reflective teacher.
❖ Update on qualities of a good teacher.
❖ New description of teacher expectations.
❖ New description of teaching styles.

Chapter 7: Teaching And Learning Nursing Digital Age (New Chapter)

Chapter 8: Classroom Management (New Chapter)

Chapter 9: Introduction to Educational Technology
❖ New description of impact of technology in teaching.
❖ New description of relationship between technology and media.
❖ New description of selecting appropriate media.
❖ New description of trends education technology.

Chapter 10: Evaluation
❖ Update on definition of evaluation.
❖ New description of components of evaluation.
❖ Update on definition of assessment.
❖ Update on summative evaluation.
❖ Update on formative evaluation.
❖ Update on difference between formative and summative evaluation.
❖ New description of continuous comprehensive evaluation.
❖ Updates on clinical evaluation.

Chapter 11: Guidance and Counseling
❖ Update on concept of guidance.

- ❖ Update on concept of counseling.
- ❖ Update on need for guidance and counseling.
- ❖ Update on purposes of guidance and counseling.
- ❖ New description of guidance functions of teachers.
- ❖ New description of issues in guidance and counseling.

*Chapter 12: Discipline*
- ❖ Update on definition of discipline.
- ❖ New description of preventive discipline.
- ❖ New description of discipline with dignity.
- ❖ New description of eclectic approach to discipline.
- ❖ New description of practical approach to discipline.

*Chapter 13: Ethics and Evidence-based Nursing Education (New Chapter)*

*Chapter 14: Communication and Human Relations*
- ❖ Update on significance of communication in nursing
- ❖ New description of principles of communication
- ❖ New description of types of communication
- ❖ New description on media and channels of communication
- ❖ New description on principles of effective communication in nursing practice
- ❖ New description on effective communication in clinical area
- ❖ New description on standardized communication tools
- ❖ New description on assertive communication
- ❖ New description on definition of interpersonal relationships
- ❖ New description on importance of interpersonal relationships in nursing
- ❖ New description on human relations skill in nursing
- ❖ New description on understanding self and nursing practice
- ❖ New description on social behavior and nursing practice

**B Sankaranarayanan**
**Sindhu Gopinathan**

# ACKNOWLEDGMENTS

We are deeply indepted to Almighty for enabling us to complete this project in a fine manner. Our humble pranams to Shri Mata Amritanandamayi Devi for all blessings and care.

We thank Dr Sunil PR, Assistant Professor, Sree Chitra Tirunal Institute for Medical Sciences and Technology (SCTIMST), Thiruvananthapuram, Kerala, India, for motivating us to go ahead with this project.

We thank our parents, teachers, brothers and sisters for their encouragement and support. We are grateful to all authors and publishers whose works we have made use of in the preparation of this publication.

We are grateful to our well-wishers especially, students and nursing faculty for their ongoing support and encouragement.

# CONTENTS

1. **Basis of Nursing Education**     1
   - Meaning of Education   1
   - Concept of Education   2
   - Definition   5
   - Principles of Education   6
   - Education as a Process   8
   - Education as a Lifelong Process   9
   - Components and Characteristics of Educative Process   11
   - Functions of Education   11
   - Aims of Education   13
   - Value Education   16
   - Transformational Education   16
   - Relationship-based Education   16
   - Competency-based Education   17
   - Education and Life   19
   - Agencies of Education   19
   - Factors Influencing Trends in Education   19
   - Current Trends in Education   20
   - Nursing Education   23

2. **Philosophy and Education**     33
   - Meaning   33
   - Definition   34
   - Branches of Philosophy   34
   - Relationship between Philosophy and Education   34
   - Educational Philosophy   35
   - Educational Philosophy and the Teacher   37
   - Educational Philosophies   37
   - Theistic Realism or Supernaturalism   49
   - Humanistic Existentialism   49
   - Eclecticism   50
   - Philosophy of Nursing Education   51
   - Eclecticism as Philosophy of Nursing Education   52

3. **Educational Objectives**     56
   - Definition   56
   - Purpose of Educational Objectives   56
   - Classification of Educational Objectives   57
   - Bloom's Taxonomy of Educational Objectives   58
   - Bloom's Taxonomy and Central Objective   62
   - Bloom's Taxonomy and Nursing Education   63
   - Revised Bloom's Taxonomy   63
   - Qualities of an Educational Objective   64
   - Criteria of Behavioral Objective   65
   - Meaningful Statement of Objectives   65
   - Components of a Behavioral Objective   66
   - Advantages of Writing Behavioral Objectives   66
   - Writing Good Objectives   66
   - Setting Learner-friendly Objectives for Teaching Nursing   67
   - Strengths of Behavioral Objectives   67
   - Weaknesses of Behavioral Objectives   68

4. **Curriculum**     70
   - Meaning and Definition   70
   - Modern Concept of Curriculum   71
   - Models of Curriculum   71
   - Components of Curriculum   72
   - Components of Nursing Curriculum   73
   - Nature of Curriculum   74
   - Nature of Nursing Curriculum   74
   - Criteria for a Desirable Curriculum   74
   - Types of Curriculum   75
   - Nature of Twenty First Century Curriculum   78
   - Responsibility of Curriculum Development   79
   - Levels of Curriculum Planning   80
   - Elements in Planning a Curriculum   80
   - Organization of Curriculum   81
   - Curriculum Development   81
   - Steps in Developing Official Curriculum   81
   - Principles of Curriculum Development   84
   - Principles Related to the Development of Nursing Curriculum   85
   - Factors Influencing Curriculum Development in Nursing Education   86
   - Aspects of Curriculum Development   88
   - Steps in Curriculum Development in Nursing Education   88
   - Formulation of Educational Objectives   89
   - Selection of Learning Experiences   90
   - Organization of Learning Experiences   92
   - Organization of Clinical Experience   95
   - Evaluation of the Curriculum   96
   - Syllabus and Curriculum   97
   - Core Curriculum   97
   - Curriculum for Excellence in Nursing Education   97

- Concept of Happiness Curriculum and Nursing Education 98
- Curriculum Revision/Changing the Curriculum 98
- Course Outline Planning 100
- Unit Planning 101
- Lesson Planning 103

## 5. Learning 109
- Definition 109
- Key Concepts of Modern Learning 110
- Characteristics of Learning 110
- Factors Influencing Learning 111
- Principles of Learning 111
- Nature of Learning 113
- Learning Theories 113
- Barriers to Learning 116
- First Principles Thinking and Learning 117
- Types of Learning 117
- Approaches to Learning 119
- Active Learning Strategies 126
- Determinants of Learning 127
- Types of Learners 129
- Characteristics of Present-day Learners 130
- Emotional Intelligence and Learning 131
- Emotions and Learning 132
- Motivation and Learning 134
- Environment and Learning 137
- Definition of Learning Nursing 139
- Principles of Learning Nursing 140
- Remembering and Forgetting 140

## 6. Teaching–Learning Methods 143
- Meaning of Teaching 143
- Definition of Teaching 144
- Teaching is a Science as Well as an Art 144
- Teaching–Learning Process 144
- Principles of Teaching 145
- Learner-centered Principles of Teaching 147
- Qualities/Marks of Good Teaching 148
- Maxims of Teaching 150
- Teaching Styles 152
- Characteristics of Effective Teaching 153
- Teaching Skills 154
- Use of Examples 156
- Questions and Questioning 157
- Qualities of a Good Teacher 159
- The Hay McBer Model of Teacher Effectiveness 161
- Reflective Teacher 162
- Teacher Expectations 162
- Teacher–student Interaction 162
- Teacher Awarenesses 163
- Feedback in Teaching–Learning Process 164
- Teachable Moments 165
- Qualities of a Good Nurse Educator 166
- Teaching–Learning Methods 166
- Lecture Method 169
- Interactive Lecture 173
- Demonstration 174
- Discussion 176
- Seminar and Symposium 180
- Seminar 181
- Symposium 183
- Simulations 184
- Role Playing 188
- Microteaching 188
- Teaching Nursing 191
- Clinical Teaching 193
- Assignment 202

## 7. Teaching and Learning Nursing in Digital Age 206
- Online Education 206
- Digital Teaching 206
- Online Teaching in Nursing Education 211
- Online Learning 218
- Evidence-based Teaching in Nursing 221
- Innovative Teaching Methods in Nursing 222
- Types of Innovative Teaching Methods in Nursing 222

## 8. Classroom Management 227
- Definition 227
- Goals of Classroom Management 228
- Principles of Classroom Management 229
- Strategies for Effective Classroom Management 230
- Importance of Classroom Management 231
- Components of Classroom Management (The Three C's of Classroom Management) 232
- Factors Influencing Classroom Management 233
- Practical Guidelines for Classroom Management 234
- Classroom Communication 234

## 9. Introduction to Educational Technology 244
- Meaning 244
- Definition 245
- Development of Educational Technology 245

- Types of Educational Technology  246
- Characteristics of Educational Technology  247
- General Objectives of Educational Technology  247
- Advantages of Educational Technology  248
- Scope of Educational Technology  248
- Significance of Educational Technology  249
- Role of Technology in Education  249
- Impact of Technology in Teaching  251
- Technology and Media  252
- Selecting Appropriate Media  252
- Trends in Educational Technology  253
- Audiovisual Aids  253
- Computers in Nursing Education  269

## 10. Evaluation  275
- Meaning and Definition  275
- Components of Evaluation  276
- Assessment  276
- Evaluation, Measurement, Assessment, and Testing  276
- Difference between Assessment and Evaluation  277
- General Principles of Evaluation  278
- Characteristics of Evaluation  279
- Purposes of Evaluation  280
- Purposes in Nursing Education  280
- Objective-based Evaluation  280
- Functions of Evaluation  280
- Types of Evaluation  282
- Continuous Comprehensive Evaluation  285
- Steps in Evaluation  286
- Techniques and Tools of Evaluation  286
- Observation  286
- Anecdotal Records  288
- Rating Scales  288
- Checklists  291
- Cumulative Record  292
- Achievement Tests  292
- Selection of Appropriate Test Item  292
- Objective Test  292
- Short Answer Items  293
- True-false or Alternative-response Items  294
- Multiple Choice Item  294
- Multiple-response Item  298
- Matching Item  299
- Essay Tests  300
- Suggestions for the Essay Tests  301
- Oral Examinations  304
- Practical Examinations  305
- Qualities of an Evaluation Tool/ Characteristics of a Good Achievement Test  305
- Construction and Administration of Achievement Test  307
- Test Administration  309
- Clinical Evaluation  310
- Clinical Evaluation Process  312
- Internal Assessment  312
- Self-assessment and Self-reporting Techniques  313

## 11. Guidance and Counseling  315
- Guidance  315
- Counseling  317
- Differentiation of Guidance and Counseling  318
- Bases of Guidance and Counseling  319
- Functions of Guidance and Counseling  320
- Purposes of Guidance and Counseling  321
- Need of Guidance and Counseling  321
- Need for Guidance and Counseling in Nursing Education  322
- Aims of Guidance  323
- Principles of Guidance  323
- Guidance Areas  325
- Educational Guidance  325
- Vocational Guidance  326
- Personal Guidance  327
- Social Guidance  328
- Avocational Guidance  329
- Health Guidance  329
- Financial Guidance  330
- Guidance and Counseling Services  330
- Admission Service  330
- Orientation Service  330
- Student Information Service  331
- Information Service  331
- Counseling Service  332
- Placement Service  332
- Remedial Service  333
- Follow-up Service  333
- Research Service  333
- Evaluation Service  333
- Guidance and Counseling Personnel  334
- Guidance Functions of Teachers  334
- What Guidance is Not?  334
- Purposes of Student Counseling  335
- When Counseling is Required?  335
- Who Should be Counseled?  335
- Class Teachers as Counselors  335
- Levels of Counseling  336

- Classification of Counseling  336
- Different Counseling Techniques/ Approaches to Counseling  337
- Phases of Counseling  337
- Counseling Interview  338
- Qualities of a Good Counselor  339
- Problems in Student Counseling  339
- Organization of Guidance and Counseling Services  341
- Forms of Organization  341
- Basic Concepts Related to Guidance and Counseling Services  342
- Requirements for Organizing Guidance and Counseling Services  342
- Guidance Committee  342
- Principles of Organization of Guidance Services  343
- Organization of Guidance and Counseling Services in Nursing Institutions  343
- Issues in Guidance Program  344

## 12. Discipline  347
- Meaning and Definition  347
- Modern Concept of Discipline  348
- Need for Discipline  348
- Functions of Discipline  348
- Aims of Discipline  349
- Principles of Discipline  349
- Types of Discipline  349
- Self-discipline  350
- Assertive Discipline  350
- Preventive Discipline  350
- Discipline with Dignity  350
- Eclectic Approach to Discipline  351
- Discipline Strategies/Approaches  351
- Specific Measures to Maintain Classroom Discipline  351
- Practical Guidelines to Discipline  353

## 13. Ethics and Evidence-based Nursing Education  355
- Ethics-review  355
- Ethical Decision Making  356
- Ethical Standards for Students  358
- Value-based Education in Nursing  358
- Value Development Strategies  358
- Evidence-based Education  359
- Student-Faculty Relationship  361
- Information and Communication Technologies in Education  361

## 14. Communication and Human Relations  365
- Communication Process  365
- Interpersonal Relationship  376
- Human Relations  379
- Information, Education and Communication for Health  383
- Using Mass Media  387

*Bibliography*  389

*Index*  403

# Educational Technology/Nursing Education

(Revised INC Syllabus for BSc Nursing, 2021)

**PLACEMENT:** V SEMESTER

**THEORY:** 2 Credits (40 hours)

**PRACTICUM:** Lab/Practical: 1 Credit (40 hours)

**DESCRIPTION:** This course is designed to help the students to develop knowledge, attitude and beginning competencies essential for applying basic principles of teaching and learning among individuals and groups both in educational and clinical settings. It also introduces basics of curriculum planning and organization. It further enables students to participate actively in team and collaborative learning.

**COMPETENCIES:** On completion of the course, the students will be competent to:
- Develop basic understanding of theoretical foundations and principles of teaching and learning.
- Identify the latest approaches to education and learning.
- Initiate self-assessment to identify one's own learning styles.
- Demonstrate understanding of various teaching styles that can be used, based on the learner's readiness and generational needs.
- Develop understanding of basics of curriculum planning and organizing.
- Analyze and use different teaching methods effectively that are relevant to student population and settings.
- Make appropriate decisions in selection of teaching learning activities integrating basic principles.
- Utilize active learning strategies that enhance critical thinking, team learning and collaboration.
- Engage in team learning and collaboration through interprofessional education.
- Integrate the principles of teaching and learning in selection and use of educational media/technology.
- Apply the principles of assessment in selection and use of assessment and evaluation strategies.
- Construct simple assessment tools/tests integrating cognitive, psychomotor and affective domains of learning that can measure knowledge and competence of students.
- Develop basic understanding of student guidance through mentoring and academic advising
- Identify difficult situations, crisis and disciplinary/grievance issues experienced by students and provide appropriate counseling.
- Engage in ethical practice in educational as well as clinical settings based on values, principles and ethical standards.
- Develop basic understanding of evidence-based teaching practices.

## COURSE OUTLINE
### T – Theory, P – Practical (Laboratory)

| Unit | Time (Hours) T | Time (Hours) P | Learning outcomes | Contents | Teaching/ learning activities | Assessment methods |
|---|---|---|---|---|---|---|
| I | 6 | 3 | Explain the definition, aims, types, approaches and scope of educational technology | **Introduction and Theoretical Foundations** <br> *Education and educational technology:* <br> ➢ Definition, aims <br> ➢ Approaches and scope of educational technology <br> ➢ Latest approaches to education: <br>   – Transformational education <br>   – Relationship-based education <br>   – Competency-based education | Lecture-cum-discussion | Quiz |
| | | | Compare and contrast the various educational philosophies | *Educational philosophy:* <br> ➢ Definition of philosophy, education and philosophy <br> ➢ Comparison of educational philosophies <br> ➢ Philosophy of nursing education | | |
| | | | Explain the teaching learning process, nature, characteristics and principles | *Teaching learning process:* <br> ➢ Definitions <br> ➢ Teaching learning as a process <br> ➢ Nature and characteristics of teaching and learning <br> ➢ Principles of teaching and learning <br> ➢ Barriers to teaching and learning <br> ➢ Learning theories <br> ➢ Latest approaches to learning <br>   – Experiential learning <br>   – Reflective learning <br>   – Scenario-based learning <br>   – Simulation based learning <br>   – Blended learning | Group exercise: Create/discuss scenario-based exercise | Assessment of assignment: Learning theories—analysis of any one |

| Unit | Time (Hours) T | Time (Hours) P | Learning outcomes | Contents | Teaching/ learning activities | Assessment methods |
|---|---|---|---|---|---|---|
| II | 6 | 6 | Identify essential qualities/attributes of a teacher | **Assessment and Planning** *Assessment of teacher:* ➢ Essential qualities of a teacher ➢ Teaching styles: Formal authority, demonstrator, facilitator, delegator *Assessment of learner:* ➢ Types of learners ➢ Determinants of learning– learning needs, readiness to learn, learning styles ➢ Today's generation of learners and their skills and attributes ➢ Emotional intelligence of the learner ➢ Motivational factors —personal factors, environmental factors and support system **Curriculum Planning** Curriculum—definition, types ➢ Curriculum design— components, approaches ➢ Curriculum development —factors influencing curriculum development, facilitators and barriers ➢ Writing learning outcomes/ behavioral objectives ➢ Basic principles of writing course plan, unit plan and lesson plan | Lecture-cum-discussion  **Self-assessment exercise:** ➢ Identify your learning style using any learning style inventory (e.g. Kolb's learning style inventory) ➢ Lecture-cum-discussion  **Individual/ group exercise:** ➢ Writing learning outcomes ➢ Preparation of a lesson plan | ➢ Short answer ➢ Objective type  **Assessment of assignment:** Individual/ Group |
| | | | Describe the teaching styles of faculty | | | |
| | | | Explain the determinants of learning and initiates self-assessment to identify own learning style | | | |
| | | | Identify the factors that motivate the learner | | | |
| | | | Define curriculum and classify types | | | |
| | | | Identify the factors influencing curriculum development | | | |
| | | | Develop skill in writing learning outcomes, and lesson plan | | | |
| III | 8 | 15 | Explain the principles and strategies of classroom management | **Implementation** *Teaching in classroom and skill lab—teaching methods:* ➢ Classroom management— principles and strategies ➢ Classroom communication - Facilitators and barriers to classroom communication - Information communication technology (ICT)—ICT used in education | Lecture-cum-discussion | ➢ Short answer ➢ Objective type |

| Unit | Time (Hours) T | Time (Hours) P | Learning outcomes | Contents | Teaching/ learning activities | Assessment methods |
|---|---|---|---|---|---|---|
| | | | Describe different methods/strategies of teaching and develop beginning skill in using various teaching methods | Teaching methods—features, advantages and disadvantages<br>➢ Lecture, group discussion, microteaching<br>➢ Skill lab—simulations, demonstration and re-demonstration<br>➢ Symposium, panel discussion, seminar, scientific workshop, exhibitions<br>➢ Role play, project<br>➢ Field trips<br>➢ Self-directed learning (SDL)<br>➢ Computer-assisted learning<br>➢ One-to-one instruction | ➢ Practice teaching/ micro-teaching<br>➢ Exercise (peer teaching)<br>➢ Patient teaching session<br>➢ Construction of game – puzzle<br>➢ Teaching in groups— inter-disciplinary | Assessment of micro-teaching |
| | | | Explain active learning strategies and participate actively in team and collaborative learning | Active learning strategies:<br>➢ Team-based learning<br>➢ Problem-based learning<br>➢ Peer sharing<br>➢ Case study analysis<br>➢ Journaling<br>➢ Debate<br>➢ Gaming<br>➢ Inter-professional education | | |
| IV | 3 | 3 | Enumerate the factors influencing selection of clinical learning experiences | **Teaching in the Clinical Setting—Teaching Methods**<br>➢ Clinical learning environment<br>➢ Factors influencing selection of clinical learning experiences<br>➢ Practice model<br>➢ Characteristics of effective clinical teacher | Lecture-cum-discussion | Short answer |
| | | | Develop skill in using different clinical teaching strategies | ➢ Writing clinical learning outcomes/practice competencies<br>➢ Clinical teaching strategies —patient assignment— clinical conference, clinical presentation/bedside clinic, case study/care study, nursing rounds, concept mapping, project, debate, game, role play, PBL, questioning, written assign-ment, process recording | Writing clinical outcomes— assignments in pairs | Assessment of written assignment |

| Unit | Time (Hours) T | Time (Hours) P | Learning outcomes | Contents | Teaching/ learning activities | Assessment methods |
|---|---|---|---|---|---|---|
| V | 5 | 5 | Explain the purpose, principles and steps in the use of media<br><br>Categorize the different types of media and describe its advantages and disadvantages<br><br>Develop skill in preparing and using media | **Educational/Teaching Media**<br>➢ Media use—purpose, components, principles and steps<br>➢ Types of media<br>*Still visuals:*<br>➢ Nonprojected—drawings and diagrams, charts, graphs, posters, cartoons, board devices (chalk/white board), bulletin board, flannel board, flip charts, flash cards, still pictures/ photographs, printed materials-handout, leaflet, brochure, flyer<br>➢ Projected—film stripes, microscope, powerpoint slides, overhead projector<br>*Moving visuals:*<br>➢ Video learning resources —videotapes and DVD, blu-ray, USB flash drive<br>➢ Motion pictures/films<br>*Realia and models:*<br>➢ Real objects and models<br>*Audio aids/audio media:*<br>➢ Audiotapes/compact discs<br>➢ Radio and tape recorder<br>➢ Public address system<br>➢ Digital audio<br>*Electronic media/computer learning resources:*<br>➢ Computers<br>➢ Web-based videoconferencing<br>➢ E-learning, smart classroom<br>*Telecommunication (distance education):*<br>➢ Cable TV, satellite broadcasting, videoconferencing Telephones—telehealth/ telenursing<br>*Mobile technology* | Lecture-cum-discussion<br><br><br><br><br><br>Preparation of different teaching aids (integrate with practice teaching sessions) | ➢ Short answer<br>➢ Objective type<br><br><br><br><br>Assessment of the teaching media prepared |

| Unit | Time (Hours) T | Time (Hours) P | Learning outcomes | Contents | Teaching/ learning activities | Assessment methods |
|---|---|---|---|---|---|---|
| VI | 5 | 3 | ➤ Describe the purpose, scope, principles in selection of evaluation methods and barriers to evaluation.<br>➤ Explain the guidelines to develop assessment tests<br>➤ Develop skill in construction of different tests<br>➤ Identify various clinical evaluation tools and demonstrate skill in selected tests. | **Assessment/Evaluation Methods/Strategies**<br>➤ Purposes, scope and principles in selection of assessment methods and types<br>➤ Barriers to evaluation<br>➤ Guidelines to develop assessment tests<br>*Assessment of knowledge:*<br>➤ Essay type questions,<br>➤ Short answer questions (SAQ)<br>➤ Multiple choice questions (MCQ—single response & multiple response)<br>*Assessment of skills:*<br>➤ Clinical evaluation<br>➤ Observation (checklist, rating scales, videotapes)<br>➤ Written communication —progress notes, nursing care plans, process recording, written assignments<br>➤ Verbal communication (oral examination)<br>➤ Simulation<br>➤ Objective structured clinical examination (OSCE)<br>➤ Self-evaluation<br>➤ Clinical portfolio, clinical logs<br>*Assessment of attitude:*<br>➤ Attitude scales<br>*Assessment tests for higher learning:*<br>➤ Interpretive questions, hot spot questions, drag and drop and ordered response questions | Lecture-cum-discussion<br><br><br><br><br><br><br><br><br><br><br>Exercise on constructing assessment tool/s | ➤ Short answer<br>➤ Objective type<br><br><br><br><br><br><br><br><br><br>Assessment of tool/s prepared |
| VII | 3 | 3 | Explain the scope, purpose and principles of guidance. | **Guidance/Academic Advising, Counseling and Discipline**<br>*Guidance:*<br>➤ Definition, objectives, scope, purpose and principles<br>➤ Roles of academic advisor/ faculty in guidance | Lecture-cum-discussion | |

| Unit | T | P | Learning outcomes | Contents | Teaching/learning activities | Assessment methods |
|---|---|---|---|---|---|---|
| | | | • Differentiate between guidance and counseling<br>• Describe the principles, types, and counseling process<br>• Develop basic skill of counseling and guidance<br>• Recognize the importance of preventive counseling and develop skill to respond to disciplinary problems and grievance among students | *Counseling:*<br>• Difference between guidance and counseling<br>• Definition, objectives, scope, principles, types, process and steps of counseling<br>• Counseling skills/techniques—basics<br>• Roles of counselor<br>• Organization of counseling services<br>• Issues for counseling in nursing students<br>*Discipline and grievance in students:*<br>• Managing disciplinary/grievance problems—preventive guidance & counseling<br>• Role of students' grievance redressal cell/committee | • Role play on student counseling in different situations<br>• Assignment on identifying situations requiring counseling | • Assessment of performance in role play scenario<br>• Evaluation of assignment |
| VIII | 4 | 2 | • Recognize the importance of value-based education<br>• Develop skill in ethical decision making and maintain ethical standards for students<br>• Introduce knowledge of EBT and its application in nursing education | **Ethics and Evidence-based Teaching (EBT) in Nursing Education**<br>*Ethics – Review*<br>• Definition of terms<br>• Value based education in nursing<br>• Value development strategies<br>• Ethical decision making<br>• Ethical standards for students<br>• Student-faculty relationship<br>*Evidence-based teaching—introduction*<br>• Evidence-based education process and its application to nursing education | • Value clarification exercise<br>• Case study analysis (student encountered scenarios) and suggest ethical decision-making steps<br>• Lecture-cum-discussion | • Short answer<br>• Evaluation of case study analysis<br><br>Quiz—MCQ |

# CHAPTER 1: Basis of Nursing Education

## LEARNING OBJECTIVES

After completing this chapter, reader will be able to:

- Explain the meaning of education.
- Explain the concept of education.
- Define education.
- Explain education as a process.
- Identify the components of educative process.
- List down the characteristics of educative process.
- Explain the functions of education.
- Recognize the aims of education.
- Identify the types of education.
- Explain transformational education.
- Explain relationship-based education.
- Explain competency-based education.
- Realize the current trends in education.
- Define nursing education.
- Explain the aims of nursing education.
- Realize the current trends in nursing education.
- Identify issues in nursing education.
- Appreciate challenges facing by nursing education.

Quest for knowledge is an innate quality of human beings which makes them distinct from all other creations by God. This everlasting affinity towards knowledge fuelled all inventions ranging from fire in the prehistoric period to the cloning in the modern times. Ancient man recognized the need of organizing the knowledge for utilizing it to the maximum extent possible. This attempt to organize the knowledge has led to the development of education system. As time passed, there occurred a tremendous increase in the human needs, many of them arised from the man's desire to tame the nature for a better living. Increase in human needs demanded a more organized and specific knowledge for supporting special ventures. This led to the refining of the organized knowledge and ultimately resulted in the formation of separate branches of knowledge, which are specialized in particular areas of human activity. This specialization eventually gave birth to professions. Today, a perfect combination of services rendered by various professions makes this planet a better place to live. In this chapter, we will discuss the basis of general education and nursing education.

## MEANING OF EDUCATION

The word education is derived from the latin word *'educare'* which means to *'lead out'*. This derivation connotes *'growth from the within'*. Thus, the root meaning of education can be given as making manifest the inherent potential in a child. (The words child and student are used interchangeably throughout this book). The term education is derived from the latin word *'educere'* meaning to *'bring up'*, to *'train"* or to *'mould'*. According to this derivation, education is the bringing up of the child in a desirable manner. Some educationists believe that the word education has been derived from the two words 'e' and 'duco', 'e' means *'out off'* and 'duco' means *'to lead'*. 'Pedagogy' is another term which is commonly used for mentioning education.

This word is derived from two Greek words, namely 'pedo' (child) and logos (discussion) which means "science of instruction for the purpose of leading the pupils".

The idea of education is not merely to impart knowledge to the pupil in some subjects but to develop in him those habits and attitudes with which he may successfully face the future. In the narrow or technical sense, education stands for deliberate instruction or training providing to the child by the society through its various institutions during a particular time in order to modify his behavior. Broadly speaking, education refers to any act or experience that is intended to modify the behavior of an individual. Education is the product of experience. It is a dynamic complex process through which the experience of the race, i.e., knowledge, skills and attitudes are transmitted to the members of the community. Every society has to fulfill diversified needs in order to achieve progress and education is regarded as one of the best ways to fulfill these needs. Education is a purposeful process aimed at the development of human beings. It is concerned with directing the child in the matter of bringing out his hidden talents. In short, education is the act or process of acquiring and imparting knowledge, is crucial to the development of a learner with a view to his or her participation in the transformation of the world for a better tomorrow.

Life involves a constant and continuous modification of experience. Ideas change, attitudes and skills undergo an alteration. Education is the process of helping the child to adjust with this changing world. Such an adjustment is not a 'somehow' one but a 'superior adjustment'. The best type of education is that which guides the immature child to live his life richly and abundantly, at the same time to contribute to social betterment. By means of education the child is subjected to certain experiences that are intended to modify his behavior in order to bring about proper adjustment with the changing environment. In fact, education is the basis of life. For leading a purposeful and ideal life education is needed.

## CONCEPT OF EDUCATION

### Earlier Concept of Education

It is difficult to explain the concept of education due to its complex nature. The nature of education is influenced by various factors. As a result, education is viewed as a dynamic process. Earlier education is viewed under three categories **(Fig. 1.1)** namely traditional education, scientific education and progressive education.

Traditional education is subject-centered. It gives more importance to the subject matter. The level of learner or the needs of society is not given due consideration. Priority is given to preparation of logical organization and presentation of subject matter. Teacher is considered as an expert in the subject matter. Education is viewed as presentation of subject matter by the teacher. Students are considered as recipients of knowledge. The relevance of subject matter in terms of societal needs is also not considered.

Societal education is society-centered. It is the result of the development in psychology tests and measurements and experimentation. Education gives a careful consideration to the need of society. No adequate consideration is given for the needs of the learner or subject matter. Focus is on the measurement of abilities of children than their needs. Aim of scientific education is to prepare learners to meet societal needs when they become adults. Thus, scientific education is also considered as an adult-centered approach.

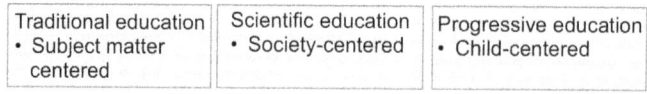

**Fig. 1.1:** Earlier concept of education.

Progressive education is child-centered education. It is based on the needs of the child. Teacher's role is that of a facilitator and guide. Teacher's duty is to observe the spontaneous actions of children and to study their emotional reactions. Subject matter and activities are selected according to the needs of the child. Experience in facing new situations prepares children for future life. Living fully and purposefully today gives practice in facing situations later in life. Rousseary, Pestalozzi, Froebel and Tolstoy recommended progressive education. In progressive education learning is an active, democratic and socialization process.

## Modern Concept of Education

Modern concept of education is a combination of traditional education, scientific education and progressive education with dominance to progressive education (**Fig. 1.2**). Modern concept is characterized by the stability and ideals of the traditional education, the accuracy and skills of scientific education and spontaneity and creativeness of the progressive education.

From the traditional education we adopt certain ideals and standards of belief and conduct such as cooperation, respect for laws, consideration for others, honesty, trust worthiness, etc.

From the scientific education we get the idea of curriculum based on the needs of public and society.

In modern concept of education dominance is for progressive education or child-centered education. Focus is on the development of the whole child and adequate understanding of the needs of the child.

Each child is unique. There is marked difference in capacity to learn, in interests, skills, habits and attitudes. Modern concept of education considers each child or student as a teaching unit instead of class. Considering each student as unique enable the student to make decisions to become self-directing, to be responsible for one's conduct, one's work and one's relation with others. Modern education contributes to effective living. Teacher's role is that of a facilitator and guide. The teacher sets the learning environment or situation that is comfortable, attractive and free from stress. A happy and constructive student-teacher relationship contributes

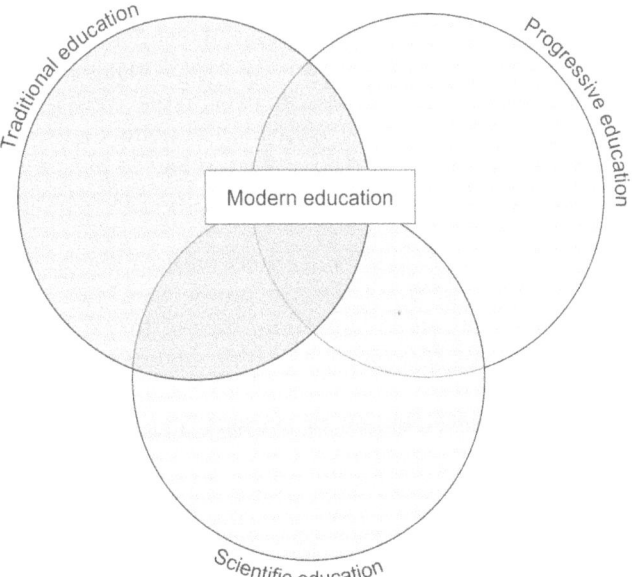

**Fig. 1.2:** Concept of modern education. Dominance to progressive education.

spontaneity and creativity. In such a situation there is more learning and less teaching, more study and action and less recitation. Moreover in such a situation, learning is considered as an active democratic and socialization process.

## 21st Century Concept of Education

Education in 21st century is perceived as a human asset that enhances knowledge, skills and potential to make human life much valuable. It is a lifelong process essential to lead a successful life. Nonformal type of education is also gaining importance due to easy access to knowledge. Modern education encourages collaboration than competition. Learning through collaboration is said to be one of the most effective forms of learning. Learning in groups enhances learning and critical thinking skills. Concept of education as an institutional process of face-to-face interaction between teacher and learner is slowly vanishing due to technological advancements. Now, educative process is possible at anytime and anywhere with the help of gadgets. Traditional roles of teacher and learner in the educative process is no longer valid. In modern education teacher is the facilitator of learning in a learner-centered context. In other words, modern education acknowledge that each student has a chance to learn outside the scope of school.

In a knowledge driven economy, need of creating valid knowledge is a concern of education. By attaining valid knowledge only youngsters can lead a fruitful life in the society. The ability of attaining valid knowledge is largely determined by the level of learners. To properly understand the level of learner, educationists need to understand the cognitive development of learners. Thus, modern education gives more importance to cognitive neuroscience for determining the learning needs of children.

In spite of all technological advancements 21st century education derives its vision from the word "educare" the word education comes from-meaning "developing oneself from within". Thus, modern education provides all encouragement to fulfill the abilities of a learner. By way of helping learners to fulfill the abilities, we can enhance their self-worth, their capabilities and their values for society as a whole.

Modern education follows a "All tech-All human" approach to achieve its aims, especially in the post COVID scenario. It utilizes all possibilities of technology to ensure easy access to knowledge at the same time utilize maximum human capital to generate knowledge, validate knowledge and impart knowledge. Technology can never replace teachers from the educative process. In this knowledge driven economy, education not only depends academicians and professionals to create valid knowledge but also all experienced personnel in the concerned field. The words "All human" denote the significance of experience in achieving the aims of education

All developments in education should be learner-centered then only aims of education can be achieved. From the **Figure 1.3** you can easily understand the concept of 21st century education. All developments related to education, related to technology, devices, media, content or subject matter teaching approaches, teaching methods, philosophical foundations, teacher–student interaction, evaluation, guidance and counseling, discipline, etc., should ultimately leads to all round development of learners. In short, 21st century concept of education is based on the following aspects:

- ❖ Education is perceived as human asset that enhances knowledge, skill and potential to make human life more valuable.
- ❖ Create valid knowledge to support a knowledge driven economy.
- ❖ **Focus on 6 C's of education like character, commitment (responsibility), communication, collaboration, critical thinking and creativity.**

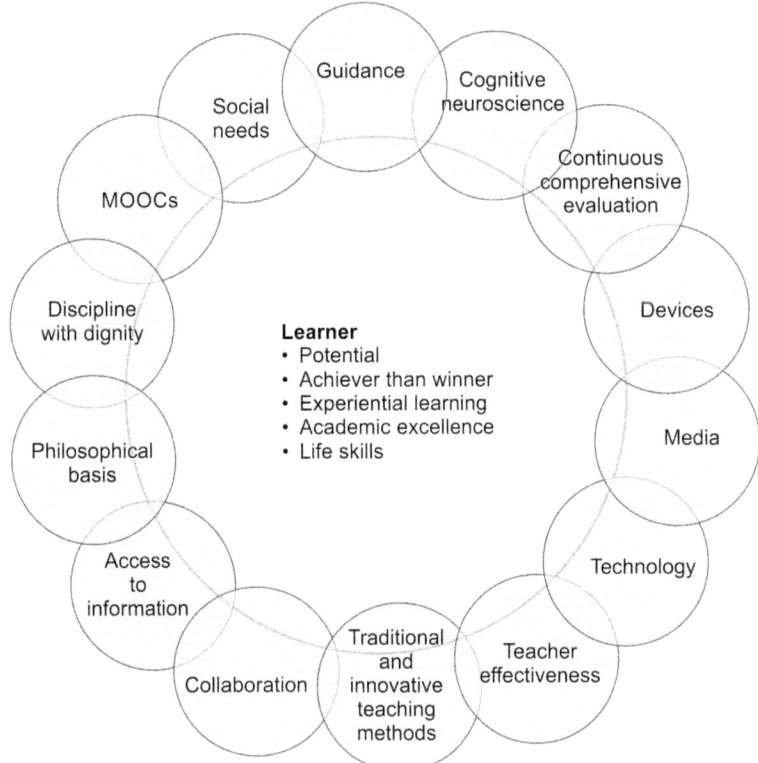

**Fig. 1.3:** Learner-centered "All human-All tech" 21st century concept of education.

- Education is a lifelong process.
- Learner should be the focus of all developments in education.
- Education should be based on a sound philosophical background.
- Human element in educative process is preserved without ignoring the role of technology in education.
- To address needs of learners all developments in education should consider recent developments in cognitive neuroscience and ways to access information.
- Aim of education is to make learner a good human being and achiever rather than winner. This can only be achieved by promoting collaboration than competition.
- Along with subject matter adequate consideration need to be given for life skills in education.
- Education should fulfil societal needs for by enabling learners to meet challenges faced by the society.
- Massive open online courses (MOOCs) influence education system in a big manner.
- Education process happens not only in institutions. It is possible at any time anywhere with the help of gadgets.

# DEFINITION

According to Pestalozzi, "education is the natural, harmonious and progressive development of man's innate powers". By virtue of birth itself man is endowed with hidden potentials or powers. This powers may be classified as physical, intellectual, aesthetic, social and spiritual powers. Education has to serve as a means for developing these powers in a harmonious manner. The term 'natural' denotes the need for considering the natural ability of the child while providing education, i.e., education has to consider the developmental needs of the child. The word 'progressive' indicates not only the steady increase in the development but also the development in the desirable direction.

As per John Dewey, "education is the development of all those capacities in the individual which will enable him to control his environment and fulfill his possibilities". This definition signifies the role of education in managing one's own immediate surroundings or environment in a productive manner. Moreover, this definition emphasize the need for providing rich and varied educational programs in order to develop different capacities of the student population. John Dewey recommends appropriate changes or innovations in the education system for preparing the youngsters to grab opportunities arising out of societal changes so that they can fulfill their possibilities in an admiring manner.

According to Mahatma Gandhi, "education is the all-round drawing out of the best in child and man—body, mind and spirit". Gandhiji believes that children are bestowed with tremendous vitality and curiosity to learn. They have within them the springs of youth, joy and vigour. 'Drawing out' the best from children by motivating or stimulating is the duty of the education rather than simply 'pouring in' information in a ready-made form. He also states that education is a process of developing three H's, i.e., head, heart and hand. By stating the development of head, heart and hand, He means the development of intellectual, spiritual and physical faculties of the child. All-round development is achieved through the proper and harmonious development of intellectual, spiritual and physical faculties. The best in man is related to three aspects, namely body, mind and spirit. All aspects should be given fair consideration because best in man is an end result of the harmonious development of these aspects. The practice of giving more attention to the intellectual ability or memory power rather than focusing on the all-round development by the present education system is cited as one of the reasons for the unrest prevailing among our youth. This problem would not have been of any significance, had we incorporated values of education envisaged by Gandhiji in our system of education properly.

## PRINCIPLES OF EDUCATION

Education is a planned and purposeful activity with several aims. In order to achieve these aims education need to be based on certain principles. As education is a complex process the following principles may not be sufficient to address all the cardinal aspects of education **(Fig. 1.4)**.

- ❖ **Learner-centered education:** This principle ensures learner participation in the educative process. The educative process is based on the needs of the learner. Each learner or child is unique. There is marked difference in capacity to learn in interests, skills, habits and attitudes. Modern education consider each child or student as a teaching unit instead of class.
- ❖ **Oriented to life:** The worth of education is measured by its contribution to the most effective living. Education should prepare the child to face the uncertainties as life in future. Education enable the student to think for oneself-the ability to make decisions to become self-directing, to be responsible for one's conduct, one's work and one's relation with others. Education prepares the child to utilize all possibilities of life. In short, education enable student to embrace life in the fullest manner.
- ❖ **Emphasis on learning by doing:** Learning is a permanent change in behavior that results from experience. As ultimate aim of education is behavior modification, emphasis should

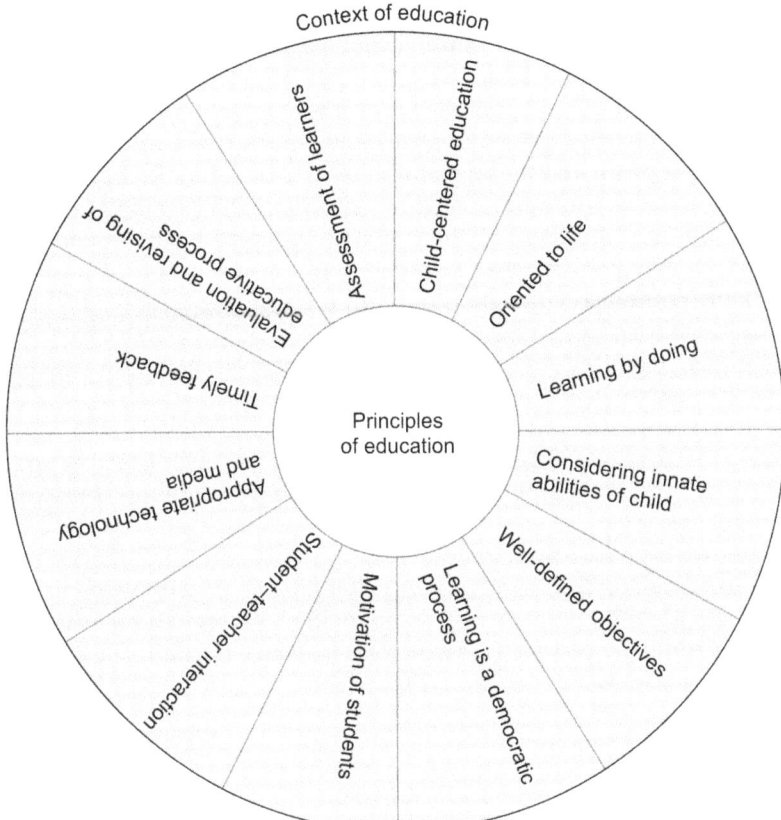

**Fig. 1.4:** Principles of education.

be given to learning from experience or learning by doing. Experience must be organized in some way to contribute to development, to facilitate learning and retention of skills. All experiences should be related to one another to form a unified whole. Learning should be active than passive. Learning situations that resembles life situations give opportunities for exploration, critical thinking and reasoning.

- ❖ **Consideration to innate potential or abilities of the child:** This principle is similar to first principle. Each child is blessed with innate potential or abilities. Education enables the child to realize his potential and utilize it properly for a good life.
- ❖ **Based on well-defined behavioral objectives:** Ultimate aim of education is behavior modification of learners. This is possible only when education is directed by well-defined educational objectives (*see* Chapter 3: Educational Objectives).
- ❖ **Learning is an active, democratic and socialization process:** The teacher sets the learning environment or situation that is comfortable, attractive and free from stress. In such as situation there is more learning and less teaching, more study and action and less recitation. In such a situation learning is considered as an active, democratic and socialization process.
- ❖ **Motivation of student is essential for fruitful learning:** The best teacher is one who inspires or motivates the students to achieve objectives of learning. Motivation is important in the teaching–learning process. Motivation arouses, sustains, directs and determines the intensity of learning effort. Learning becomes effective and pleasant only when children are motivated. Motivating the students is essential to make classroom instruction effective.

- **Positive student–teacher interaction is an integral part of educative process:** Teacher-student interaction is a two way communication process intended to bring out behavioral modification of the learner. A happy and constructive relationship between student and teacher is essential for fostering spontaneity and creativity among students. Positive student-teacher interaction contribute to constructive relationship between teacher and student.
- **Selection of appropriate technology and media:** No media can replace good teaching. Even then, selection of appropriate technology and media assists in achieving the aims of educative process. Affordability and quality of education can be enhanced by using appropriate technology and media.
- **Provide timely feedback:** Good feedback improves student learning. Timely feedback helps to correct shortcomings and reinforce good behaviors. When learner performance is not good frequent feedback sessions are essential. Feedback also helps teacher to analyze her own performance.
- **Assessment of learners:** Proper conduct of formative and summative evaluation is essential for achieving the aims of education. Formative evaluation is for learning and summative evaluation is of learning. Proper assessment also helps in finding shortcomings in the education process.
- **Evaluate and revise educative process:** Educative process is influenced by a variety of factors. We cannot predict what all factors will influence the education in what all ways. Thus, education is a multipolar as well as a dynamic process. Hence, periodic evaluation and revising of educative process is essential for making education relevant in accordance with the changing context of education **(Fig. 1.5)**.

# EDUCATION AS A PROCESS

Education is considered as a process as well as a product. From the above said definitions and meaning, it is clear that education is a process through which a child attains knowledge, skills, attitudes and other abilities required for leading a productive life in the society. As a product, education is the aggregate of what is acquired through learning, i.e., the knowledge, skills, ideas and values. Educative process mainly depends on the inherent potential of the child.

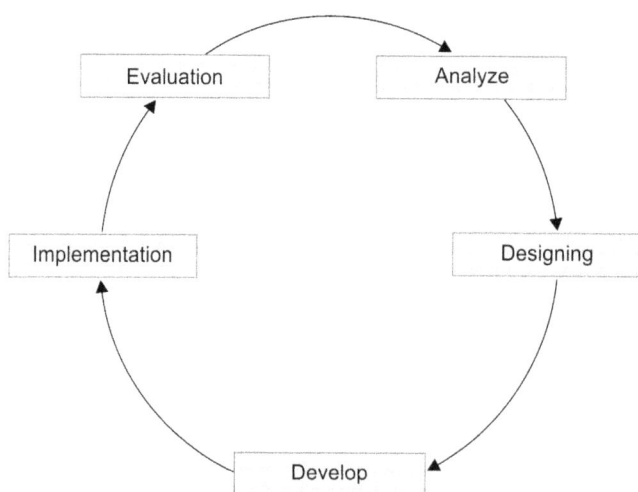

**Fig. 1.5:** Evaluation and revising of educative process.
*Source:* Aggarwal JC. Theory and principles of education. Vikas Publications;1993.

It is hoped that through the educative process teacher can bring out the hidden talents in the child by way of creating a conducive environment. Based on factors involved in the educative process, it can be viewed as a bipolar process, tripolar process or a multipolar process.

## Education as a Bipolar Process

Some educators view education as a bipolar process and believe that education is an end result of the interaction between the educator or teacher and the educant or student. Teacher imparts knowledge to the student with an intention to change latter's behavior. Educationists like Adams and Ross believe that education is essentially a bipolar process and recommends close cooperation and better understanding between the teacher and student for achieving the aims of education. Teacher should always consider the level of students. Even though teacher–student interaction is a vital component of the educative process, we cannot ignore the influence of social environment and technological advancements on the education system. In this sense, it is difficult to view education as a bipolar process.

## Education as a Tripolar Process

A considerable proportion of educationists believe that education is a tripolar process involving the interaction between the student, the teacher and the social environment. John Dewey believed that education is essentially a tripolar process. This view motivated educationists to consider the societal changes and social environment while constructing the curriculum. Tripolar process justifies the bilateral relationship between the society and education. Without undermining the contributions of the tripolar approach for the progress of education in the past, we have to say that it is incompetent to address the current issues in the educative process as it ignores the role of media and technology in the field of education.

## Education as a Multipolar Process

In order to cope with the fast changing and competitive nature of the world, one has to take up the responsibility for his or her own education. This new self-learning concept of education is influenced by several factors along with the teacher, student and the social environment. Easy access to knowledge due to the technological advancements and the increased acceptance of nonformal and informal types of education (*see* types of education) has reduced the importance of the teacher and school when compared to the past. Different from the past, present day education is flexible, more student-centered, focused on creativity than mere spoon-feeding by the teachers and depend heavily on technological advancements. In the present context, it is difficult to predict precisely what all factors will influence the education in what all ways. From the above said points, it is evident that the educative process is neither a bipolar process nor a tripolar process but a multipolar process only.

# EDUCATION AS A LIFELONG PROCESS

Education is now interpreted not as referring to an initial period of training of youth, but to a continual and lifelong process. It is not something that concerns itself with certain aims or philosophies nor does its responsibility end with devising some classroom techniques for the teacher. Education today aims at elevating itself to the level of a complex and comprehensive science with broader objectives. It now attempts to relate itself not merely to pedagogy but is conceived as andragogy, which according to Pierre Furter, is the science of training man throughout his life span.

According to J Deler, lifelong education is concerned about work and life, success in work that benefits the community, especially the younger generation. In a deeper level, lifelong education is about knowing oneself better and gaining a kind of self-esteem that helps one to deal effectively with problems of life. In short, lifelong education enable us to take control of our own lives irrespective of the circumstances.

Education as a lifelong process is based on four pillars of education:

1. **Learning to know:** During one's lifespan immense knowledge is generated and effective learning skills are needed to acquire this knowledge. Learning to know is concerned with developing effective learning skills or **"learning how to learn".**

   According to UNESCO, "Learning to know implies learning how to learn by developing one's concentration, memory skills and ability to think". Effective learning skills helps in acquiring knowledge for understanding the complexities of the modern world. Moreover, adequate knowledge provide a strong foundation for further learning.

   As a result of learning the children are transformed—they are more enlightened, more empowered and more enriched. In short, by learning how to learn throughout life, we can utilize the opportunities education provides throughout our life for a better living.

   This pillar of education demands more self-motivation, effort and critical thinking.

2. **Learning to do:** Learning to do is concerned with developing competence, attitude and aptitude for leading a productive life, Competence is much more than skill. Competence involves achieving mastery in a variety of skills. It is essential to perform skills with accuracy and speed. Skills can be broadly classified as occupational or professional skills and life skills or soft skills.

   An individual with competence and desirable attitude can easily achieve success in life. Competency helps to think creatively, critically and holistically. Moreover, competency helps to deal effectively with different situations in life. In short, a competent person can lead a successful life by possessing good problem solving skills, decision making skills and team building skills.

3. **Learning to be:** Learning to be focus on achieving the maximum overall development in the life span of an individual by utilizing opportunities with the help of education. The foremost aim of education is the development of innate potential of child or student. Learning to be is the way to become a good human being by fully developing innate potential and understanding oneself better. By becoming a good human being he can fulfill his commitment as individual, family member and a citizen.

   'Learning to be' is interpreted in one way as learning to be humane, by way of acquiring knowledge, skills and values essential for personality development. Personality development involves development of the intellectual, moral, cultural, emotional and physical capabilities of an individual. Learning to be is also concerned about the development of critical thinking, independent judgement power, personal commitment and responsibility. In effect, learning to be enables us to grow from within by understanding ourselves throughout life.

4. **Learning to live together:** As there exists lot of opportunities due to globalization, modern education promotes collaboration than competition. The aim is to be make the student an achiever than a winner. Education helps to understand others and realize the importance of shared purpose throughout life.

   Learning to live together aims development of understanding of oneself and others, empathy, cooperative social behavior, appreciation of diversity of human race and ability in working towards common objectives.

## COMPONENTS AND CHARACTERISTICS OF EDUCATIVE PROCESS

From analyzing the concept of education and the multipolar approach we can easily make out the below mentioned components and characteristics of the educative process. Components of educative process are knowledge, application of skills, understanding, comprehension, expression, appreciation, teaching, learning, initiation, instruction, training and indoctrination.

Among the components, knowledge enjoys a dominant position. Directly or indirectly all other components are involved in the transmission of knowledge. Education has its own ways and means to impart knowledge either in the ready-made form or motivating the child to hunt for knowledge by utilizing his inherent potentials.

### Characteristics

- **Education is a purposeful activity:** Irrespective of its formal, informal or nonformal nature, education is carried out with a purpose. The purpose may vary according to the needs of the child or demands by the society. Considering the alarming increase in the educational expenditure, educationists have to design cost-effective ways for achieving the purposes of education.
- **Education is a deliberate process:** Education is a process of deliberately guiding the development of pupils by the communication and manipulation of knowledge, which in its wake fosters needed skills and attitudes. We can also say that education is a deliberate process of transmitting all the resources and achievements of a complex society to the coming generations.
- **Education is a planned activity based on objectives:** This characteristic is somewhat similar to the first one. By and large education is a planned activity based on predetermined objectives. This is the most important feature of educative process. Unfortunately, this is the most neglected aspect also. Proper planning with short-term and long-term objectives are essential for developing a viable and fruitful education system. This characteristic highlights the need for a vision regarding the education so that it can contribute substantially for the national development. In order to react promptly to social changes and technological advancements in an effective manner, flexibility should be maintained while formulating objectives.
- **Educative process is influenced by the society, social changes and technological advancements:** Education and society are maintaining a bilateral relationship. Societal changes can influence education, at the same time education leads to social changes also. Success of any education system lies in understanding this reciprocative relationship between education and society. Technology of education is being developed not only with the aim of making education more widely available but also for improving the quality of education. Developments in technology will bring about changes and shifts in educational goals, which in turn result in the emergence of newer techniques.

## FUNCTIONS OF EDUCATION

Philosophers and educationists propose the following functions of education:
- **To complete the socialization process:** The main social objective of education is to complete the socialization process. With the emergence of nuclear families, the role of school and other institutions in the socialization process has increased considerably. The school trains the child to develop honesty, consideration for others and ability to distinguish between right and wrong. Socialization process also enables the child to cooperate with others and to

grow as a good citizen by respecting the laws framed by the society. Socialization is achieved through textbooks and learning experiences intended to develop social skills.

- **To transmit the cultural heritage:** All societies are proud to uphold or highlight their cultural heritage and ascertain that the culture is preserved and transmitted through social organizations to future generations. All types of education and all agencies of education have to carry out the function of cultural transmission in an earnest way by teaching the elements of culture like literature, history, art, philosophy, etc.
- **Formation of social personality:** Personality of individual members in a society shares some common features of the culture. Along with the process of transmitting culture, education also contributes to the formation of social personality. Formation of social personality helps man to adjust with his environment and flourish himself in cooperation with others.
- **Reformation of attitude:** In the developmental process, child may have incorporated some undesirable attitudes, beliefs and disbelief, loyalties, prejudices, jealousy, hatred, etc. It is the duty of the education to reform the undesirable attitudes and other negative aspects by means of removing the wrong beliefs, illogical prejudices and unreasoned loyalties from the child's mind. A collective effort by the school and home will bring out spectacular results in the matter of reforming attitudes.
- **Education for occupational placement—an instrument of livelihood:** Nowadays, this is regarded as the first and foremost function of education by a large section of people. This function is related to the practical aim of education and receiving more attention due to the diversified needs of the society. Education should prepare students not only to foresee the future occupational position but also enable them to attain it in an impressive way. The relevance of this function is evident from the importance we are giving to vocational training.
- **Conferring of status:** It is understood that an individual's status in the society is determined by the amount and type or kind of education he has received. In the current situation, the kind of knowledge one is gaining is important than the amount. For example, a graduate nurse or a diploma nurse can flourish anywhere in the world compared to a person holding PhD in a traditional subject.
- **Education trains in skills that are required by the economy:** Economy and education always enjoy a bilateral relationship. For example, the number of well functioning hospitals is directly related to the number of qualified and competent nurses passing out from the nursing institutes. More patients will be admitted to a hospital which is providing quality nursing care. This will lead to more money transactions and ultimately results in the economical development of the nearby areas of the hospital.
- **Fosters participant democracy:** In participant democracy, ordinary citizen is aware about his rights and duties and participates actively in the democratic process. Literacy is essential to nurture participant democracy and literacy is the product of education. Thus, education fosters participant democracy.
- **Education imparts values:** Education help the students to realize the role of values in leading a good life as a social being. Through various activities education imparts values, such as cooperation, team spirit, obedience, etc.
- **Education act as an integrative force:** Education act as an integrative force in society by communicating values that unite different sections of the society. By and large students learn social skills from the educational institutions. In India, through education we are teaching the concept of 'unity in diversity' as a part of developing this integrative force.

❖ **Values and orientation which are specific to certain professions are also provided by education:** This function deals mainly with the professional education. For example, in nursing institutes, nursing students are educated in a particular way to meet the health needs of the society.

## AIMS OF EDUCATION

Direction is important than speed. Aims of education are concerned with providing the much needed direction for the educative process. The aims stand for the goals, targets or broader purposes that may be fulfilled through the process of education.

Factors determining educational aims are philosophy of life, elements of human nature, religious factors, political ideologies, socioeconomic factors and problems, cultural factors, knowledge explosion and scientific and technological advancements.

The main aim of education was interpreted to be the preservation of knowledge. But in the modern society, knowledge in every subject is cumulative so that as each year passes there is more to be learnt. One of the main tasks of education in the modern society is to keep pace with this knowledge explosion. In such a society, knowledge cannot be received passively. It is something that has to be actively discovered. Education should focus on the nurturing of curiosity, stimulation of creativity, development of proper attitudes and values and the building of essential skills such as independent study and capacity to think and judge for oneself.

❖ **From human being to being human:** Education enables the child to become a good human being by nurturing good qualities and differentiating between right and wrong in life. Ongoing behavior modification through educative process enables the child to develop good qualities essential to become a good human being.

❖ **Developing life skills recommended by WHO:** Developing life skills recommended by WHO helps to achieve above said aim. Life skills are abilities for adaptive and positive behavior that enable humans to deal effectively with the demands and challenges of life. One of the aim of education is to assist child in developing essential life skills identified by WHO such as decision making, problem solving, creative thinking, critical thinking, effective communication, self-awareness, assertiveness, empathy, equanimity, interpersonal relationship, stress management and resilience.

❖ **Utilitarian aim:** Utilitarian aim is concerned with providing knowledge and skill required by the child for leading his day to day life. Fulfillment of this aim will enable him to make use of the knowledge and skill in a fruitful manner. This aim makes the educative process a purposeful one and depicts the relationship between education and life. To enhance or update the knowledge, students should be given enough opportunities for widening and deepening their knowledge through exploration. They should also be motivated to think and answer the why, what, how and when of their each learning activity. Encouraging students to express ideas in their own words will help them to acquire more knowledge.

❖ **Vocational aim:** Education should prepare the child to earn his livelihood so that he can lead a productive life in the society. Dignity of labor and respect to the labor have to be developed or inculcated by means of education.

❖ **Social aim:** Every individual is considered as a productive member of the society. Through education the individual child should be provided with the required assistance to become a useful member of the society, irrespective of the socioeconomic status. Keeping this aim in mind, educationists have to help learners to develop a healthy, purposeful, productive, exploratory and controlling adjustment with the environment. Society is the result of the interrelations of individuals. It consists of big and small groups and there are subgroups within each group. Education helps the child to understand this interrelations of individuals and the possibilities of various groups. Peaceful existence of society is determined by a phenomenon of balancing and counter-balancing between various social forces. By creating a social order, education ensures the effective functioning of this phenomenon and prepare students to safeguard the peaceful existence of the society. Education not only helps in the formation of social norms and their implementation but also trains the learner to follow them. Effective utilization of social resources is essential for the progress of the society and education equip the learners to harness the social resources in an ecofriendly as well as people friendly manner. By way of education, students realize the importance of social values like justice, fair play, healthy competition, harmony, etc. In short, education instils a sense of obligation and loyalty towards the community and its needs. By means of social aim, education gives direction in the development of the society.

- **Intellectual aim:** Intelligence is essential for acquiring knowledge, thinking, reasoning, judgment and generalization. Education provides enough opportunities to develop the innate intellectual capacity of the students. Development of intelligence through education will enable the child to lead an independent life with confidence.
- **Citizenship:** Education enables the children to grow as productive citizens by following the social and moral standards set by the society. Education should motivate the child to perform his duties and responsibilities as a citizen, for the welfare of the society. All countries in general and democratic countries in particular have to uphold this aim of education.
- **Physical health and well being:** Education prepare the child to lead a healthy life through providing the knowledge required for a healthy living and helping him to develop a positive attitude towards health. Education should also help the child to develop a health conscience and respect towards his or her own health.
- **Character development:** According to Mahatma Gandhi, the end of all knowledge must be the building up of character. Education assists the child to develop certain human values, attitudes and habits which are essential for building a desirable character. Many educationists share the view of Mahatma Gandhi and regard character development as the supreme aim of education.
- **Moral development:** Moral values like honesty, truthfulness, justice, goodness, purity, courage, reverence, dutifulness, punctuality, self-confidence, discrimination between good and bad, observation of rules, belief in systematic organization, etc., are inculcated through education. These qualities contribute to the development of morality and sound character.
- **Cultural development:** By undergoing education child becomes cultured and civilized. Cultural development is manifested through the development of an aesthetic sense and respect for others' culture.
- **Education for leisure:** Leisure is the time meant for enjoyment and recreation. Leisure plays an important role in recharging our depleted energy levels. Leisure time should be utilized in such a way that the individual as well as the society should benefit from it. Education prepares the child to use his leisure time for doing something useful.
- **Self-realization:** What we are is God's gift to us and what we become is our gift to God. Child is born with tremendous potential and education should help the child to become what he has to become by assisting to realize his potential and then equipping him to utilize the identified potential to the maximum extent possible. Self-realization also helps the child to realize his strengths, weaknesses, opportunities and threats so that he can exert a good control over his life by strengthening the weakness.

- **Mental and emotional development:** In this fast changing world, good mental health is a must to cope with the changing lifestyles and societal needs. Education should train the child by giving adequate opportunities for mental and emotional development. Nowadays, lot of research is taking place to gather more information regarding the role of emotional development on education and life. Research studies conducted by Holman in 1998 shows that emotional development is very important for attaining success in life. His study reveals that more individuals with higher intelligence quotient and lower emotional quotient (EQ) have failed to reach higher positions in life corresponding to their IQ when compared to individuals with normal IQ and high EQ. Individuals with normal IQ and high EQ have managed to reach higher positions which usually demands a very high IQ and leading a very satisfied and happy life. Based on his study, Golman suggests that instead of IQ, EQ should be considered as the parameter of achievements in life. According to him, placing challenges in front of a person with lower EQ is just like serving a delicious diet to a person who is not having the appetite. Of course, more research is needed before replacing IQ with EQ. Recent studies also show that emotional development is essential to conduct proper self-appraisal, control unhealthy emotions, develop an aim in life, attain emotional maturity, etc. In fact, emotional development is a must for leading a happy and content life. It is earnestly hoped that this aim will receive more attention in the coming years.
- **Autonomous development:** Percynunn believes that main aim of education is autonomous development of the individual. An individual child has to develop in total by seeking assistance and direction extended by the education. Total or all-round development enables the child to adjust with the life situations and include development of personality, character, leadership, maturity, mental health, physique and intelligence. Percynunn recommends formal education for the autonomous development. She believes that activity oriented curriculum enriched with varied learning activities, teaching methods, facilities for guidance and counseling, discipline and proper direction will contribute to the autonomous development of the child.
- **Physical literacy:** Education should enable learners to follow a healthy lifestyle by incorporating exercise, balanced diet and other desirable habits.
- **Self-education aim:** As education is considered as a lifelong process, it should prepare the child to adopt a proactive role towards the learning process (*see* Chapter 5: Learning). Education has to properly harness the natural curiosity and urge present in the child while imparting knowledge. This aim is gaining importance in this era of knowledge explosion where students are expected to take a leading role in the teaching-learning process than the teacher. Teachers should make sure that students are learning as a result of the internal motivation rather than a reaction to the compulsion exerted by others.
- **International understanding:** Education is a universal process and it helps in creating universal understanding. The progress we achieved in the field of education is the result of the combined efforts of people from different countries, the scholars of all periods, the followers of all religions and members of all the races. Education is the common heritage of mankind and it is not an exclusive property of any particular nation, race or community. All educationists, irrespective of their caste, color and creed worked devotedly towards the development of education. The man-made boundaries or restrictions cannot check the free flow of information and cooperation among educationists. As the world has reduced to a global village due to the advancements in the information technology, the aim of international understanding has conquered new dimensions.
- **Harmonious development:** Ultimately the overall aim of education is to ensure harmonious development through the achievement of the above mentioned aims. Harmonious

development will enable the child to deal effectively with the problems and uncertainties of life.

## VALUE EDUCATION

Value education is the process of enabling children to develop values essential for leading a successful life by way of educative process. Values are essential for the proper development of personal, social, moral and spiritual behaviors along with academic excellence.

Considering the major role of technology in education and influence of social media among youngsters special attention is needed to inculcate values among children.

Values influence behavior and attitudes. Values help us to distinguish between good and bad. Thus, values are essential for making good choices in life. Good choices in turn create success in life.

Value education motivates students to become more proactive in learning. This is evident by spending more time on learning, increase in attendance and reduction in the unhealthy use of mobile phones and social media. Proper faculty development programs enable teachers to provide value education in an appropriate manner.

Curriculum of value education focuses on personal, social, moral and spiritual development of children along with other aims of education. Curriculum should include provision for developing values like responsible behaviors, loyalty, empathy, passion, honesty, reliability, dependability, optimism and commitment along with subject matter. A sound system of values helps children to grow and live as good human beings as well as responsible citizens. Quality of education can be improved by making it more value oriented one.

## TRANSFORMATIONAL EDUCATION

Transformational education refers to the educative process that enables learners to realize their full potential as a human being by adhering to ethical and social values.

In transformational education learning encourages learners to seek solutions to problems they face. It also fosters learners' emotional connection, person well-being and reverence for the natural world. Transformational education is authentic, purposeful and engaging. It also prepares to face the future boldly and become lifelong learners.

**Transformational education enables learners to:**
- Develop genuine concern and love for the world around them.
- Consider themselves as capable and competent in bringing out positive change in society.
- Become lifelong learners and learn with intention and purpose.
- Enhance their capacities for learning creativity and problem solving.

## RELATIONSHIP-BASED EDUCATION

Relationship-based education is based on a holistic approach and consider each student as a teaching unit rather than the whole class. When teacher consider each learner as a teaching unit it fosters better teacher–student relationship. This will in turn foster physical and mental health of learners. One important aspect of relationship-based education is that it encourages collaboration than competition among learners. Relationship-based education believes that true teaching involves facilitating learning and not only in the classroom, but everywhere else in school. It ensures students active engagement in learning. Thus, learning outcomes can be achieved in a better manner.

**Relationship-based education involves**
- Know the individual learner (strengths, weaknesses, passion, etc.)
- Identify student needs.
- Work to meet those needs.

## COMPETENCY-BASED EDUCATION

According to CBSE, competency-based education (CBE) is an approach to teaching, learning and assessment that focuses on the learners demonstration of learning outcomes and attaining proficiency in particular competencies in each subject. Teaching which uses a CBE methodology works to empower students and provide them with a meaningful and positive learning experience. It is learner-centered and actively engages them in the learning process. It emphasizes real world applications of knowledge and skills and the authenticity of the learning experience.

### Key Features of CBE Approach
- Equity for all students
- Differentiated support based on students individual learning needs
- Student progress or achievement is based on evidence of mastery rather than time spent in this classroom.
- Emphasis on formative assessment or ongoing assessment, particularly peer and self assessment, where students are encouraged to reflect on their own work and identify areas for improvement.

## TYPES OF EDUCATION

Education can be classified into formal, informal and nonformal types.

### Formal Education

Formal education is based on certain rules, customs and procedures. It involves a direct face to face interaction with the teacher and rendered through educational institutions in a pre-planned and organized manner. Formal education is conducted for a prescribed period of time and is based on a well defined curriculum. It is very systematic in nature and given by specially qualified personnel.

### Informal Education

Informal education is not systematically planned and has the following characteristics: (a) no formal agencies like school or college is involved and provided by informal agencies, such as home, family or community; (b) no prescribed schedule or well defined curriculum and takes place mainly as a result of experiences gaining from day to day life or interactions with others; (c) no specially qualified personnel to teach or no evaluation system like examinations and conferring of certificates; and (d) emphasis is on habits, ideals, attitudes, and skills.

### Nonformal Education

Nonformal education adopts a midway between formal and informal types of education. The characteristics of nonformal education are: (a) very flexible without rigid rules, regulations and fixed stages or time frame; (b) systematically planned, organized and implemented; (c) integrated with the life and work of the learners; and (d) designed to meet the learning needs of different categories in the society.

According to KL Kumar, nonformal education is based on the following concepts, such as (a) equality of opportunity, (b) students' desire of learning and progress, (c) faith in the dignity of an individual, (d) freedom of time, place and pace of learning, (e) ability to learn at any age in life, (g) autonomy of style and technique of learning, and (h) facility to acquire knowledge in new areas.

Nonformal education provides more opportunity for personal development compared to formal education. The main advantage of nonformal education is its flexibility and adaptability to learner's needs and changing needs of society. There is a marked difference between formal and nonformal education. Simkin's differentiate nonformal and formal education in terms of purposes, timing, content, delivery system and control **(Table 1.1)**.

Depending on the means of communication and state of art in educational technology, KL Kumar classifies nonformal education into (a) correspondence education; (b) distance education; (c) open learning/open program; (d) continuing education program; and (e) telelecturing/teleconferencing.

A new type of distance education namely massive open online courses (MOOC) is gaining acceptance all over the world **(Fig. 1.6)**. A massive open online course (MOOC) is an online course aimed at unlimited participation and open access via the web. In addition to traditional course materials, many MOOCs provide interactive user forums to support community interactions among students and teachers. MOOCs are a recent and widely researched development in distance education which were emerged as a popular mode of learning in 2012.

**TABLE 1.1:** Difference between formal and nonformal education.

| Characteristics | Formal | Nonformal |
| --- | --- | --- |
| Purposes | Long-term and generally credential based | Short-term and specific non-credential based |
| Timing | Long cycle/preparation/full-time | Short cycle/recurrent/part-time |
| Content | Standardized/input centered/theory based | Individual output centered skill based |
| Delivery system | Entry requirements select learners | Learners select entry requirement |
| | Institutional based, rigidly structured, teacher-centered and resources intensive | Community based, flexible learner-centered and resource saving |

*Source:* Kumar KL. Educational technology. New Age Publishers; 1996.

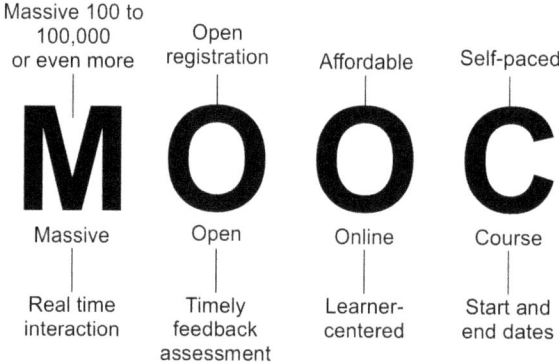

**Fig. 1.6:** MOOC, the preferred distance education program.
*Source:* Bates T. Teaching in digital age. Center for open education; 2015.

# EDUCATION AND LIFE

Herbert Spenser says education is complete living. According to John Dewey education is not just a preparation for life, but it is life itself. Education helps to achieve survival skills like literacy, numeracy, communication and building relationships. Education is a lifelong journey. As adults we learn when there is a problem to solve or a crisis to overcome. We all learn from our experiences. Thus, education is something that gives meaning to life through experiences. Jeferson's words "All graduated are not educated but all educated are graduated" clearly explains the relationship between life and education. Graduation alone is not enough to attain success in life. Many philosophers and world's richest individuals have only basic education. They achieved success because of their learning form life experiences.

When we say education is a lifelong process it does not mean acquiring knowledge from books only. It is the knowledge we gain from experiences and by observing life of others. Mahatma Gandhi is not a PhD holder, but one can take PhD by studying life of Mahatma Gandhi. This is a best example of relationship between life and education. Education is much more than earning degrees. It is what we gain from our life experiences. Real education helps us to rebuild life even if our life is shattered like a rain drop caught in the eye of a cyclone.

# AGENCIES OF EDUCATION

Agency of education is the medium through which education is carried out. Educational institutions are commonly referred as agencies of education. Educational agencies fall into any one of the four types, namely formal, informal, active and passive agencies. Formal agencies are mainly concerned with providing formal education, for example, schools, colleges, etc. As name indicates, informal agencies are providing informal education, for example, home, family, play groups, etc. Active agencies facilitate human interaction through a two-way communication process, for example, family, school, religious organizations, etc. Passive agencies lack the provision for interaction while transferring information, for example, television, newspapers, etc.

According to FJ Brown, educational agencies can be classified as formal institutions, group organizations, commercial agencies and noncommercial agencies. Formal institutions and group organizations are synonymous with formal and informal agencies of the first classification. Commercial agencies are profit oriented ones, like press, cinema, etc. Noncommercial agencies are service-oriented ones such as governmental organizations, voluntary agencies, etc.

# FACTORS INFLUENCING TRENDS IN EDUCATION

According to confederation of industries three factors such as: (1) development in cognitive neuroscience, (2) change in job market, and (3) access to information determines the trends in education.

1. **Development in cognitive neuroscience**: Cognitive neuroscience is the study of the biological process and aspects related to cognition with specific focus on role of brain in cognition. It is a combination of psychology and neuroscience. Cognitive neuroscience explains the role of brain in cognition, including perception, attention, language understanding, memory, problem solving and decision making. Cognitive neuroscience finds how neurons process information and how learning occurs. Thus, any development in cognitive neuroscience influences education.

2. **Changes in job market:** Vocational aim is one of the aims of education. Education prepares youngsters to find suitable job according to their capabilities and needs of the society. When there is a change in job market, it naturally influences trends in education.
3. **Access to information**: Teacher and textbooks as the main source of information is rapidly changing due to technological advancements in education. Easy online access to information transformed the education process in a big manner. Best example is the increased acceptance of MOOCs or massive open online courses in education.

## CURRENT TRENDS IN EDUCATION

The changes that are occurring in the social and cultural life of the society as a result of the impact of advancements in the science-based technology are broadly described as modernization. Since education is a multipolar process, it is influenced by the modernization in different ways. Due to gobalization and liberalization, changes occurring in other parts of the world will also influence the education pattern of a country. Even though certain aspects in the new trends are painful to those who view education as a noble process, they are irresistible in the current context. Let us see some of the current trends in education.

❖ **Pedocentric:** Student is the focus of present day education system. The interest is shifted from the subject matter to the student and the teaching–learning process is largely directed by the nature and needs of the learner. This basic shift in emphasis from the subject of instruction to the nature and needs of the learner is based on the *mathetic principle*. The term mathetics is derived from the Greek word *mathein* which means to learn. Mathetics is the science of behavior of the pupil undergoing the process of learning. Mathetics is in contrast to pedagogy whose main interest is in the behavior of the teacher while instructing pupils. The teacher today does not consider the child as a vessel waiting to be filled up with facts; nor as a pliable plastic material which can be transformed into any shape enabling him to project his ideas on it. The modern teacher considers each child as akin to a plant and helps the child to grow according to his abilities and aptitudes. Teacher helps the child to learn. Progressive educationists like Rousseay, Pestalozzi, Froebel, Montessori, John Dewey and others have contributed to the development of a child-centered education. As a result, education has become more interested in the *'whole child,'* all the thoughts, feelings and actions of the individual pupil, in his mental and social development rather than presenting some information to him in a ready-made form. In accordance with this trend, student is motivated to participate actively in the teaching–learning process. This way of teaching by eliciting maximum student participation is called *participatory approach* in teaching.

❖ **Teacher's role:** The shift in emphasis from the teacher to the pupil in the process of education and the carrying out of instructional activities with the realization of specific and clear-cut learning outcomes has inevitably led to a reassessment of teacher's role in the classroom. The model of teacher as the pivotal and dominant figure in education, presenting a variety of information to pupils has practically disappeared. Modern education transformed the teacher's role from a dictator to a friend of students. Teacher of today is considered as a facilitator of learning, whose main duty is to prepare students for learning by enabling them to actively participate in the teaching-learning process rather than simply spoon-feeding. The less the pupils rely upon the teacher, the better: a successful teacher must enable his pupils to do without him. The changing role of the teacher in education has been the result of a plurality of intertwining influences like philosophical, psychological, social, technological and educational. Psychological studies have clearly revealed the influence of classroom climate and atmosphere in the creation of a fertile learning environment. In the creation of such an environment, the nature of teacher–pupil relationship, teacher's personal attitude towards his students, his professional philosophy and life values plays an important role. As said earlier, teacher of the past functioned as an authoritarian figure. But with the changing goals of education and newer psychological discoveries related to effective learning, such a style of teacher functioning is not only unproductive but even detrimental to learning. The classic study of Lewin, Lippift and white has demonstrated the long-term benefits of a democratic classroom set up as compared to the authoritarian or laissez-faire teacher behavior. There have been criticisms of this study but other investigations have also indicated the importance of the emotional component in learning and have generally tended to support the view that a warm, humane and responsive teacher attitude has a stimulating effect on the pupil learning. Even though the role of teacher have changed, we cannot ignore them because the future of education directly depends upon the quality of the intermediary inventive minds of teachers and their ability to invent and innovate.

- **Activity-centered:** Modern education is activity-centered. We are currently giving more emphasis to learning by doing. Curriculum of today is organized in terms of the tasks to be performed and goals to be reached rather than in terms of lessons to be learned. This will provide knowledge and skills essential for leading a good life. Teachers have to motivate the children to do experiments, search out facts for themselves and undertake projects.
- **Creative education:** One of the most significant trends in today's school is the encouragement of creativity. Human advances come through original thought and intervention. Creative education is a good medium to develop original thought and intervention.
- **More focus on life skills:** Education now give more importance to life skills recommended by WHO. Life skills are abilities for adaptive and positive behavior that enable humans to deal effectively with the demands and challenges of life. Life skills recommended by who includes skills such as decision making, problem solving, creative thinking, critical thinking, effective communication, self-awareness, assertiveness, empathy, equanimity, interpersonal relationship, stress management and resilience.
- **Promotion of value education:** Value education is the process of enabling children to develop values essential for leading a successful life by way of educative process. Now education is giving more importance to value education for grooming youngsters as good citizens and human beings.
- **Emphasis on collaboration than competition:** In modern education emphasis is on collaboration or cooperation than competition. This helps children to become good human beings with a mindset to help others.
- **More attention to Finnish model of education:** Finland education focuses on grooming children as good human beings with a mindset to help others. Emphasis is on cooperation rather than competition. It also gives more importance to psychological counseling and individual guidance. Many countries including India is adapting good features of Finnish model to improve quality of education system.
- **More flexible options:** Now, students can choose a program suitable to their aptitude and interest. This will help student to find alternative career paths than traditional ones.
- **Promotion of critical thinking:** Modern education follows critical pedagogy to promote critical thinking among children. Critical thinking is essential for proper judgment and proper judgment is needed for taking good decisions. By making good decision only one can build a desirable future and achieve success in life.
- **Preference to experiential learning:** Experiential learning is a method of educating through firsthand experience. Experiential learning allows children to discover and understand

through their own effort. Activity-based learning environment promote experiential learning. In experiential learning, knowledge, skills and experience are acquired mainly outside the traditional academic classroom setting and may include internship, field trips, field research and project.

- **Ability-based learning:** In ability-based learning, students are allowed to learn at their own pace. When students with same skill levels and ideas are grouped together, the stress lowers and they can learn more easily.
- **More acceptance to MOOCs:** Massive open online courses (MOOCs) are free online courses available for anyone to enroll. MOOCs provide an affordable and flexible way to provide quality education to masses.
- **Outcome-based education:** With the implementation of standards and new assessment practices education is now more outcome oriented than before.
- **More freedom to teachers in instructional design:** Teachers now enjoy more freedom in developing suitable and relevant instructional methods. Teachers can follow innovative teaching methods that enhance the all round development of students.
- **More community participation:** Considering the reciprocative relationship between education and society, this is an expected trend. Education is seeking more community participation for solving its problems. The presence of parent–teacher association in all most every educational institute is a good example for the community participation. Parents' participation can also be elicited through socialized projects and programs. The result is that parents and the teachers meet in small and large groups to discuss their common problems. Funding of various projects in the technical institutes by the industrial sector is also an example of this trend.
- **More reliance on technology:** Technology exerts great influence on education as a tool for teaching and learning. Judicious use of educational psychology in the development and practice of educational technology has increased its user friendly nature considerably. Cost-effectiveness of technology-based educational programs is good when compared to the cost of traditional programs. Education system is preferring technology not because it simplifies the teaching-learning process, but because technology empowers new solutions. Technology will help the teachers to solve the emerging educational problems created by factors like growing school population, heterogeneity of pupils in schools, divergent and even confusing needs of learners, rapid development of new information, expanding curriculum and the social changes arising from modernization. Developments in educational technology bring about changes and shifts in educational goals which in turn stimulate the emergence of newer techniques. Technology of education is being developed with the aim not only of making education more widely available but also of improving the quality of education. As stated earlier, the nature of emerging techniques of education has been influenced by modern psychology. The facility for online education through information technology enabled services has redefined the concept of nonformal education. With the wide spread use of computers in education, computer-assisted learning and computer-assisted instruction are becoming common even in the lower levels of education. Nowadays, universities are changing to virtual universities by fully utilizing the technological advancements for imparting knowledge.
- **Increased acceptance of nonformal type of education:** Universities and other elite educational organizations has come out from glass towers for providing nonformal education through study centers and regional centers. Some of them are generating more revenues through providing nonformal education than the formal education. As said earlier, information technology enabled services has redefined the concept of nonformal education.

Different from the past, various forms of nonformal education like correspondence education, distance education, etc., are gaining acceptance among the youth.

- **Restructuring traditional programs:** In order to meet the challenges of globalization, education system is restructuring the traditional programs by integrating and correlating various subjects, for example, traditional BSc botany program has converted to applied botany in many institutes by way of integrating some aspects of biotechnology.
- **Increased opportunities for higher studies:** In the present situation, a talented student can do higher studies irrespective of the economic status. Doors of all elite universities in the world are kept open for the talented young people and flexible educational loans are available for meeting the expenses of education.
- **Methods of appraisal:** Because of multiple educational goals, a comprehensive system of evaluation is being evolved. The child's progress is judged by the comparison of his own work and achievements. Latest methods of evaluation are based on a vision of learning and well-defined performance indicators. In addition to the cognitive abilities, other abilities are also evaluated in a more objective manner.
- **Innovation in teaching and learning:** Lot of innovations are taking place in teaching and learning on a regular basis. These innovations will help in the intellectual development, personal development and career development of the youth.
- **Educational quality assurance:** Present day education system is more concerned about quality, cost-effectiveness and accountability. Educational quality assurance is a process of monitoring and evaluating efficiency and effectiveness of educational provision and to institute remedial measures as and when needed.
- **Emergence of individual as a teaching unit:** Class as a unit of teaching is disappearing. As a result of the advancements in instructional planning and evaluation of learning, teachers realize the existence of widely different backgrounds, differences in student abilities and interests. Hence the teachers of today realize the need for presenting learning experience to suit individual difference existing among pupils by using the media and methods generated by educational technology. In short, advancements in educational technology motivated the teachers to view education as an individual activity rather than a classroom activity.
- **Commercialization of education and presence of foreign universities:** Due to misappropriation of funds and scarcity of resources, government is finding it difficult to meet the educational demands of the society, thereby denying opportunity for education to a vast majority of people. This has motivated the government to concentrate more on the basic education. Now, government is withdrawing slowly from providing higher education and allowing private sector to play a major role, subjected to certain social control measures. If the government implement the social control measures properly, this approach would bring spectacular changes in an otherwise gloomy educational scenario. Foreign universities are now attracting Indian students by offering job-oriented programs. Since Indian universities are still continuing the age old programs and very much reluctant to change according to the new trends in the international level, India has become a gold mine for the foreign universities.

# NURSING EDUCATION

## Definition

Nursing education is a professional education which is consciously and systematically planned and implemented through instruction and discipline and aims the harmonious development of the physical, intellectual, social, emotional, spiritual and aesthetic powers or abilities of the student in order to render professional nursing care to people of all ages, in all phases of health and illness, in a variety of settings, in the best or highest possible manner.

## Aims of Nursing Education (Fig. 1.7)

- **Harmonious development:** Nursing education aims the harmonious development of the physical, intellectual, emotional, social, spiritual and aesthetic powers or abilities of the student. Harmonious development is essential for achieving the qualities required for leading a successful professional and personal life. In short, nursing education aims to prepare students as good human beings with qualities of a professional nurse.
- **Inculcating the right attitude:** Right attitude towards nursing forms the basis of nursing career. Right attitude helps to adjust with the student life and motivate to achieve excellence in the upcoming professional life. Nursing education offers a variety of learning experiences with an aim to inculcate proper attitude among students.
- **Knowledge and skill aim:** Nursing education provide the much needed knowledge and skill required to practice the profession in a successful manner. Technological advancements in the field of education helps nurse educators to fulfill this aim in a meticulous way.
- **Emphasis on high-tech high-touch approach:** High-tech high-touch approach in nursing care was devised to preserve the human component of nursing care without undermining the advantages of the technological advancements in the field of patient care. Nurse educators have to motivate the students to maintain the human element of nursing while rendering care with the help of sophisticated gadgets.
- **Prepare students to take up a proactive role in learning:** The model of teacher as the pivotal and dominant figure in education, presenting a variety of information to pupils has

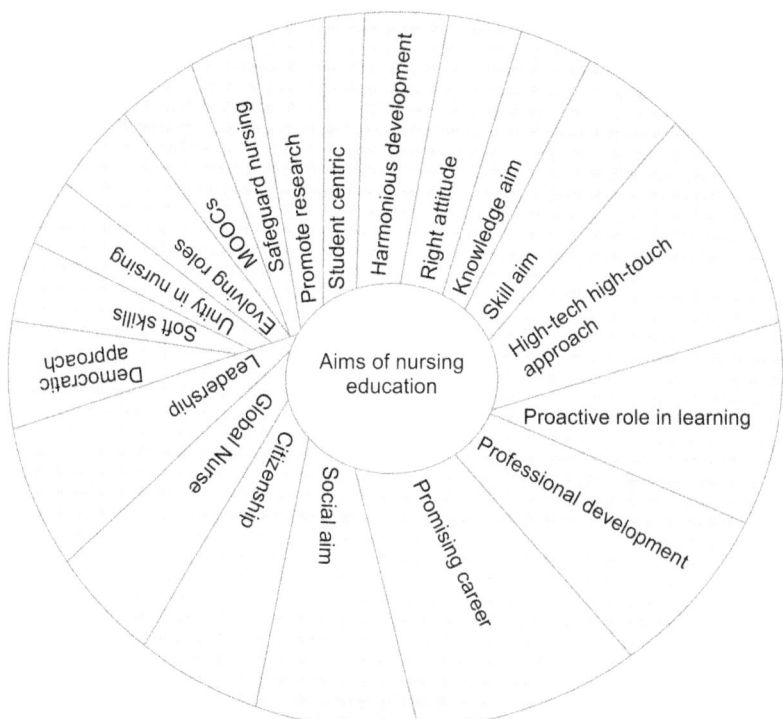

**Fig. 1.7:** Aims of nursing education.

practically disappeared. To a certain extent this is applicable to nursing education also. Nurse educator of today is considered as a facilitator of learning, whose main duty is to prepare students to adopt a proactive role in learning so that they will actively participate in the teaching-learning process.

- **Professional development:** Nursing education prepares the student to render professional nursing care in the best or highest possible manner. Nurse educators can fulfill the professional aspirations of the students by way of providing guidance, arranging adequate learning experiences and serving as role models. The need of professional development in this era of competition and knowledge explosion should be explained properly to the students. Easy access to information, availability of staff development programs and increased opportunities for higher education will help nurses to maintain the professional development.
- **Assist to build a promising career:** Nursing profession offers a variety of career opportunities. Helping students to realize their potentials and interests will enable them to build a promising career.
- **Social aim:** Nursing education prepares the student to become a useful member in the society. This will in turn help them to interact effectively with the people and render dedicated care without any discrimination.
- **Citizenship:** Nursing education should motivate the student to perform his or her duties as a citizen for the welfare of the fellow human beings.
- **To prepare global nurses:** Globalization and liberalization has created world wide opportunities for professional nurses ever than before. Today, a competent nurse with good knowledge in English can easily build a career in other nations. Considering the high demand of Indian nurses in the international context, we can add one more aim, namely preparation of global nurses.
- **Leadership aim:** Since nursing profession is experiencing a shortage of eminent leaders, leadership aim is very important. Nursing education has to nurture leadership abilities among students.
- **Student-centric teaching-learning process:** In student centric teaching process, students are the center of all activities of the nursing institutions. This can be achieved by following student-centered teaching methods, providing good clinical supervision, simulation exercises, etc.
- **Safeguard role of nursing in health care:** Many hospitals, especially corporate one's are trying to replace nurses with less trained people through national skill development mission programs. It is the duty of nursing education to convince the society about the consequences of such initiatives shortage of professional nurses cannot be solved by replacing nurses with nonprofessionals.
- **Preparation for evolving roles:** New roles arising due to technological advancements in patient care can be called as evolving roles than extended or expanded roles. It is the duty of the nursing education to prepare students to identify evolving roles and fulfill them properly.
- **Promoting research:** Promoting research is a priority of nursing education. Research is viewed as a part of professional life than tool for acquiring higher qualification.
- **Promote affinity towards professional organization:** Many of our issues can be solved if strengthen our professional organizations. Nursing education should promote affinity towards professional organization.

- **Bridge the gap between nursing education and service sector:** Nursing service can contribute to the development of nursing education and vice versa. Unfortunately, collaboration between two sectors is not adequate. Nursing education need to take a proactive role in uniting two sectors.
- **Preparation of MOOCs:** Many nurses are willing to update themselves if flexible distance education courses are available. MOOCs are the best suitable distance education program. Hence, it is the duty of nursing education to prepare MOOCs, suitable for nursing profession.
- **Promote democratic approaches in nursing education:** This aim is an extension of the student centric aim. Social changes and influence of modern social media demands a more democratic approaches in nursing education.
- **Development of soft skills:** Soft skills are a part of nursing curriculum in addition to unique skills of nursing. Even then, development of soft skills is considered as an aim of nursing education.
- **Entrepreneurship aim:** Dynamic changes in healthcare system offers lot of opportunities for nurses to start healthcare related firms. Nursing students need to be trained for developing entrepreneurship qualities for utilizing these opportunities.

## Trends in Nursing Education

A profession is a dynamic integration of various faculties of knowledge. Since nursing education is a professional education, it is dynamic by its own nature and thereby giving rise to trends. Let us see some of the current trends in nursing education.

- **Curriculum changes:** Flexible curriculum designs are evolving to facilitate diversity of educational opportunity and overcome barriers of distance and time. These curricula are often competency based, focused on outcome and emphasize student participation and responsibility for learning.
- **Innovations in teaching and learning:** In nursing education, lot of innovations are taking place in the areas of teaching and learning. Invariably, these innovations lead to intellectual development, personal development and career development.
- **Educational quality assurance:** Educational quality assurance is a process for monitoring and evaluating efficiency and effectiveness of educational provision and to institute remedial measures as and when needed. In India, nursing education is flourishing in an unprecedented manner; naturally this will lead to dilution in the quality of nursing education in the absence of proper quality control measures. Motivated by this situation, accrediting bodies and nurse educators are expressing deep concern regarding the quality of nursing education. It is high time to prepare a quality index of nursing institutions all over the country by categorizing them into different grades based on the infrastructure and faculty profile.
- **More reliance on technology:** Technology exerts greater influence on nursing education as a tool for teaching and learning. Judicious use of educational psychology in the development and practice of educational technology has increased its user-friendly nature considerably.
- **Emphasis on high-tech high-touch approach:** High-tech high-touch approach in nursing care was devised to preserve the human component of nursing care without undermining the advantages of technological advancements in the field of patient care. Present day nursing education is preparing the students to maintain the human element of nursing while caring the patients with the help of sophisticated gadgets.
- **Preparation of global nurses:** Nursing education is all set to reap benefits created by globalization and liberalization by way of preparing global nurses. Many institutions are

preparing students with a global perspective through providing learning experiences to enrich students' knowledge in English along with the attainment of other objectives.
- **Transnational acceptance:** Nursing educational programs in one nation is widely accepted by other nations. In fact, this transnational acceptance is the main reason for the development of nursing education in the countries like India.
- **Ensuring a promising career:** Unlike many other professional education programs, nursing education ensures a promising career either in India or abroad. A study conducted by Johnson and Johnson reveals that nursing education will maintain this status at least for the coming ten years.
- **Emergence of new specialities:** In par with the developments in the medical and allied fields, nursing education is also offering new specialities to meet the needs of the community.
- **Increased opportunities for higher studies:** Different from the past many institutions are offering programs such as post certificate BSc nursing, MSc nursing, MPhil and PhD. An eligible candidate can easily pursue higher education without much time lag.
- **Diminishing government role:** Shortage of funds coupled with certain policy decisions has prevented the government from investing further in the field of nursing education. Now, the private sector is playing a dominant role for the development of nursing education.
- **Uniformity and standardization:** Various universities and nursing boards are conducting nursing programs in a different manner. Even though efforts are on the way to bring about the much needed uniformity and standardization, nothing significant has been achieved so far.
- **Coping with the impact of globalization:** As a result of the impact of globalization, the status of nursing shifted from that of a caring profession to a rewarding profession. Very few students are trying to inculcate the traditional values of nursing profession during their student period. Majority consider nursing education only as a means for securing a rewarding career. Nursing education sector is trying hard to cope with this worrisome impact of globalization.
- **Enhanced student status:** In the past, students joining for nursing educational programs were viewed as student nurses rather than nursing students. Increased career opportunities offered by the nursing as well as the tremendous increase in the number of nursing institutions prompted society and other healthcare professions to consider nursing students as nursing students.
- **Emergence of democratic and student-centered campus:** Social changes and influence of social media led to the emergence of democratic and student-centered nursing institutions.
- **Proactive apex bodies:** Apex bodies like universities and nursing councils are taking active steps with the help of technology to maintain standards of nursing education.
- **Dominance of skill aim over knowledge aim:** Service sector offers better prospectus than education sector. For securing job in service sector competence in nursing practice is essential. This motivated nursing students to refine skills through deliberate practice. Students put more effort to acquire skills than theoretical knowledge.
- **Preference to degree program:** Preference to BSc nursing program is increasing due to various reasons. One reason is the diminishing global demand of GNM Program. Issues related to multiple entry levels to nursing profession is another reason.
- **Simulation as preferred method of teaching:** Simulation is gaining importance as a method for skill training. Hundred percentage accuracy is needed in performing skills related to patient care. Hence, simulation is the best way to acquire skills in a fool proof manner.

- **More quality conscious institutions:** Many nursing colleges are voluntarily seeking accreditation than mandatory requirements. Many colleges now have National Assessment and Accreditation Council (NAAC) accreditation. National Accreditation Board for Hospitals and Healthcare Providers (NABH) accreditation to parent hospital also improve quality of teaching.
- **Consideration to soft skills:** So far soft skills are considered as a part of nursing curriculum and considered less important than unique skills of nursing practice. Now, soft skills have equal importance as unique skills.
- **Shortage of competent nurse educators:** Prospects of service side is better than education. Hence, nurses prefer service side. This will lead to the shortage of competent nurse education.
- **BSc nursing as entry criteria to the profession:** The trend is now favoring for BSc nursing as less takers for diploma programs. Global trends are also in favor of BSc nursing program.
- **Unique status for nursing education:** Now, nursing education is considered as a unique professional education program. Earlier nursing education was included among paramedical programs.
- **Establishment of nursing universities:** Many states are in the process of establishing nursing universities to empower nursing education sector. This is a welcome move if implemented in the proper manner.
- **Autonomous institutions:** In the near future, nursing colleges with excellent facilities and academic performance may be awarded with autonomous status by considering them as centers of excellence.
- **Innovative distance education programs:** Innovative distance education programs are needed for enabling vast majority diploma holders to acquire degree equivalent programs. Meticulous distance education programs can be developed by following innovative curricular designs and utilizing developments in educational technology.
- **More indigenization of learning content:** Different from the past, nursing education is depending more on Indian study materials. This also promote implementation of institutional curriculum and there by more student participation in the teaching–learning process.

## Issues in Nursing Education

As higher education is influenced by various factors, issues or challenges is an integral part of it. Nursing education is also not an exception. Addressing issues or challenges is essential for nurturing professionalism. Some of the issues include:

- **Multiple level entries to profession:** One can enter to nursing profession by successfully completing ANM, GNM or BSc nursing. Earlier, this was not an issue due to demographic and social reasons. But, now this is an issue need to be addressed properly. Phasing out Diploma programs and choosing degree as single level entry to profession is a real challenge to all stakeholder of nursing profession.
- **Challenges from new educational programs:** Different from the past, students now can choose from a variety of programs for higher education. New programs require only less commitments and training compared to nursing. Nursing education need to take proactive steps to retain its preference.
- **Technology driven teaching process:** No media or technology can replace good teaching. Many teachers are ignoring the human component of teaching. For them teaching is a simple presentation of downloaded 3D animated videos. Naturally, aims of nursing education is not achieved properly.

- **Inadequate collaboration with service sector:** Education sector need to collaborate more with service side for the benefit of nursing profession. Nursing education can prosper only through a fruitful collaboration with service sector.
- **Less correlation between theory and practice:** This issue is mainly due to the lack of ideal clinical situation. Good clinical supervision and setting up an ideal teaching ward in parent hospital helps to solve this issue.
- **Shortage of middle level faculty members:** Middle level faculty members like associate professors form the backbone of nursing colleges. The success a government nursing colleges is an example of this. Unfortunately, in private sector there is shortage of middle level faculty members. Middle level teachers are experienced than first level teachers and not busy with administrative matters like seniors. Thus, middle level teachers can guide students in a proper manner.
- **Curriculum related issues:** As nursing education is influenced by many main problem is an overloaded curriculum. Curriculum related issues can be solved by periodic curriculum revisions.
- **Nursing students as staff nurses:** This is a major issue. This issue even questions the professional status of nursing. On the pretext of clinical posting nursing students are posted to compensate the shortage of staff nurses.
- **Inadequate representation in health universities:** Nursing colleges are the main sources of income for health universities. But, health universities are not giving adequate representation to nursing faculty members.
- **Less assertive in safeguarding nursing profession:** Corporate hospitals are trying to replace professional nurses with less trained people under nation skill development mission program. Unfortunately, nursing education sector is not highlighting the consequences of this worrisome issue.

## Challenges Before Nursing Education

As Nursing education is a dynamic process, it has to confront challenges for further growth. Following are some as the challenges nursing education need to address properly:
- **Correlating theory and practice:** Very often it is finding difficult to practice what is taught in the classroom. One reason is blindly following foreign textbooks for teaching without understanding available clinical facilities. By setting up a model teaching ward in the parent hospital we can address this challenge properly. Building state of the art simulation labs also help to overcome this issue.
- **Preparing students for evolving roles:** As healthcare sector is changing rapidly, no specific role can be assigned to nurses in the future. The roles arising differently from traditional ones are commonly known as evolving roles. Students can be prepared to take up these evolving roles by assisting them to develop proper attitude towards change and update themselves as required.
- **Replacing GNM program with BSc nursing:** Deciding BSc nursing as the entry criteria to profession has its own challenges. Nursing education need to address this challenge by effectively utilizing technological advancements in education.
- **Safeguarding nursing from new generation healthcare professions:** Many roles earlier performed by nurses are taken away by new healthcare professions. For example, physician assistants now brief about patient condition to doctors in some hospitals even though nurses taking care of patients round the clock. Nursing education by way of helping nurses maintain competency can safeguard the role of nurses in healthcare system.

- ❖ **Ensuring adequate nurse educators:** This is a big challenge for nursing education. Providing adequate remuneration and other facilities is one way to ensure adequate faculty members.
- ❖ **Maintaining autonomy of nursing education:** Nowaday's, many others are involving in the policy decisions related to nursing education. This will lead to dilution in the quality of nursing education. Nursing education need to safeguard its autonomy as a professional education.
- ❖ **Appreciating developments in cognitive neuroscience:** Understanding developments in cognitive neuroscience is essential to develop proper teaching-learning methods. It will also help in developing nursing specific teaching-learning process.
- ❖ **Implementing discipline with dignity:** Rigid discipline has no role in modern education. This is applicable to nursing education also. Implementing discipline with dignity is the preferred way in nursing education
- ❖ **Promoting judicious use of social media:** Harmful use of social media can result in various problems and results in low academic performance by students. Promoting judicious use of social media is a challenge to nurse educators. Students need to be motivated to follow **"Disconnect and learn more"** principle to avoid unnecessary use of social media.
- ❖ **Sharing of resources:** Nursing institutions can jointly set up state of the art simulation labs for the purpose of training students. As the cost is very high institutions can jointly develop these kind of facilities. But difference in viewpoints, philosophy, etc., are creating problems in sharing resources.

## SUMMARY

Education is a purposeful process aimed at the development of human beings. It is concerned with directing the child in the matter of bringing out his hidden talents. Educative process is best considered as a multipolar process. Components of educative process are knowledge, application of skills, understanding, comprehension, expression, appreciation, teaching, learning, initiation, instruction, training and indoctrination. Education is a planned activity and based on objectives. Educative process is influenced by the society, social changes and technological advancements.

Completing the socialization process, transmission of cultural heritage, formation of social personality, reformation of attitude, occupational placement, conferring of status, encouraging the spirit of competition, training the skills that are required by the economy, fostering participant democracy and imparting values are some of the functions of education. Aims of education is concerned with providing the much needed direction for the educative process. Aims of education include utilitarian aim, social aim, intellectual aim, citizenship, physical health and well being, character development, moral development, cultural development, mental and emotional development, autonomous development, self-education aim, international understanding and harmonious development.

Formal education, informal education and nonformal education are the types of education. Agencies of education can be classified mainly into formal, informal, active and passive agencies. Modern education is child centered and teacher is considered as a facilitator of learning. Modernization has given rise to many trends in education.

Nursing education is a professional education meant to prepare professional nurses. Aims of nursing education are harmonious development, inculcating right attitude, knowledge and skill aim, emphasis on high-tech high-touch approach, professional development, leadership development, social aim, citizenship and assisting to build a promising career.

Nursing education enjoys a rich tradition. Goldmark report published in 1923 contributed considerably to the development of nursing education. Recent trends in nursing education include curriculum changes, innovations in teaching and learning, quality assurance, reliance on technology, emphasis on high-tech-high-touch approach, uniformity and standardization, preparation of global nurses, transnational acceptance, high chance of a promising career, emergence of new specialities, preference to short-term clinical programs, increased opportunities for higher studies and potential shortage of nurse educators.

## MULTIPLE CHOICE QUESTIONS

1. **Education is considered as a:**
   a. Bioplor process
   b. Tripolor process
   c. Multipolor process
   d. None of the above

2. **Modern education favors:**
   a. Collaboration
   b. Competition
   c. Mutual understanding
   d. Independent learning

3. **The meaning of word "educare" is to:**
   a. Lead
   b. To bring up
   c. To train
   d. To mould

4. **Who said education is life itself?**
   a. John Dewey
   b. Jeferson
   c. Aristotle
   d. Mahatma Gandhi

5. **"Learning to be" is focused on development of:**
   a. Potential
   b. Knowledge
   c. Skill
   d. Attitude

6. **Who told education is the "all round drawing out of the best in child and man-body mind and spirit"?**
   a. Mahatma Gandhi
   b. John Dewey
   c. Pestalozzi
   d. Aristotle

7. **Modern education is:**
   a. Learner-centered
   b. Teacher-centered
   c. Subject-centered
   d. Technology-centered

8. "Learning to do" is mainly concerned with development of:
   a. Knowledge
   b. Teacher-student relationship
   c. Competency
   d. Positive learning environment
9. **Physical literacy is concerned with:**
   a. Well being
   b. Learning
   c. All round development
   d. Teaching
10. **MOOC is an example of:**
    a. Nonformal education
    b. Formal education
    c. Informal education
    d. None of the above

## ANSWER KEY

| 1. c | 2. a | 3. a | 4. a | 5. a | 6. a |
| 7. a | 8. c | 9. a | 10. a | | |

# CHAPTER 2

# Philosophy and Education

## LEARNING OBJECTIVES

After completing this chapter, reader will be able to:

- Define philosophy.
- List down the branches of philosophy.
- Identify the relationship between philosophy and education.
- Define educational philosophy.
- Explain idealism as an educational philosophy.
- Explain pragmatism as an educational philosophy.
- Explain realism as an educational philosophy.
- Explain theistic realism as an educational philosophy.
- Explain humanistic existentialism as an educational philosophy.
- Explain eclecticism as an educational philosophy.
- Explain the philosophy of nursing education.

In the history of mankind, civilization did not bring happiness to his life. In his search for happiness, perfection and truth, he was forced to find answers to certain vital questions related to his existence in nature, value of life and universe. This attempt by man to solve his worries through seeking solutions to many unaddressed issues led to the development of a new discipline namely philosophy.

## MEANING

The word *"philosophy"* has been derived from two Greek words *"Philos"* and *"Sophia"*. Philos means "Love of" and Sophia means "Wisdom". Thus, philosophy means love of wisdom. Philosophy is search for wisdom and truth. Knowledge is a constituent of wisdom and wisdom helps us to analyze the facts in the process of finding relationships. Wisdom, which is a combination of intelligence, knowledge and initiative helps us to recognize the value of life and to identify our place in this world. In the simplest form we can say philosophy is the values and beliefs every individual has in his life.

Philosophy is love of wisdom. Love is a strong desire to achieve something. Wisdom is the right application of knowledge. Thus, philosophy motivates to acquire knowledge and its right application. We can grow properly only through acquiring knowledge and its right application. Philosophy helps us to develop good values that are essential to lead a successful life. Philosophy makes one responsible for his own life. It also helps us in making ethical choices and realizing our potential.

Philosophy helps us to know who we are by "Inquiring within". By doing introspection we can easily find the meaning of our life and thereby our place on earth. Philosophy helps us to solve problems in life by finding suitable solutions. Advice and wisdom comes down to us through philosophy. We have little control over our circumstances but have complete control over our way (attitude and ability) of reacting to a circumstance. Philosophy helps us to choose the right way of reacting to a situation. We are finding the meaning of our life by reacting to a situation in a proper manner. Thus, philosophy is good at explaining abstract ideas, it helps us to understand **"what is"** and **"what is to be".** In short, philosophy helps us to lead a successful life by understanding present and preparing for the future.

## DEFINITION

- According to Brightman, "philosophy is an attempt to think truely about human experience or to make out whole experience intelligible". This definition correlates philosophy with the thinking process and thereby explaining rationale behind the human experiences. Moreover, this definition indirectly highlights the need of philosophy for a better understanding and living.
- Henderson says that philosophy is a search for comprehensive view of nature, an attempt at a universal explanation of nature of things. This definition focuses on reality and truth.
- In Raymond's opinion, "philosophy is unceasing effort to discern the general truth that lies behind the particular facts, discern also the reality that lies behind appearances". This definition more precisely deals with the reality of life and truth.

## BRANCHES OF PHILOSOPHY

A discussion on the branches of philosophy will help you to follow the forthcoming discussion with minimum effort. As a discipline, philosophy has got five branches, namely *epistemology, logic, metaphysics, esthetics and axiology.* Epistemology deals with the origin and sources of knowledge. Logic is concerned with the systematic study of knowledge and its inter-relationships. Metaphysics deals with the ultimate true nature of things. Esthetics studies about the beauty and harmony in life. Axiology is concerned with the nature of morality and value.

## RELATIONSHIP BETWEEN PHILOSOPHY AND EDUCATION

Philosophy is the science of knowledge and knowledge is the antidote to ignorance. By eliminating ignorance, we can bring about behavioral modification. Education is a planned and purposeful activity with several aims, but the ultimate aim is to bring about the behavioral modification of the learner. To bring about behavioral changes, we have to formulate certain predetermined objectives of education based on values, ideas, beliefs, attitudes and social needs. Philosophy as the science of sciences, philosophy as the mother of all arts, provides the prerequisites required to formulate the objectives of education. Education is always directed by predetermined objectives, thus philosophy directs education. Education without philosophy is blind and philosophy without education is meaningless. According to Ross, education and philosophy are the two sides of a coin, presenting the views of the same thing. Hence philosophy and education are closely related. Philosophy deals with the abstract actions of life and education deals with the active actions of life. Any system of education is influenced by a philosophical viewpoint. Philosophy explains the nature as well as the sources of knowledge and how to validate it. Philosophy guides the educationists in the selection of valid knowledge. The contributions of philosophy in determining the nature of educative process, the nature of learner and the nature of teacher-student relationship is widely appreciated. Previously discussed five branches of philosophy is providing a sound basis for the curriculum development, development and practice of teaching methodology and character development of students. The concept of morality and value system are also influenced by philosophy.

Educational philosophy provides a vision for education. If philosophy is the love of knowledge then education is the acquisition of knowledge. Traditionally education was viewed as a disciplinary process. Philosophy only guided education from the disciplinary process to the present child-centered education. Educational philosophy clarifies concept and analyses propositions, beliefs and theories of education. A philosophy-based vision is essential to understand the new trends in the educational system, especially the contemporary educational movement.

The educational process depends on four fundamental aspects: The educational institutions, teachers, curriculum and the students. Correlation between these four aspects is essential for educational process. Philosophy helps to bring out correlation between these four aspects. Philosophy is concerned with generating knowledge and education is concerned with acquiring or imparting knowledge.

Education may be regarded as the practical aspect of philosophy and philosophy is the intellectual aspect of education. Both philosophy and education go hand in hand. Education depends on philosophy for its guidance and philosophy depends on education for explaining its concepts in a meaningful manner.

## EDUCATIONAL PHILOSOPHY

Philosophy is search for wisdom and truth. Philosophy directs education by providing certain guidelines. In a way, education is the application of philosophy or philosophy of education is applied philosophy. In short, educational philosophy is the application of philosophy, in an attempt to meet the challenges faced by the education system.

### Definition

According to Beth Lewis, "educational philosophy or philosophy of education is a system of thinking about what education is for and how it should be done". According to this definition educational philosophy helps us to find answers for the following questions.
1. What is education?
2. What is the purpose of education?
3. Who should be educated and how?
4. What should be taught?
5. Why should some subjects be taught and not other subjects?
6. How student should be taught?
7. How should students be evaluated and disciplined?

In other words, educational philosophy try to answer questions related to all aspects of education like curriculum, valid knowledge, teaching methods and social considerations such as need for equity, freedom, authority and democracy in education.

In day-to-day educative process, "educational philosophy is the belief or guiding principles a teacher possess about "big picture" of education which include learner, classroom, school and society". As per this definition, every teacher needs to develop a philosophy of education and comes to the classroom with a unique set of principles and ideals that promote learning. In short, teacher need to be aware of her own educational philosophy.

### Functions of Educational Philosophy

From the above discussion, we can summarize the functions of educational philosophy as follows:
1. Assist in determine various aspects of education like aims, purpose, curriculum, teaching-learning process, etc.
2. Contribute in defining the role of teacher, learner, school and society in the educative process.

3. Assessing properly the influence of crucial factors affecting modern education. Crucial factors affecting modern education are developments in cognitive neuroscience, access to information and change in job market.
4. Preserving core values of education.
5. Assist education system in addressing challenges effectively.
6. Assist teachers to perform effectively by developing a suitable educational philosophy.
7. Prepare youngsters to use the power of philosophy in life.

A sound philosophy of education is based on an adequate philosophy of life. Philosophy serves as the source of objectives required by education. Education and philosophy reciprocate each other. Different philosophers, based on their view regarding the life, developed different types of educational philosophies namely idealism, naturalism, pragmatism, realism, theistic realism, eclecticism, etc. In one way or other these philosophies are serving the purpose of guiding the education system. In order to enrich the forthcoming discussion, let us briefly discuss the influence of philosophy in the cardinal areas of education like aims of education, nature of the learner, teacher-pupil relationship, curriculum, teaching methodology, discipline and the role of teacher in education.

- **Philosophy and aims of education:** Role of philosophy in determining the aims of education is a widely-accepted fact and different philosophies have formulated different aims of education.
- **Philosophy and curriculum:** Curriculum is the sum total of all the activities and experiences provided by the school to its pupil in order to achieve the aims of education. To a great extent, content of the curriculum is determined by the philosophy and various philosophies recommend different contents for the curriculum.
- **Philosophy and methods of teaching:** A teaching method will help the teacher to conduct teaching activity in an agreeable, student friendly and successful manner by initiating and maintaining a link between the subject matter and the student. A method is essential for the construction and organization of knowledge. Critical thinking is essential to device a method. As philosophy is a way of thinking, definitely there exists a relationship between philosophy and methods of teaching. Based on their respective beliefs, different philosophers recommend different teaching methods.
- **Philosophy and teacher:** Teacher enjoys a significant role in the educational process as a facilitator of learning. It is the duty of the teacher to help the child to develop a philosophy of life, which embraces the body, mind, career and relationships. Nothing will come out of nothing, so a talented teacher should be oriented to the philosophy and apply this philosophy in the thinking process and in the teaching activity. Each philosophy is maintaining its own reservations regarding the qualities of a teacher.
- **Philosophy and discipline:** In the simple sense, discipline is the conduct of the pupil and most of the philosophers are very much interested in this particular aspect of education. Philosophy determines the nature and types of the discipline.

For convenience, while discussing individual philosophies in detail, the above mentioned aspects are categorized under a major heading, namely "educational implications".

## Importance of Education Philosophy

From the above discussion itself we can understand the importance of educational philosophy. Philosophy provides vision for education. It also helps in formulating definition, goals and meaning of education. Educational philosophy is needed to determine aims of education, formulate curriculum, device methods of teaching, explaining the nature of learners and teacher and selecting the type of discipline.

Educational philosophy helps to understand the educational process. It explains concepts and assumptions related to educational theories. Philosophy explains the role of student in educational process. Traditionally, education is viewed as a disciplinary process. Educational philosophy only helped education to move from the traditional view to the present child-centered education.

Philosophy is concerned with generating knowledge and education aims at imparting knowledge. Educational philosophy synthesizes various types of information and experiences to generate knowledge. Generating knowledge is a philosophical activity without which no education is possible. Thus, we can say the philosophical basis of education is rooted in the branch of philosophy known as epistemology. Epistemology deals with the origin and source of knowledge.

Perry says "As far as education is concerned philosophy is neither inevitable and normal". His words underlines the importance of educational philosophy.

## EDUCATIONAL PHILOSOPHY AND THE TEACHER

Teacher should have his own philosophy of education. Then only he can fulfill his responsibilities as a teacher. Educational philosophy helps the teacher to find solutions for problems related to teaching. It is only through a philosophy of education one can determine the curriculum, the textbooks, the methods of teaching, methods and standards of evaluation and methods of maintaining discipline, etc. Hence, the teacher should have an educational philosophy.

The study of educational philosophy helps the teacher to critically evaluate his teaching and make necessary changes in his teaching. Philosophy has the potential in provoking for changing and rejects some of our beliefs, develops analytical and logical skills and reasoning. Educational philosophy clarifies concept and analyzes propositions, beliefs and theories of education. A philosophy-based vision is essential to understand the new trends in the educational systems especially the contemporary educational movements.

Relationship between educational philosophy and teacher will be more clear from the upcoming discussion of individual educational philosophies.

### Philosophy of a Teacher

The best teacher is one who inspires the students. Thus, educational philosophy of best teacher is his beliefs about best ways to inspire students. Some of such beliefs are: (a) learning is a basic need of student like, food, shelter and clothing; (b) students need to be active participants in learning; (c) learning is a physiological activity involving the whole body; (d) students need timely feedback to improve; (e) each student is unique and has his own pace of learning; (f) exciting learning environment is a must for learning; (g) students need information, knowledge and skills and (h) students need tools and resources for effective learning.

## EDUCATIONAL PHILOSOPHIES

### Idealism

Idealism is the oldest philosophy. The word *ideals* is derived from the Greek word *"Iden"* which means *"to see"*. Plato is the father of idealism. Idealism believe that man is a combination of spiritual and material aspects, of which the spiritual aspect is more real and important. According to an idealist, spiritual nature is the essence of life and physical world is a visible evidence for the presence of a greater spirit invisible for us. Idealist gives more importance to mind and self rather than matter and body. Idealism regard spirit and intellect are of supreme value than physical matter. As per the idealism, individual experience is valid than the material world and man lives in the world of ideas rather than facts. Idealist also believes that the purpose of life is to know the ultimate truth and mind is not dependent on physical reality. As a spiritual being, man is the most beautiful and superior creation by God. The development of personality has been given priority in idealistic philosophy and believes that ultimate aim of life is the exaltation of the personality. The goal of learning and living is to transform the natural man into an ideal man by attaining physical, intellectual, emotional, moral and spiritual perfection. Idealism highlights the need for inculcating moral and cultural values in human life and advice effective utilization of moral and cultural values along with the spiritual value for controlling the physical environment.

## Principles of Idealism

Idealists put forward the following principles to substantiate the validity of their viewpoints.

1. **Presence of universal mind:** Idealist believes that there is a universal mind and symbolize this universal mind as God. All knowledge and human life originated from this universal mind or God. Being a beautiful creation by God, ultimate aim of human life is the realization of God or universal mind. Even now this principle holds true as most of us thank God for giving a chance to live in this world and seek God's blessings for a smooth and successful living.

2. **Regards man as a spiritual being:** According to idealism, man is a combination of spiritual and material aspects, of which spiritual or mental aspect is more real and important. This spiritual nature of man is the essence of his existence and makes him distinct from other creations by God. Idealists believe that mind or spirit is not merely brain and its activity but it is a real thing with a separate entity. This statement is now inviting criticisms as more and more evidences are emerging from recent research works to support the relationship between brain and the concept of mind.

3. **The world of ideas and values are superior than the materialistic world:** Idealism believe in the worth of ideals or higher values. Higher values, which makes the human life more meaningful are not created by man. They have a prior existence as a gift from God to the mankind. The foremost aim of man should be the realization of these higher values. According to Plato, these higher values are truth, goodness, glory and beauty. Idealist also believes that attainment of these higher values will be possible only through the realization of God. This principle is really an antidote to varied problems prevailing in our highly materialistic and consumer-driven modern society. Addition of higher values to the day-to-day life will enliven our lives by avoiding problems.

4. **The real knowledge is perceived in mind:** According to idealists, knowledge attained through activity and creativity of mind is valid than the knowledge acquired through senses. This principle is against simple mugging up of bookish knowledge and recognizes the importance of critical thinking and activity in gaining knowledge or skill. Modern educationists consider critical thinking as an integral part of problem solving and problem solving is the most widely accepted method of learning, especially in nursing. The drawback of this principle is that it misjudged the role of senses in acquiring knowledge.

## Educational Implications of Idealism (Fig. 2.1)

Idealism considers student as an individual with immense potential. Education should help the student to realize these potential. Curriculum should consist of those knowledge and experiences which help the student to attain development. The child should be taught the

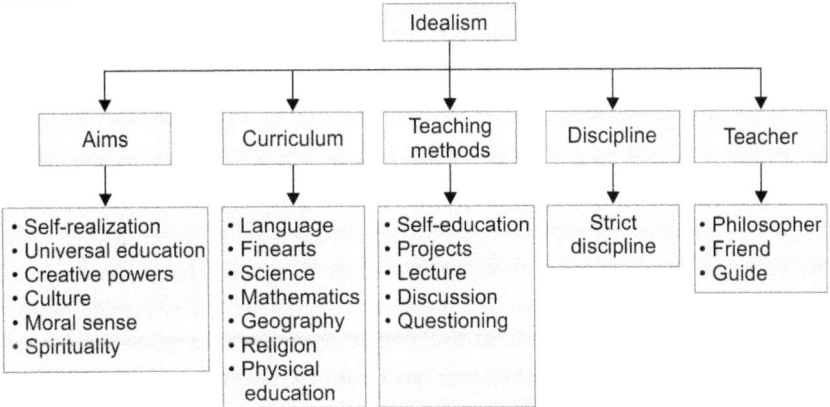

Fig. 2.1: Educational implications of idealism.

ways and means to acquire and verify knowledge. The teacher should impart essentials of knowledge and assist to develop moral and esthetic values in the child. As said earlier, idealism stresses more on the spiritual development of the child. Let us see these aspects in detail.

*Idealism and Aims of Education*

- **Self-realization:** Self-realization or development of self-image is facilitated by attaining full knowledge about the self. Human being is a wonderful creation by God and human life is the greatest or grandest work of God. JS Ross says that the education in idealism refers to the development of highest potential of the self. Education should help the child to develop the self-image or self-realization. This aim is widely admired due to its relevance in the present-day competitive world. In one or other way all human beings are blessed with enormous powers and potential. It is the duty of the education to assist the child to identify and nurture these innate hidden potential to the maximum level. Self-realization help us to find a place to settle and flourish in this world. In short, self-realization is a prerequisite for a dedicated and successful living.
- **Exaltation of personality through self-realization:** Education is for the exaltation of personality. In the words of an idealist, "education is for the exaltation of human personality and the exaltation of personality is based upon the concept of realization of the highest potential of the self in a social and cultural environment". Education aims to build a healthy personality, which is very adjusting with our immediate surroundings.
- **Universal education:** According to idealism, human race is one and every individual in the society need to be educated irrespective of the caste, creed, color and social status. Even in those days itself idealism recognized the importance of education in the socioeconomic development of nations. Low literacy rate in developing countries and nearly cent-percent literacy rate in developed countries justifies this aim of education. Major contribution of this aim to the education system is that it motivated many nations to accept the right for education as a birth right or a fundamental right.
- **Development of inventive and creative powers:** Idealism encourage man to change or modify the environment according to his needs and mould nature to suit his purposes through his inventive and creative skills. According to idealism, education must nurture the inventive and creative powers of man. Even though this aim sounds good, it is inherent with some deficiencies. Creative and constructive practice of this aim helped the mankind to survive by overcoming many challenges and fuelled all major inventions and achievements.

Now, forgetting the judicious use of this aim, greedy modern man is using this aim in a destructive manner even by endangering the existence of the nature. If practised properly, this aim is really a blessing in the context of new challenges and misuse of it can lead to major disasters.

- **Conservation, promotion and transmission of cultural heritages:** Culture is very essential for the development of human potential and making culture prevail is the duty of education. Education helps the child to become aware about the culture and feel proud of it. Education also equip the child to contribute something to the cultural enrichment and its transmission to the future generations. Based on this aim, nations incorporate essence of their cultural heritage in the curriculum.
- **Bringing out or the enrichment of the cultural environment:** Let us see much about this aim from the words of an idealist, "idealism believe that man is responsible for the environment, especially for his immediate environment. The child can grow only, if the environment is suitable for his growth. Hence, preservation and enrichment of the cultural values in the environment should be the aim of education."
- **Development of moral sense:** The development of moral sense will help the child to lead a healthy life and to differentiate between right and wrong, good and evil. Moral sense will also help the child to admire truth, goodness and beauty. Considering this aim of education, many schools have included moral science in the curriculum.
- **Cultivation of spiritual values:** Idealism believe that man is essentially a spiritual being and gives prime importance for cultivating spiritual values through education. In idealism, eternal and unchanging spiritual values are considered as fundamental values of life. Education should help the child to lead a spiritual life so that he will be able to respect the spiritual worth and dignity of other people.

## *Idealism and Curriculum*

Overall development of child is the aim of idealistic curriculum. To achieve this overall development, subjects which assist the child to develop morally, esthetically, intellectually and physically are included in the curriculum. Subjects like poetry, fine arts and religion promote moral and esthetic development, whereas subjects like language, science, mathematics and geography foster intellectual development. Invariably, physical education leads to physical development.

## *Idealism and Methods of Teaching*

According to idealists, classroom is a spiritual setting where human minds interact and unite and students develop spiritually. Pestalozzi and Froebel are the two well-known idealist educationists contributed to the teaching methodology. Pestalozzi recommends self-education or self-activities of children. Froebel developed the popular method of teaching namely *"Kindergarten".* Kindergarten method regard school as a garden, the teacher as gardener and students as tender plants intended to grow to beauty and perfection. Questioning, discussion and lecture method for teaching language, projects and imitation are some of the methods suggested by idealism. Idealism believe that by employing these teaching methods, students can receive knowledge and develop learning abilities with the help of the teacher.

## *Idealism and Discipline*

According to idealism, self-realization is the prime aim of education and recommend strict discipline for the attainment of self-realization. Thus, idealism is against free discipline.

Teacher has to impose strict discipline. Idealist believes that a disciplined mind only can attain the highest values of life namely truth, goodness and beauty.

## Idealism and Teacher

Idealism reserves a high place for the teacher and recognize teacher as a philosopher, friend and guide. According to idealism, the best teacher is one who always inspires the students and serves as a role model to them. Idealistic concept regarding the inspiring teacher is genuine, as an inspiring teacher is considered as the best teacher by the modern students. Just like oxygen in the inspired air, inspiring thoughts and words are really inevitable to survive in this competitive word. An idealistic teacher has to guide the student for achieving the all-round development.

# Naturalism

Rousseau and Aristotle have been the proponents of naturalism. Naturalism is concerned with natural self and believes that reality and nature are identical and beyond nature there is no reality. For naturalists, nature is everything and nothing exists superior than nature so they separates nature from God and allot no place for supernaturalism and spiritualism. With the help of physical and chemical laws naturalism explains the universe, the physical world, life and mind. This nature is governed by its own laws and man is regarded as a child of nature. External or heavenly values have nothing to do with the development of the child, whereas child grows and develop by himself as a result of brain function and contributions from the physical and biological nature of the world. Naturalists also believe that all our activities, whether it may be biological, psychological or social are initiated by our instincts. It considers matter as superior to spirit and gives importance to scientific method of observation and verification. Naturalism stresses the need to return to the nature from artificiality.

## Definition

According to Hayward Joyce, naturalism is a system of which the salient characteristic is the exclusion of whatever is spiritual or indeed, whatever is transcendental of experience. This definition straightaway denies whatever is spiritual and supernatural.

## Different Forms of Naturalism

Physical naturalism, biological naturalism and mechanical naturalism are the three different forms of naturalism. Physical naturalism believes that laws of physical nature govern the laws of human life and adherence to natural laws is essential for human existence. Biological naturalism strongly agrees with the theory of evolution and according to this philosophy, man being a descendant of ape possess animal nature and is devoid of any element of spiritualism. Mechanical naturalism views man as a mere machine devoid of spirit and soul and aims at training man as a good machine.

## Principles of Naturalism

1. **Child-centered education:** In naturalistic point of view, prime importance has to be given to the child than teachers and others. This is the major contribution of naturalism to the educational system. The present-day education system is neither teacher centered nor subject matter centered but child centered only. Today, teacher's role is limited to a facilitator of learning.

2. **Education as the natural development of the child's power and capacities:** Education pattern should coincide with the natural development and learning capacity of the child. To achieve this, education has to be planned according to the laws of growth and development.
3. **Negative education in early childhood:** In the early life of a child, simple persuasion is enough to initiate learning instead of forcing him to learn. This simple persuasive way of initiating learning instead of using force is known as negative education.
4. **Education should be based on child's psychology:** This principle advocates the need for considering individual difference among students. Individual difference in intelligence, temperament and emotions among students should be identified and taken into account while implementing the educative process. This principle is very much appreciated by the modern educationists. Nowadays the validity of educative process is determined by how well it is catering to the individual needs of students.
5. **The role of teacher should be that of a guide:** This principle is somewhat similar to the first one. Instead of passively transferring knowledge, the teacher has to arrange an environment with necessary opportunities and materials required for the personal development of the child and guide the child as and when needed. Qualities like love, sympathy and understanding for the child are essential for good teaching. In short, child should take an active role in the teaching-learning process than the teacher.

## *Educational Implications of Naturalism (Fig. 2.2)*

Applied to education, naturalism considers child as a gift of nature with potential for natural growth according to the laws of nature. The child is an active individual capable of self-development. The aim of education is to develop the child as a healthy and active personality in a natural setting. The growth process must be natural and real without any interference from outside. The powers of the child should be developed in a natural way by allowing the child to freely interact with the nature. The curriculum should provide concrete and real experiences in a natural context. The child should be exposed to a variety of sensory and physical activities. The child learns by interacting with nature. Morality and character are learned indirectly with the help of natural consequences of behavior. Discipline is developed as a result of consequences of behavior of the child. The teacher plays the role of guiding the child in learning from nature. Using several methods, the teacher creates a congenial situation for the child to learn from nature. Importance is given to the development of individuality and a sense of freedom. Let us see these aspects one by one.

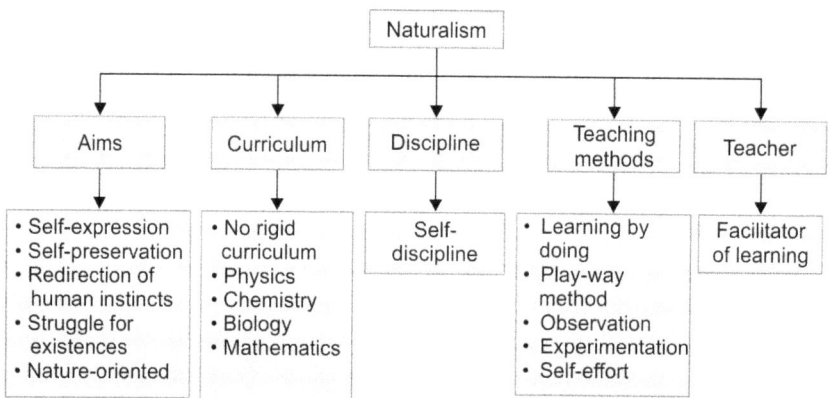

**Fig. 2.2:** Educational implications of naturalism.

## Naturalism and Aims of Education
According to naturalism, education should strive to attain the below mentioned aims:
* **Self-expression:** Naturalist believes that children should be provided with an opportunity to express their ideas and talents. The best photograph in the world is of no good, if it is still in camera, like that the talents of children cannot be judged and directed properly to reap results, if they are not expressed.
* **Self-preservation:** In naturalistic point of view, self-security or self-preservation is an unavoidable aspect in life and education should enable the child to develop these qualities. Self-preservation is the power to be ourselves but it is not self-centered. A person who respects and value himself is much more likely to be able to do the same for others. Self-preservation involves a sense of direction and helps us to identify the right direction in life.
* **Redirection of human instincts:** Naturalist believes that each child is born with certain instincts, which are the guiding force behind all human conduct. These instincts may develop improperly if they are self-directed by the child. Hence through education the human instincts have to be redirected for achieving socially desirable results.
* **Struggle for existence:** Naturalist says that individual child may have to face several painful and stress laden situations in the physical world. Hence children have to be educated in such a way that they will be able to struggle for their existence and able to adjust themselves with the environment.
* **Education according to nature:** While educating the child, his whole nature, i.e., tendencies, developmental status, capacities, instincts, likes and dislikes should be considered.
* **Perfect development of individuality:** Education should aim at developing the child into joyous, rational, balanced, useful and mature person.

Most of the above-said aims matches with the aims of modern education system but ignoring the spiritual and moral development of the child is considered as a major drawback of naturalism.

## Naturalism and Curriculum
Naturalist maintains a unique view regarding the curriculum. As per naturalism, there is no need for a rigid curriculum and consider nature as a grand book from which children can learn everything to become an individual. Naturalist believes that subjects like physics, chemistry, botany, zoology, geography, history and mathematics should be taught to children with special importance to experience. These subjects should be correlated with the life around the child so that he can acquire most of the knowledge from the natural setting itself.

## Naturalism and Methods of Teaching
* **Learning by doing:** Naturalism appreciate direct experience and believe in the principle of learning by doing.
* **Play-way method:** Play-way method is the brain-child of Caldwell Cook. He recognized that good learning is more often the result of spontaneous effort and free interest rather than compulsion and forced application. Since spontaneous effort and free interest are two main features of play, this method of teaching is called play-way method. Play-way approach enhances the quality of teaching by offering elements of freedom, interest, reality and spontaneity.
* **Observation and experimentation:** Observation is regarded as a direct experience and a yielding method when employed by a talented teacher. Observation simplifies the learning process and help the student in retaining the learned skills and facts. As naturalism believe in conducting experiments, children have to be provided with practical experience.

- **Self-education or self-effort:** This is a classical contribution of naturalism. Now, more or less education is viewed as a lifelong process. Educationists all over the world unanimously agree that self-education or self-effort is inevitable in this era of knowledge explosion. The concept of self-education have motivated the modern educationists to consider education as a lifelong process. Thus, self-education is a classical philosophical thought of naturalism and recommend different kinds of assignments and activities for attaining all-round development through self-education or self-effort.

### Naturalism and Discipline
Naturalism favors total freedom and oppose punishment or external discipline. Rousseau believes that child should be allowed to face the natural consequences of his actions and this exposure to consequences will naturally result in the development of self-discipline.

### Naturalism and Teacher
In naturalism, teacher's place is behind the scene. Instead of passively transferring information, the teacher has to arrange an environment or stage with necessary opportunities and materials required for the personal development of the child and guide or direct the child as and when needed by adopting the role of a director or facilitator.

## Pragmatism

Pragmatism adopt a midway between idealism and naturalism. The word pragmatism is derived from the Greek word *"Pragma"* means action. Pragmatism is otherwise known as instrumentalism or functionalism. Since emphasis is given to learning by doing and learning by experience, it is also called experimentalism.

Pragmatism originated in ancient Greece. Modern pragmatism originated in America and proponents of modern pragmatism include Charles Saunders Pierce, William James and John Dewey.

### Definition of Pragmatism
According to Ross, pragmatism is essentially a humanistic philosophy maintaining that man creates his own values in course of activity, that reality is still in making and awaits its part of completion from the future. This definition emphasis on creation through continuous activity and states that certain values are essential for growth and development of the individual.

### Forms of Pragmatism
- **Humanistic pragmatism:** According to this ideology, that which satisfies the needs, requirements, aspirations, objectives of the human beings and cater to the welfare of mankind only can be considered as true and real.
- **Experimental pragmatism:** As per experimental pragmatism, whatever can be experimentally verified is true or what worked is true.
- **Biological pragmatism:** According to this ideology, power and capacity possessed by human beings is valuable and enables him to adjust with his environment or change the environment according to his needs.

### Principles of Pragmatism
Principles of pragmatism are: (a) Man is considered as essentially a biological and social organism; (b) Knowledge should be experimentally verified and it should be useful to the learner; (c) Pragmatism has faith in man's capacity to shape his destiny; (d) There are no

absolute values. All values are relative. What works as useful becomes a value; (e) Only those theories which can work in practical situations are true; (f) Pragmatist is more concerned with the present and immediate future; (g) Pragmatism accepts only the knowledge which is empirical, i.e., which can be experienced at sensory level; (h) Only those ideas which can be realized in life are real.

## Educational Implications of Pragmatism (Fig. 2.3)

In fact, pragmatism revolutionized the education system. Pragmatic trend in education is known as progressivism in education and the school based on pragmatic ideas was known as progressive school. Pragmatism considers the learner as a growing biological and social being ready to adjust to the environmental demands. The aim of education should be to prepare the individual to face the challenges of life, to face the problems and to solve them. Education must prepare the child to become an effective member of the community. It should also try to develop competencies in the child. Hence the curriculum should include those subjects and experiences which are suitable to the child's interests and needs. The curriculum should develop an attitude of inquiry, facilitate artistic expression, encourage constructiveness and sustain interest in the child. Deway suggests that curriculum should include varieties of activities of real life. The pragmatism advocates observation and experiment as methods of teaching. Deway advocates "learning by doing", which encourages the child to learn through activities. Deway considers discipline as a function of the teaching-learning situation. If the learning is made joyful and interesting, there is no need to use external rewards and punishments. A pragmatic teacher helps in organizing learning activities and guides the learner in his activities. Instead of providing knowledge in the ready-made form, teacher should encourage the learner to learn through active interaction with the learning situation. Let us discuss these aspects in detail.

### Pragmatism and Aims of Education

* **Harmonious development of the individual:** Pragmatist believes that various growth-oriented experiences and different learning situations are essential for the harmonious development of the child. More and more growth accompanied by inculcation of new values will enhance the overall development of the child. Harmonious development includes physical, emotional, intellectual, social, spiritual and esthetic development. Harmonious

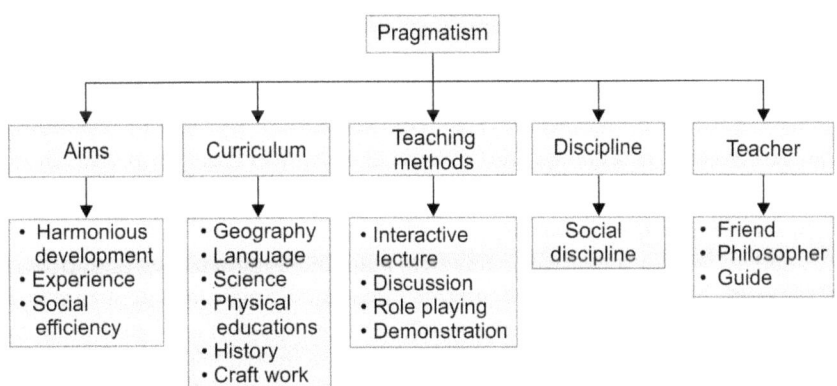

**Fig. 2.3:** Educational implications of pragmatism.

development will prepare the child to face the challenges of life, to face the problems and to solve them.
- **Continuous experience:** Pragmatist recommends continuous and varied experiments to children in a graded way for enhancing the competency. Continuous and varied experiences can be provided only by reconstructing the experiences according to the capacity, interest and need of the child. Cumulative effect of all these experiences will influence the growth and development of the child.
- **Social efficiency:** Appropriate education helps the child to lead a productive life in the democratic society. Belief in democracy, flexibility, social efficiency, active participation in changing social order are the social dimensions of individual growth and these social dimensions are nurtured by quality education.

### *Pragmatism and Curriculum*

Pragmatism suggest broad field curriculum and advocate underlying principles for curriculum construction.
- **Principle of utility:** Based on this principle those subjects, experiences and activities which can satisfy the present and future needs or expectations of the child should be included in the curriculum. Subjects like language, physical training, science, history, geography, agriculture and home science for girls should be included in the curriculum. This principle also recommend vocational and technical education. A curriculum which gives significance to practical knowledge and experience assists the child to acquire knowledge, proper activity and skills. Thus, utilitarian form of curriculum helps the child immensely in his growth and development.
- **Principle of interest:** Curriculum should be based on the child's interest. Subjects, activities and experiences that suits to the interest, aptitude, attitude and needs of the child should be included in the curriculum. Child's interest can be categorized into interest in conversation, interest in creation and expression, interest in investigation and interest in construction. Reading, writing, counting, art, craft work, natural science and other practical works will satisfy the varied interests of the child.
- **Principle of experience:** This principle focuses on the child's activity, vocation and experience. Student achieves experiences from the activities in the library, classroom, laboratory and playground. Co-curricular activities also form an integral part of the curriculum. Provision for various types of productive learning experiences in the curriculum will foster thinking capacity in addition to the development of social and purposeful attitudes.
- **Principle of integration:** This principle deals with the integration of various subjects and experiences. Pragmatist considers knowledge as a single unit. As a single unit, knowledge cannot be divided into watertight compartments or as separate subjects, not connected with one another. In order to develop the right concept and for proper understanding, various units have to be closely connected and correlated. Whatever is taught in the previous classes may have to be integrated with the new classes so that the child can sustain his development.

### *Pragmatism and Methods of Teaching*

In fact, pragmatism revolutionized the concept of teaching. Pragmatist gives importance to the child than the book, teacher and subject matter. Pragmatistic methods are dynamic, vary from class to class and time to time. Pragmatism deny any outdated, lifeless and rigid methods of teaching. As students differ in their innate capabilities, no fixed or single method of teaching is suitable to entire students. For the first time, pragmatism recommended *participatory approach* of teaching, which is considered as an excellent approach by the current education system.

In participatory approach, irrespective of the method of teaching, students are allowed and motivated to participate actively in the teaching-learning process. Teaching method should provide opportunities for practical work, activities and productive experiences. Interactive lecture, discussion, role playing, demonstration, return demonstration, experiment method and activity-oriented teaching are some of the methods suggested by pragmatism. Following principles developed by pragmatism will help us in the selection and formulation of teaching methods.

1. **Principle of progressive learning:** This principle states that a child's initiative to attain a goal depends on his natural interests, aptitudes, abilities and experiences. Pragmatism oppose simple bookish knowledge in favor of self-learning through self-effort. Method of teaching should provide growth-oriented experiences and productive practical activities in order to equip the child to face and overcome the challenges associated with the modern life.
2. **Principle of learning by doing:** Pragmatism favors activity and experience than thoughts and ideas. According to this principle, aim of education should be achieved through experiences, preferably though real-life experiences and real-life situations. Hence, this principle insists to provide more and more creative experiences and experimental activities to the child so that he learns from his own experience.
3. **Principle of integration:** As knowledge is considered as a whole, integration of different subjects is essential to develop a unified view.

*Pragmatism and Discipline*

Pragmatists does not believe in strict and rigid discipline. They believe in social discipline. Social discipline may develop in child from experiences and help which the child receives from the society, school and home. Purposeful cooperative activities may help the child to develop mutual interest, initiative, self-reliance, tolerance and consideration for others.

*Pragmatism and Teacher*

Pragmatism consider teacher as a friend, philosopher and guide to the children. Ability to maintain a close relationship with children for understanding their interests and awareness regarding the social condition are the two important qualities needed for a teacher. The pragmatist teacher teaches his pupils to think and act for themselves rather than to know or to react.

# Realism

First valid explanation regarding this ideology was given by Aristotle and later modified by Gemore, Russel and John wild. According to this philosophy, things we see and perceive are real and knowledge acquired through senses only is true.

## Definition

- ❖ In JS Ross's opinion, "the doctorine of realism asserts that there is a real world of things behind and corresponding to the objects of our perception". This definition deals with the reality of things in this world and the nature of our perception.
- ❖ According to Butter, "realism is the reinforcement of our common acceptance of this world as it appears to us". This simple definition justifies the statement that seeing is believable.

## Forms of Realism

- ❖ **Humanistic realism:** According to humanistic realism, only education can bring out human welfare and success. Erasmus, Rabelias and Milton support this view. Erasmus believes that knowledge seems to be of two kinds, that of things and that of words. That of words come first but that of things is more important. Rebelias recommends liberal education by giving significance to religious, social and moral values. Milton favors complete and generous education for the all-round development of human beings.

- **Social realism:** Social realism propose an education system which can promote the working efficiency of individuals. Attainment of real knowledge will make human life happy and successful through fulfilling the needs of the society.
- **Sense realism:** Sense realism originated in the 4th century and has got immense applications in the modern education system. Sense realism believe that knowledge primarily comes through the senses and not from words. In the process of educating the child, his ears, mouth, skin and limbs should be freely used to the maximum. All knowledge originates from the external nature. Hence education should adopt real and effective methods instead of artificial techniques. Sense realism recognize the importance of observing the nature, study of scientific subjects, practical education and research.
- **Neorealism:** This ideology is more inclined towards science than education. Moreover, lack of authentic literature pertaining to the contribution of neorealism to education limits the possibility for a detailed discussion.

## Principles of Realism

Principles of realism can be summarized as follows. (a) Worldly realities of everyday life are true; (b) It does not believe in the existence of any absolute truth; (c) It accepts only sensory experiences of the external world as real; (d) It looks at man like a physical being controlled by rules and laws; (e) Real knowledge is obtained by analyzing and experiencing sensations; (f) It advocates the methods and principles of physical science for acquiring knowledge.

## Educational Implications of Realism

Realism considers the child as a dynamic and growing entity ready to face the realities of life. The laws of nature control the child. The aim of education is to prepare the child to face the realities of life and to solve the problems. The knowledge and experiences given in the school should be appropriate to achieve this aim. Hence the realist suggests that the curriculum should be broad based and includes varieties of subjects, especially science subjects. While selecting the subject, the learners background and social demands should be considered. Realism suggests objective method of teaching. Importance must be given to observation, experimentation and activities. According to realism, discipline is developed by properly controlling the environment. A realist teacher should encourage the pupil to make discoveries and learn through interaction with the external world. The teacher should know the psychological nature of the child for effective teaching.

### Realism and Aims of Education

Realism suggest six main aims of education, they are: (a) Prepare the child for a real life; (b) Prepare the child for a happy and successful life; (c) Fosters mental and physical powers of child; (d) Developing and training of senses; (e) Providing vocational education; (f) Make the child familiar with the nature and social environment.

### Realism and Curriculum

Realistic curriculum prefers subjects and activities which can prepare children for day-to-day living. Science and vocational subjects enjoy predominant position in curriculum followed by arts, literature and languages.

### Realism and Methods of Teaching

Realism opposes bookish knowledge as it failed to prepare the child for real life. Since realism believes that knowledge comes through senses and words, it justifies the use of appropriate audiovisual aids in teaching. Realism recommends objective method of teaching. Importance must be given to observation, experimentation and activities.

### Realism and Discipline

Realism believes in self-discipline and advocate moral and religious education for the development of self-discipline among children.

### Realism and Teacher

In realism, an honorable position is reserved for teachers. A realist teacher is well versed in content and aware about the needs of the children. He is also interested in research and transferring knowledge in a clear and intelligible way by employing psychological and scientific principles.

## THEISTIC REALISM OR SUPERNATURALISM

Theistic realism originated as a Christian philosophy and according to this philosophy there is a personal God. God is the author or creator of nature and man. God has created this universe and placed man in the universe as His child. God helps His children to attain the eternal destiny—that is union with God. Man is made up of a body and soul. Man is created to serve the God on earth and man will achieve eternal health and happiness with the God in heaven. Education is regarded as an active social process and can take place in the family, school and church. Teacher has to provide an environment and opportunities to the child conducive for acquiring the ideas, attitudes and habits required for leading a social life. Teacher should also help the child to recognize the social nature of man, identify the social needs of man and provide needed assistance to man.

## Educational Implications of Theistic Realism

### Theistic Realism and Aims of Education

The aims of education are social development, economic competency, moral development, spiritual perfection and physical development.

### Theistic Realism and Curriculum

In curriculum, high ranking is given to spiritual and moral values, social sciences, behavioral sciences and biological sciences.

### Theistic Realism and Methods of Teaching

Theistic realism prefer discussion method, lecture method and practical experiences as teaching methods.

### Theistic Realism and Discipline

Theistic realism is against rigid discipline and favors self-discipline. Teacher's role is very important in fostering self-discipline among children.

### Theistic Realism and Teacher

Theistic realism believes that guidance is essential for the all-round development of the child and consider teacher as a guide. Bringing out the child's hidden potentials and nurturing leadership qualities are regarded as primary functions of the teacher.

## HUMANISTIC EXISTENTIALISM

Humanistic existentialism is the youngest philosophy. Existentialism may be described as a modern philosophy which is primarily build upon the work of the scholars of the twentieth century.

### Main Assumptions

- **Man's existence:** Existentialist believes that man is most important, has inherent dignity and is worthy of respect and care simply because he exists. Man cannot accept the ready-made concepts of existence forced upon him. He is a free agent capable of shaping his own life and choosing his own destiny.
- **Self-knowledge:** Man has an inherent creative drive towards higher and more positive levels of existence and self-actualization. Social responsibility and individual worth are given due importance in existentialist philosophy.
- **Freedom and responsibility:** The most basic and irrefutable freedom is the freedom of choice; the options may be limited but choices always exists. Man's freedom to choose gives man an element of unpredictability. Because man makes his own life choices, he is accountable for the consequences of those choices. Individual uniqueness and personal accountability for one's action are the ultimate products of existentialist philosophy.
- **Man is not complete:** According to existentialist philosophy, man is not complete. He has to face many challenges in the process of becoming a complete man.

### Educational Implications of Existentialism

The educational implications of humanistic existentialism are (a) According to existentialism the primary aim of education is the making of individual as one who lives and makes decisions about what he will do; (b) School should provide an environment where the individuals find security, encouragement and acceptance by teachers; (c) All school subjects and activities should provide situations for the development of human beings; (d) Teacher has to facilitate development or originality and creativity by providing necessary materials and opportunities; (e) The teacher has to be very active and equip students to face challenges; (f) School should nurture democratic ideas; (g) Concern and respect for the individual student should be the main concern of the school.

## ECLECTICISM

Irrespective of other differences, all educational philosophies view education as a dynamic process and this dynamic nature is essential for meeting the diversified and ever increasing needs of the society. No single educational philosophy alone can help the education to maintain its dynamic nature. This motivated educationists to create a new educational philosophy by pooling all the good and relevant features from different educational philosophies. This newly created educational philosophy is named as *eclecticism*. It is earnestly hoped that through eclecticism or eclectic tendency we can maintain the dynamic nature of education in order to meet the demands of the society.

### Need for Eclecticism in Education

Education is always driven by societal needs and these needs are changing from time to time. Efficient education systems promptly foresee the future needs of the society and reprioritize its aims accordingly. This reprioritization helps the education system to meet the demands of the society. As said earlier, education always depends on philosophy to derive its objectives, but no educational philosophy is complete in itself. Moreover, sometimes certain aspects of an educational philosophy get outdated while some other aspects of the same philosophy remain valid. This motivated the educationists to identify valid and relevant ideas from various philosophies and pool them to formulate an agreeable philosophy of education namely eclecticism. In broad sense, eclecticism is a harmonious combination of recent tendencies in education and agreeable features of different philosophies. Based on this harmonization, eclecticism is otherwise known as eclectic tendencies in education. As eclecticism is helpful in solving various problems related to present-day education system, it is graded as the best philosophical approach.

## Salient Features of Eclecticism

(a) Aim of education is to prepare good citizens; (b) Recommends broad and flexible curriculum; (c) Emphasis coordination of various subjects; (d) Importance to co-curricular activities; (e) Ensuring availability of subject experts and better teachers; (f) Suggest scientific teaching methods based on the principles of learning by doing, learning by play and learning by observation; (g) Consider education as a tool for social control; (h) Recommends professional status for teaching job; (i) Importance to self-discipline; (j) Highlight responsibility of governments in providing education, especially in the primary level and for handicapped children; (k) Emphasis on adult and social education; (l) Harmonious relationship among school, home and society.

## PHILOSOPHY OF NURSING EDUCATION

By definition, "philosophy of nursing education is the written statement of the believes, values, attitudes and ideas which the faculty as a group agreed upon in relation to the nursing educational program, such as health, disease, nursing, nurse, nursing as a profession, education, learner, society, patient, nursing education and preparation of nurses."

Philosophy of nursing education is a perfect combination of philosophy of nursing and philosophy of education, more precisely, philosophy of nursing education is the application of the fundamental belief of nursing and education in the field of nursing education.

In the philosophy of education, importance is given to the student. The objectives formulated with a philosophical basis of education focus on the student life and the all-round development of the student. In the philosophy of nursing, emphasis is placed on the patients. Objectives may have to be formulated to provide comprehensive nursing care by identifying the patient needs, meeting those needs and evaluating the care.

Philosophy looks at whole and nursing education prepares the student to react to a situation as a whole rather than fragments. For example, while caring a patient with cerebrovascular accident, nursing student has to consider the protective, curative and rehabilitative aspects rather than concentrating in any one aspect.

Nursing is a healing science and as a belief construct, philosophy decides the healing approach. For instance, behavior of a nursing student while discharging a recovered patient is different from the behavior exhibited while caring a critically ill patient. *In short, the philosophy of a nursing institute should be enriched with value statements regarding the practice of nursing and teaching of nursing.*

Since the objectives, policies, academic and administrative control of the institution is based on the already stated philosophy, statement of philosophy is regarded as the foundation for starting a nursing institute or a nursing educational program. To formulate the philosophy, staff may have to hold several discussions and reach a consensus regarding what is feasible and reliable in relation to the interest of students, institution, society and profession.

The faculty of an institute enjoy all rights to formulate the philosophy based on their beliefs, but a thoughtfully coined philosophy usually addresses the philosophical issues like learner, society, man, nursing education, health and institution (philosophical statement concerning institution explain its aims and objectives, commitment of the institute, etc.).

The philosophy will decide the nature of student selection process, objectives of the educational programs, curriculum development, type of practical experiences provided to the students, selection and placement of staff, teaching methods and evaluation system.

Nursing prepares its members professionally through a variety of educational programs and these programs differ from each other in multiple aspects like entering criteria, duration, specialization, program evaluation, etc. Each educational program in turn depends upon the philosophy for rationalizing its various aspects. Hence, philosophy enjoys much importance in nursing education. Considering the diversity of nursing educational programs, *the philosophical statement explaining the expected outcome of an educational program deserves more attention.*

Eventhough every phase of nursing education is influenced by the philosophy, the most significant and everlasting influence of philosophy is noticed in the development and nurturing of proper attitude among nursing students towards the patient, community, fellow human beings and professional development. Through cultivating proper attitude, philosophy plays a dominant role in uplifting the professional image of nursing.

In the beginning, nursing and nursing education was solely under the influence of supernaturalism, but the changes in the education system, socioeconomic condition, scientific and technological advancements, innovations in the healthcare sector and knowledge explosion motivated the nursing education to consider other philosophies also. **Following an eclectic tendency by adopting the good features of various philosophies is also common now.**

## Factors Influencing Philosophy of Nursing Education

*Philosophy of nursing education is influenced by the following factors:* (a) Beliefs and values of faculty members regarding God, man, life, health, disease, nursing, etc; (b) The philosophical values and believes of the institution; (c) The environment where the education takes place; (d) The student and the life activities; (e) Health needs of the society; (f) The culture and background of the people; (g) Developments in nursing, medicine and allied fields; (h) Philosophy of nursing service administration; (i) The goals and objectives of the healthcare delivery system; (j) The disease pattern, the health awareness and health facilities available; (k) The available resources in terms of man, money and materials.

## ECLECTICISM AS PHILOSOPHY OF NURSING EDUCATION (FIG. 2.4)

### Meaning of Eclecticism

Eclecticism has been derived from the verb 'elect'. To elect means to choose and pick up. The good ideas, concept and principles from various philosophies have been chosen, picked up and blended together to make a complete philosophy. Thus, eclecticism is a philosophy of choice. Eclecticism is nothing but fusion of ideas from all sources. It is a peculiar type of educational philosophy which combines all good ideas and principles from various philosophies.

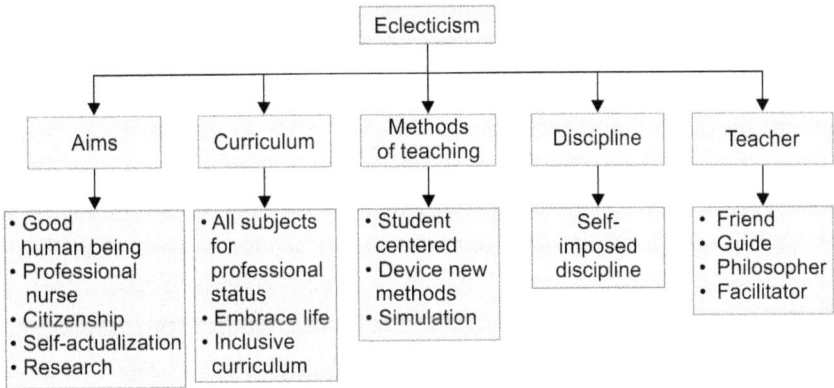

Fig. 2.4: Eclecticism as philosophy of nursing education.

## Need of Eclecticism

Considering the dynamic nature of nursing education, it is foolish to follow a particular philosophy or nursing theory. Many factors affect nursing education. We cannot predict what all factors influence nursing education in what all ways. We need to accept what is appropriate for a given time. A philosophy that explains student behavior in classroom may not be able to explain student behavior in the clinical area.

Learners always like something new and exciting. Eclectic approach is broad and includes every kind of learning activity. This approach gives a chance to nurse educator to device his or her own methods of teaching according to the circumstances and available teaching aids. Thus eclectic approach is most suitable for teaching nursing, especially in the clinical area. This approach also helps nursing students to acquire good ways of learning.

When a nurse educator believes in one philosophy it is difficult for him or her to adopt student centered teaching practices. To teach effectively nurse educator need to establish new ideals, values and standards. As a fusion of different philosophies eclecticism helps nurse education to establish new ideals, values and standards.

Eclecticism is also essential to safeguard the professional status of nursing. A profession is a dynamic integration of various faculties of knowledge. As a profession, nursing need to integrate knowledge from different faculties like sociology, psychology, etc. Belief in a single philosophy may restrict this dynamic integration. Hence, eclecticism only can bring out fruitful integration and thereby safeguard the professional status of nursing.

## Aims of Nursing Education

Aims of nursing education as per eclecticism is to educate student to become a good human being as well as a professional nurse. Citizenship is also an aim, self-actualization is another important aim of eclecticism. Promoting research is also an important aim.

## Curriculum

Subjects required for maintaining the professional status of nursing need to be included in the curriculum. Curriculum should be relevant, flexible and activity centered. Inclusion of subjects required for maintaining professional status should be done without overloading the curriculum. Eclecticism also suggests to seek opinion from all stakeholders while preparing curriculum. It is better to publish a draft proposal of curriculum in the website of university and seek opinion form all stakeholders. This will help to develop an inclusive curriculum suitable for nursing education.

## Methods of Teaching

Eclecticism gives an opportunity to nurse educator to device his or her own methods according to the circumstances and available teaching aids. Any method that is suitable to imparting knowledge and transfer of skills can be followed. Preference should be given to student centered teaching methods. Simulation is considered as the best method to teach nursing skills. As said above, teacher can device his or her own methods also discipline.

## Discipline

Self-discipline is important. As students are trained to safeguard life of human beings, importance of self-discipline need to be emphasized. A higher level of self imposed discipline is expected from nursing students. Self-discipline achieving through personality development is suitable for nursing education.

## Teacher

Nurse educator is the facilitator of learning, especially in the clinical area. The role of teacher as a friend, guide, philosopher, facilitator of learning, arranger of experiences, etc., is appreciated by eclecticism.

## Self-actualization as an Aim

When compared to other professions, we come across less politicians, artists, singers, public figures, etc., in nursing. What happens to the fire brand students after getting the degree? Why they are not nurturing their dreams apart from becoming a professional nurse. We need more nurses who contribute to the society in a larger role as a nurse. Then only we can improve our public image. It is a welcoming trend that some nurses are selected to the prestigious Indian administrative service. Being a nurse is not a limitation to fulfill our possibilities as a human being. Curriculum should emphasize the need of embracing the life fully. Nurse educators need to be more receptive to the feelings of students and encourage attaining self-actualization in life.

## SUMMARY

Philosophy is a belief construct or a value statement. Education and philosophy are the two sides of a coin, presenting the views of the same thing. Educational philosophy is the application of philosophy, in an attempt to meet the challenges faced by education system. Various educational philosophies like idealism, naturalism, pragmatism, realism, theistic realism, humanistic existentialism and eclecticism are serving the purpose of guiding the education in a meticulous way. Philosophy of nursing education is the combination of the value statement about the practice of nursing and teaching of nursing.

## MULTIPLE CHOICE QUESTIONS

1. **Which branch of philosophy deals with origin of knowledge?**
   a. Epistemology
   b. Logic
   c. Metaphysics
   d. Axiology

2. Which branch of philosophy deals with ultimate nature of things?
   a. Epistemology
   b. Logic
   c. Metaphysics
   d. Axiology
3. Which is the oldest philosophy?
   a. Pragmatism
   b. Idealism
   c. Naturalism
   d. Realism
4. Who developed "kindergarten" model of teaching?
   a. Pestalozzi
   b. Plato
   c. Froebel
   d. Aristotle
5. Who is the main proponent of naturalism?
   a. Rousseav
   b. Plato
   c. Froebel
   d. Pestalozzi
6. Which philosophy give importance to "self-expression"?
   a. Pragmatism
   b. Naturalism
   c. Realism
   d. Idealism
7. Which philosophy consider man as a social organism?
   a. Pragmatism
   b. Idealism
   c. Naturalism
   d. Realism
8. Which philosophy consider teacher as a philosopher to students?
   a. Pragmatism
   b. Idealism
   c. Naturalism
   d. Realism
9. Which philosophy is more suitable for nursing education?
   a. Pragmatism
   b. Naturalism
   c. Eclectism
   d. Idealism
10. Which is the youngest philosophy?
    a. Humanistic existentialism
    b. Idealism
    c. Pragmatism
    d. Naturalism

## ANSWER KEY

| | | | | | |
|---|---|---|---|---|---|
| 1. a | 2. c | 3. b | 4. c | 5. a | 6. b |
| 7. a | 8. a | 9. c | 10. a | | |

# CHAPTER 3

# Educational Objectives

## LEARNING OBJECTIVES

**After completing this chapter, reader will be able to:**

- Define educational objective.
- Classify educational objectives.
- Explain Bloom's taxonomy of educational objectives.
- Recognize the implications of Bloom's taxonomy of educational objectives.
- Describe the qualities of an ideal educational objective.
- Explain the different ways of stating objectives.
- Describe the components of behavioral objective.
- State behavioral objectives correctly.
- Explain the advantages of behavioral objectives.
- Identify the strengths and weaknesses of behavioral objectives.

Education is concerned with the modification of behavior. The desired behavior modification cannot be achieved in a haphazardous way. A guided and scaled down approach is required to bring out desirable behavior modifications. Educational objectives will serve the purpose of guiding teachers and students in the achievement of desirable behavior modifications in a phased manner, ultimately leading to the attainment of entire behavior modification prescribed by the educational program.

## DEFINITION

- ❖ Educational objectives are the statements of those desired changes in behavior as a result of specific teaching-learning activity or specific teacher-learner activities.
- ❖ Behavior is what the student should know or be able to do after the teaching-learning activity, i.e., the knowledge, ability, skill, attitude, appreciation and interest which the student develops as a result of the teaching-learning activity.
- ❖ Educational objectives depict what the student should be able to do at the end of a learning activity that they could not do beforehand. In broad sense, educational objectives spell out what should a learner be able to do or do better, after the successful completion of an educational program that he or she was unable to do or could not do so well before. As educational objective is focused much more on the learners' performance, it is also known as 'learning objective'.
- ❖ According to Anderson, "Learning objectives are statements that define the expected goal of a curriculum, course, lesson or activity in terms of demonstrable skills or knowledge that will be acquired by a learner as a result of instruction".

## PURPOSE OF EDUCATIONAL OBJECTIVES

The purpose of educational objectives can be summarized as follows.

- **Provide guidelines or planning for teaching-learning process:** Learning objectives clearly mention the outcome of teaching-learning process. This will motivate teachers and students to work together for the achievement of learning outcomes. Objectives provide guidelines to teachers in the selection of appropriate teaching methods. At the same time objectives help students choose the relevant and meaningful learning activities.
- **Creating a learner-centered classroom:** All inspiring teachers prefer learner-centered objectives. This is possible by considering the cognitive development and other aspects of learners in the selection of content and teaching activities to achieve learning objectives. This will in turn result in the creation of a learner-centered classroom.
- **Ensure continuity of teaching in a systematic manner:** When follow objectives teacher need to conduct teaching activities in a planned manner and according to sequence. For example, while teaching based on the objectives, teacher teaches simple lessons before proceeding to complex lesson.
- **Judicious use of resources:** Objectives clearly mention about the attainment of learning outcomes in a time bound manner. This will help avoid duplication of efforts and save precious resources.
- **Assist in good course design:** Preparing learning objectives helps in identifying appropriate content in accordance with the learning outcomes. Well defined actionable learning objectives helps avoid contents and activities not relevant to the course. This will in turn results in good course design.
- **Ensure proper placement of courses in curriculum:** Preparing educational objectives help teachers gain more insights regarding the subject matter. This will help in the proper placement of courses in curriculum. In curriculum point of view, an educational program consists of several courses. For example, nursing program consists of several courses like, medical nursing, surgical nursing, etc.
- **Provide a foundation for authentic assessment:** A well phrased objective clearly explains the performance criteria or performance standard. This will provide a foundation for authentic assessment.

## CLASSIFICATION OF EDUCATIONAL OBJECTIVES

Educational objectives are classified differently. In one classification, educational objectives are categorized into institutional or general objectives, intermediate or departmental objectives and instructional or specific objectives.

1. **Institutional or general objectives:** These objectives are generally followed by all institutions offering the same educational program. Institutional objective is usually formulated in consensus with the general curriculum objectives of the educational program by the curriculum committee of the institute. Well-constructed institutional objectives are the foundation for a relevant educational program. They are written down for the attainment of overall aim or objective of a particular educational program. It is very broad and focuses on what the institution is aimed at. For example: students acquire knowledge and able to provide comprehensive care to the clients in institution and community; in health and sickness.
2. **Intermediate objectives:** Intermediate objectives are the derivatives of institutional objectives and related to a particular learning experience or subject matter. They are formulated by the curriculum committee. For example, students acquire knowledge and able to provide comprehensive care to the patients with eye, ear and nose conditions or diseases.

3. **Instructional objectives:** Instructional objectives are specific, precise, attainable, measurable and corresponding to each specific teaching-learning activity. They are formulated by the teacher at the instructional level. For example, instructional or specific objectives for a class on peptic ulcer can be formulated as follows: Student: Defines peptic ulcer, lists down the etiology of peptic ulcer, explains the medical management of peptic ulcer, list down the nursing diagnoses of a patient with peptic ulcer. Performs nursing care of a patient with peptic ulcer and lists down the complications of peptic ulcer. From the above said examples, it is clear that the specific or instructional objectives are written in a way to cater the individual learning needs of the students, whereas the institutional and intermediate objectives are written for the entire student body without any individual consideration. In short, Instructional objective is a clear and unambiguous description of teacher's educational expectations for each student in the class.

In another classification, educational objectives are classified into central objective, contributory objective and indirect objective.

1. **Central objective:** Central objective is written for every topic or lesson. This is of supreme importance in any teaching activity. Central objective provides the basis for formulating the subsequent contributory objectives. If the teacher wishes to teach the students about the lecture method, she can formulate the central objective as follows; "by the end of the class, students acquire knowledge regarding lecturing techniques, discriminate the merits and demerits of lecture and able to practice it in an effective way by minimizing the demerits." (See Bloom's Taxonomy of Educational Objectives also).

2. **Contributory objectives:** Contributory objectives are synonymous with specific objectives. They are the derivatives of central objective. The attainment of central objective is possible only through the attainment of contributory objectives. They have to be written more specifically in terms of the knowledge, abilities, skills, attitude, appreciation and interest which will develop in the student as a result of the specific teaching-learning activity. For example, student: Defines lecture method, lists down the merits of lecture method and lists down the demerits of lecture method are some of the contributory objectives that will assist the teacher in attaining the central objective while taking a class on lecture method.

3. **Indirect objective:** Indirect or concomitant objectives are the by products of the attainment of other objectives. They have to be written down in order to bring out certain understandings, ideals and attitudes along with the attainment of contributory objectives and central objective. For example: appreciate the value of lecture method. Attainment of this indirect objective along with other objectives like central objective and contributory objectives will motivate the students to honour the value of lecture method in the future by practicing it with adequate preparation and employing suitable techniques.

## BLOOM'S TAXONOMY OF EDUCATIONAL OBJECTIVES

Bloom and his associates developed a system of classification of objectives called the *taxonomy of educational objectives.* Taxonomy of educational objectives classifies objectives into three main domains and each of these is further categorized according to the level of behavior, progressing from the most simple to the highly complex. The levels are arranged in the form of a hierarchy so that the behaviors at any given level will incorporate those of the levels below. The three domains are *cognitive,* which is concerned with knowledge and intellectual abilities, *affective,* which is concerned with attitudes, values, interests and appreciations and *psychomotor domain* is concerned with motor skills. Bloom presented the taxonomy of cognitive domain, Karath is related to affective domain and Harrow developed the taxonomy for psychomotor domain.

## Cognitive Domain

The cognitive domain consists of six levels of objectives, each of which is divided into subcategories. Let us see the six levels in brief **(Table 3.1)**.

**Level 1—Knowledge:** Knowledge is defined as recall of specifics and universals, recall of methods and processes or the recall of a pattern, structure or setting. Specifics stands for definite things like terminologies and specific facts. Universal means all-reaching or all-embracing, for example, theories and generalizations are applicable to all situations. This level is related to the remembering of previously learned material and represents the lowest level of learning outcomes in the cognitive domain. Knowledge of specifics include: knowledge of terminology and knowledge of specific facts. Knowledge of specifics include: (a) Knowledge of conventions. (b) Knowledge of trends and sequence. (c) Knowledge of classifications and categories. (d) Knowledge of criteria. (e) Knowledge of methodology. Knowledge of the universals and abstractions in a field include: (a) Knowledge of principles and generalizations. (b) Knowledge of theories and structures. Action verbs related to this level of objective are define, state, list, name, outline, write, recall, recognize, label, underline, select, measure, describe, identify, etc. Please note that some verbs associated with one level may be used to indicate other levels also. Examples: (a) Defines immunity. (b) States the four steps in curriculum development. (c) Describes the healing process.

**Level 2—Comprehension:** Even though this level represents the lowest level of understanding, the learning outcomes go one step beyond simple understanding as evidenced by the learners ability to make limited use of information in the form of translation, interpretation and extrapolation. Using other words to communicate something said or printed without altering

**TABLE 3.1:** Verbs to help in writing objectives in cognitive domain.

| Knowledge | Comprehension | Application | Analysis | Synthesis | Evaluation |
|---|---|---|---|---|---|
| Know | Restate | Translate | Distinguish | Compose | Judge |
| Define | Discuss | Interpret | Analyze | Plan | Appraise |
| Memorize | Describe | Apply | Differentiate | Propose | Evaluate |
| Repeat | Recognize | Employ | Appraise | Formulate | Rate |
| Record | Explain | Use | Calculate | Arrange | Compare |
| List | Express | Demonstrate | Experiment | Assemble | Value |
| Recall | Identify | Dramatize | Test | Collect | Revise |
| Name | Locate | Practice | Compare | Construct | Score |
| Relate | Report | Illustrate | Contrast | Choose | Select |
| Review | Operate | Criticize | Create | Assess | |
| Tell | Schedule | Diagram | Design | Estimate | |
| | Shop | Inspect | Setup | Measure | |
| | Sketch | Debate | Organize | Construct | |
| | | Inventory | Manage | Choose | |
| | | Question | Prepare | Assess | |
| | | Relate | | Estimate | |
| | | Solve | | Measure | |
| | | Examine | | | |

the meaning is called translation. Interpretation is the ability of the students to explain the meaning or significance of an information in their own words. Extrapolation is the ability to work out or estimate unknown information from the known information. Typical verbs used at this level are identify, justify, select, indicate, illustrate, represent, name, formulate, explain, judge, contrast, classify, paraphrase, translate, convert, etc. Examples: (a) Classifies cirrhosis of liver based on the etiology. (b) Identifies the importance of good nutrition during the antenatal period. (c) Explains the role of pulse polio in eradicating poliomyelitis.

**Level 3—Application:** This is the ability to use learned material such as rules, principles, concepts, etc. to new and real situations. The learning outcomes in this area require a higher level of understanding than those under comprehension. Verbs used at this level are predict, select, assess, explain, choose, find, show, demonstrate, construct, compute, use, perform, discover, prepare, produce, relate, etc. Examples: (a) Demonstrates correct use of pulse oximeter. (b) Applies the guidelines for the selection and practice of suitable teaching methods. (c) Formulates diet plan for patients with diabetes mellitus

**Level 4—Analysis:** This refers to the ability to breakdown information into its component parts, which may be elements of information, relationships between elements or organization and structure of information. Analysis helps separate the important aspects of information from the less important, thus clarifying the meaning. Learning outcomes here represent a higher intellectual level than comprehension and application because they require an understanding of both the content and structural form of information. Action verbs at this level are analyze, identify, conclude, differentiate, select, separate, compare, contrast, justify, resolve, breakdown, criticize, differentiates, discriminates, distinguishes, etc. Examples: (a) Distinguishes between marasmus and kwashiorkor. (b) Identifies the warning signs of myocardial infarction. (c) Differentiates the pain of myocardial infarction from that of angina pectoris.

**Level 5—Synthesis:** At this level learner is expected to combine various parts to form a new whole. Learning outcomes in this area stress creative behaviors with major emphasis on the formulation of new patterns or structures. Verbs that represent this level are combine, restate, summarize, precise, argue, discuss, organize, derive, select, relate, generalize, conclude, compile, compose, create, devise, plan, etc. Examples: (a) Devices a care plan for a patient with myocardial infarction. (b) Derives a solution for the hospital waste problem. (c) Summarizes the impact of consumer protection act on the nurse-patient relationship.

**Level 6—Evaluation:** This level is concerned with the ability to judge the value of material for a given purpose. Judgments are to be based on definite criteria. Typical verbs are judge, evaluate, determine, recognize, support, defend, criticize, identify, avoid, select, choose, compare, contrast, justify, appraise, etc. For example: Compare and contrast any two definitions of education.

## Affective Domain

The affective domain consists of five levels of objectives, each of which is divided into subcategories. Francis M Quinn describes the affective domain and its five levels in the following way **(Table 3.2)**. As feelings, attitudes, values and interests are components of the caring functions, this domain has particular significance in nursing. 'Values' refer to the person's concept of what he or she considers desirable and so has a large emotional component. A person's values may include sincerity, compassion, respect, etc. 'Attitudes' are positive or negative feelings about certain things and consists of both cognitive and affective aspects.

**Level 1—Receiving (attending):** At this level learner is sensitive to the existence of something and progresses from awareness to controlled or selected attention. It is difficult to tell when a

**TABLE 3.2:** Verbs to help in writing objectives in affective domain.

| Receiving | Responding | Valuing | Organization | Characterization |
|---|---|---|---|---|
| ➢ Observe | ➢ Willing | ➢ Initiate | ➢ Alter | ➢ Revise |
| ➢ Realize | ➢ Comply | ➢ Enable | ➢ Arrange | ➢ Acts |
| ➢ Attend | ➢ Obey | ➢ Feel | ➢ Combine | ➢ Display |
| ➢ Listen | ➢ Engage | ➢ Justify | ➢ Modify | ➢ Discriminate |
| ➢ Discriminate | ➢ Display | ➢ Examine | ➢ Regulate | ➢ Listen |
| ➢ Prefer | ➢ Practice | | ➢ Judge | ➢ Examine |
| ➢ Assume | ➢ Respond | | | |
| ➢ Cooperate | ➢ Accept | | | |
| ➢ Contribute | ➢ Devote | | | |
| ➢ Volunteer | ➢ Consider | | | |
| | ➢ Participate | | | |
| | ➢ Extend | | | |
| | ➢ Enrich | | | |
| | ➢ Explore | | | |

learner is receiving or attending to something, so the best indicator is verbal behavior. Typical verbs used at this level are asks, chooses, selects, replies, etc. For example, asks right questions by honouring the dignity of the patient during history collection.

**Level 2—Responding:** This is concerned with active response by the learner, although commitment is yet to demonstrate. The range is from reacting to a suggestion through to experiencing a feeling of satisfaction in responding. Verbs represent this level include answers, assists, complies, conforms, helps, etc. For example, assists the patient in carrying out activities of daily living.

**Level 3—Valuing:** Objectives at this level indicate acceptance and internalization of the values or attitudes. The learner acts out these in everyday life in a consistent way. The verbs used in this level are initiates, invites, joins, justifies, etc. For example, initiates the building of interpersonal relationship with the patients during clinical postings.

**Level 4—Organization:** Having internalized the value, the learner will encounter situations in which more than one value is relevant. This level is concerned with the ability to organize values and to arrange them in appropriate order. Verbs represent this level are alters, arranges, combines, modifies, etc. For example, combines various interaction skills to nurture interpersonal relationship with patients.

**Level 5—Characterization:** This is the highest level and having attained this level the learner has an internalized value system which has become their philosophy of life. Verbs applicable to this level are acts, displays, discriminates, listens, etc. For example, displays confidence while caring patients with myocardial infarction.

Affective domain not only guides in the inculcation of new attitudes but also assists in modifying the students' existing attitudes in a way favorable to the nursing profession. Some more action verbs like respond, cooperate, react, receive, participate, appreciate, permit, contribute and interact are also used to represent this domain.

## Psychomotor Domain

Psychomotor domain consists of seven levels. According to Francis M Quinn, these seven levels can be explained as follows:

**Level 1—Perception:** This basic level is concerned with the perception of sensory cues that guide actions and ranges from awareness of stimuli to translation into action. Action verbs are chooses, differentiates, distinguishes, identifies, detects, etc. For example, detects the early signs of decubitus ulcer.

**Level 2—Set:** This is concerned with the cognitive, affective and psychomotor readiness to act. Typical verbs are begins, moves, reacts, shows, starts etc. For example, reacts promptly to emergency situations during trauma care postings.

**Level 3—Guided response:** These objectives refer to the early stages in skill acquisition where skills are performed following demonstration by the teacher. Typical verbs are carries out, makes, performs, calculates, etc. For example, performs bed making correctly as demonstrated by the teacher.

**Level 4—Mechanism:** At this level, the performance has become habitual, but the movements are not so complex as the next higher level. Verbs used are similar to level 3. For example, calculates the volume of fluid required in the first day for a patient admitted with 60 percentage burns and weighing 50 kilograms.

**Levels 5—Complex overt response:** This level typifies the skilled performance and involves economy of effort, smoothness of action, accuracy and efficiency, etc. Again verbs are similar to level 3. For example, performs endotracheal intubation correctly.

**Level 6—Adaptation:** Here, the skills are internalized to such an extent that the students can adapt them to cater for special circumstances. Typical verbs are adapts, alters, modifies, reorganizes, etc. For example, modifies sterilization techniques according to the article to be sterilized.

**Level 7— Origination:** This is the highest level and concerns the origination of new movement patterns to suit particular circumstances. Typical verbs are composes, creates, designs, originates, etc. For example, designs a splint to restrain the forearm of a child who is on IV infusion.

Insert, remove, dissect, Palpate, inject, operate, auscultate, prepare, etc., are some of the verbs commonly used in the clinical area to denote psychomotor domain.

## BLOOM'S TAXONOMY AND CENTRAL OBJECTIVE

From the above discussion, it is clear that nursing students have to develop cognitive, affective and psychomotor abilities in order to pursue a good career. Teacher has to keep this in mind and extreme care should be taken to incorporate cognitive, affective and psychomotor domains while framing central objective. Irrespective of the criticisms levelled against Bloom's taxonomy, it still continues to help nurse educators in bringing about desirable behavior modifications among nursing students. Moreover, it is easy to derive specific or instructional objectives from such worded central objectives. For example, the central objective to teach nursing management of patients with myocardial infarction can be stated as follows, "by the end of the class, students acquire in-depth knowledge regarding the nursing management of myocardial infarction, appreciate the role of nursing care in the management of myocardial infarction and able to perform nursing care meticulously as demanded by the patient's condition". In this objective, acquire in-depth knowledge stands for cognitive domain, appreciate the role of nursing care represents affective domain and able to perform nursing care meticulously as demanded by the patient's condition denotes psychomotor domain. As demanded by the patients' condition signify the students' ability to render nursing care for a patient with myocardial infarction in the critical as well as in the stable condition.

# BLOOM'S TAXONOMY AND NURSING EDUCATION

Bloom's taxonomy is compatible with nursing education. It helps achieve aims of nursing education. By applying Bloom's taxonomy nurse educators can easily formulate educational objectives. Major aims of nursing education is to impart knowledge, transfer skills and develop proper attitude and values essential for nursing practice. The domains of Bloom's taxonomy also aims the same **(Box 3.1)**. Teacher can impart knowledge and transfer skills to students. But attitude and values cannot be transferred to students. Students themselves should caught attitudes as attitude, cannot be taught **(Box 3.2)** Bloom's taxonomy contribute much in preparing students to develop proper attitude.

# REVISED BLOOM'S TAXONOMY

In 2001, Anderson and Krathwal have slightly modified Bloom's taxonomy by adding one more level namely "creating" new knowledge in cognitive domain. According to revised version there are six levels of cognitive learning. Each level is conceptually different. The six levels are remembering, understanding, applying, analyzing, evaluating and creating.

- **Level 1—Remembering:** Remembering is the retrieving, recalling or recognizing relevant knowledge from long-term memory. Appropriate learning outcome verbs for this level include: cite, define, describe, identify, label, list, match, name, outline, quote, recall, report, reproduce, retrieve, show, state, tabulate and tell.
- **Level 2—Understanding:** Understanding can be defined as demonstrating comprehension through one or more forms of explanation. Appropriate learning outcome verbs for this level include: abstract, arrange, articulate, associate, categorize, clarify, classify, compare, compute, conclude, contrast, defend, differentiate, discuss, distinguish, estimate, exemplify, explain, extend, extrapolate, generalize, give examples of, illustrate, infer, interpolate, interpret, match, outline, paraphrase, predict, rearrange, reorder, rephrase, represent, restate, summarize, transform and translate.

**Box 3.1:** Bloom's taxonomy and nursing education.

> Bloom's domains → Aims of nursing education
> Cognitive → Knowledge
> Affective → Attitudes and values
> Psychomotor → Skills

**Box 3.2:** Attitude and nursing education.

Attitude is caught by students and not taught to them.
    Attitude and values are caught by students and not taught to them. This statement underlines the difficulty in developing proper attitude among students. Instead of measuring attitude teacher help students inculcate proper attitude. Easiest way of a nurse educator to escape from the responsibility of teaching is passing the comment, "She is not having proper attitude toward nursing". A teacher can help students to develop proper attitude by explaining the need of a proper attitude to build a promising career. Student friendly behavior in the clinical area is the best method of developing a proper attitude. Being a role model by displaying good attitude toward nursing is also important.
A nurse educator never express a negative attitude toward nursing. Moreover, never encourage discussions about nursing that have a negative impact among students. No profession is perfect. Nurse educators need to emphasis the need of 'empathetic' behavior toward patients than 'sympathetic' behavior. It is more worth to help a student develop proper attitude than securing high marks. If proper attitude is there naturally learning also take place.

- **Level 3—Applying:** Applying is the ability to use information or a skill in a new situation. Appropriate learning outcome verbs for this level includes: apply, calculate, carry out, classify, complete, compute, demonstrate, dramatize, employ, examine, execute, experiment, generalize, illustrate, implement, infer, interpret, manipulate, modify, operate, organize, outline, predict, solve, transfer, translate and use.
- **Level 4—Analyzing:** Analyzing is the ability to separate a thing or idea into its parts and determining how the parts relate to one another and to the whole idea or purpose. For example, analyze the relationship between lifestyle and diseases. Appropriate learning outcome verbs for this level include: analyze, arrange, break down, categorize, classify, compare, connect, deconstruct, detect, differentiate, discriminate, distinguish, divide, explain, identify, integrate, order, organize, relate and separate.
- **Level 5—Evaluating:** Evaluating is making judgments based on criteria and standards. Appropriate learning outcome verbs for this level include: appraise, argue, assess, compare, conclude, consider, contrast, convince, criticize, critique, decide, determine, discriminate, evaluate, grade, judge, justify, measure, rate, recommend, review, select, standardize, test and validate.
- **Level 6—Creating:** Creating is the ability to put elements, together to form a new coherent or functional whole; recognize elements into a new pattern or structure. Appropriate learning outcome verbs for this level include: arrange assemble, build, collect, combine, compile, compose, constitute, construct, create, design, develop, devise, formulate, generate, hypothesize, integrate, invent, make, manage, modify, organize, perform, plan, prepare, produce, propose, rearrange, reconstruct, recognize, revise, rewrite, specify and synthesize.

## QUALITIES OF AN EDUCATIONAL OBJECTIVE

An educational objective should be relevant, feasible and achievable, measurable, unequivocal, observable, logical, specific, action oriented and time bound. If an educational objective fails to meet any one of these qualities, it is regarded as invaluable or poor objective.

- **Relevant:** Educational objectives should have a direct relationship with the aims of learning, in other words educational objectives should be based on the needs of the learner.
- **Feasible and achievable:** Students should be able to do what is envisaged by the objective, within the allotted time and available resources.
- **Measurable:** In addition to communicating the expected behavior modification, there should be a provision in the objective to evaluate the end result, i.e., the extent of behavior modification occurred as a result of the teaching-learning activity.
- **Observable:** The qualities of measurable and observable are closely related. In the statement of objectives there should be some means to observe the progress toward the achievement of desired behavioral modifications as stipulated by the objective.
- **Unequivocal:** Equivocal words bear more than one or two meanings. Equivocal words should be avoided while framing objectives in order to provide a uniform direction in achieving learning aims by avoiding ambiguity. The words like to know, to understand, etc. are equivocal, whereas the words like to write, to solve, etc., are unequivocal. As unequivocal words are very clear there is only less chance for misinterpretation.
- **Logical:** The objectives which are written down must be agreeable or reasonable in relation to the teaching-learning activities, i.e., objectives should be internally consistent with the educational activities.
- **Specific:** Learning objectives should specify the skill going to be achieved.

- **Action-oriented**: All educational objectives should include action verbs that indicate performance as a specific task.
- **Time-bound**: All objectives should outline specific time frame they need to be met by learners.

## CRITERIA OF BEHAVIORAL OBJECTIVE

In Jerebrophy's words, "A behavioral objective is a learning outcome stated in measurable terms, which gives directions to the learner's experience and becomes basis of student evaluation".

As said earlier objectives may be general or specific, concrete or abstract, cognitive, affective or psychomotor.

The criteria of good behavioral objective resembles qualities of a good objective. The criteria includes the following:

- **Good behavioral objective is student centered**: A good behavioral objective clearly states expected student performance after the teaching-learning activity. Emphasis is on what students is going to achieve than teacher's performance. This will help teachers focus on level of students and their previous knowledge.
- **Good behavioral objectives explain learning outcomes**: Now, education is more outcome oriented. Once the outcomes are identified and described it is easy to achieve them. Hence, good behavioral objectives should explain learning outcomes.
- **Good behavioral objectives are clear and understandable:** The first prerequisite for a clear and understandable objective is explicitness. It should contain a clearly stated verb that describes a definite action or behavior.
- **Good behavioral objectives are observable:** The evaluation of learning outcomes depends on the ability to observe the outcomes. The most important aspect of an observable objective is an observable verb. The verb must describe an observable action or an action that justifies the achievement of the outcome.
- **Good behavioral objectives are stated in a time bound manner:** There should be a time frame for achieving the stated outcome. Students should be able to do what is expected by the objective within the allotted time and available resources.

## MEANINGFUL STATEMENT OF OBJECTIVES

Objectives can be stated in four different ways namely teacher-centered objective, subject-centered objective, learner-centered objective and behavior-centered objective.

- **Teacher-centered objectives:** These objectives are written down in relation to the teacher activity, which enables the teacher to bring about desirable changes in the behavior of students. For example, teacher lists down the predisposing factors of myocardial infarction and students recognize them.
- **Subject-centered objectives:** Subject centered objectives are the objectives which are written down by giving significance to the subject matter with an intention to produce some behavioral modifications among students. For example, identifies the symptomatology of myocardial infarction.
- **Learner-centered objectives:** Learner-centered objectives can be stated either in terms of activity performed by students or outcomes attained by the learner as a result of the teaching-learning activity. For example, student prepares care plan.
- **Behavior-centered objective:** Objective stated in terms of behavior modification expected is called behavioral objective or behavior-centered objective. As education is concerned with the modification of behavior, behavior-centered way of stating objective is considered

as the best way to state objectives. Forthcoming discussion will give you the required information pertaining to behavioral objectives in a condensed form.

## COMPONENTS OF A BEHAVIORAL OBJECTIVE

When written in behavioral terms an objective will include three components namely *condition of performance, student behavior and performance criteria or standard.*

- **Condition of performance** indicates the conditions or contexts under which the student will perform the behavior. A statement of objective will always begin with a condition of performance. For example, after attending the demonstration on intramuscular injection, students will be able to perform intramuscular injection correctly. Here, 'after attending the demonstration on intramuscular injection' denotes the condition of performance.
- **Student behavior** describes the behavior that the teacher want the student to perform, i.e., the knowledge to be gained and the action or skill the student is able to do. In the above mentioned example, 'student will be able to perform intramuscular injection' stands for student behavior.
- **Performance criteria or standard** specifies the level of performance that the teacher will accept as successful attainment of the objective or describes how well the behavior is to be done in comparison with predetermined standard or criteria. In the previously mentioned example, the word 'correctly' represents the standard or criteria.

## ADVANTAGES OF WRITING BEHAVIORAL OBJECTIVES

The advantages include: (a) It provides an opportunity for the teacher to examine the content which she is going to teach and motivates her to present the content in a student-friendly manner. (b) Helps the teacher determine whether or not he had actually taught what is intended to teach. (c) The use of behaviorally stated objectives motivates the teacher to consistently evaluate a student's performance, this will ultimately helps her individualize instruction in a better way. (d) Justifies the selection of content, learning experiences and teaching-learning methods. (e) Behavioral objectives can be written for cognitive, affective and psychomotor domains. This will allow nurse educators to frame objectives in a realistic way suitable to the aims of nursing education. (f) Objectives help students know what they are supposed to learn. Thus, objectives give direction to learning. (g) Objectives makes learning a purposeful process by explaining expected outcomes. (h) As students know what to learn, objectives reduces anxiety of students. (i) Help students set personal learning objective, this will in turn help develop intrinsic motivation. (j) Helps teachers provide continuous feedback to students regarding their progress of learning.

## WRITING GOOD OBJECTIVES

Following measures will help in writing good objectives. (a) Always try to prepare learner centered objectives. This will create a learner-centered classroom. (b) Familiarize with blooms taxonomy. This will help in communicating learning outcomes to students in a clear manner. (c) Ensure three components or characteristics in objective like expected performance or task, conditions under which student perform the task and criterion-how well a student must perform. (d) Use behavioral verbs that are observable and measurable in objectives. Bloom's taxonomy provides a list of such verbs. (e) Prepare only a manageable number of objectives. The number of objectives should be reasonable for the students to focus on what they should be learning and attainable through instruction within a given time period. (f) Objectives should always based on course contents instruction and assessment. (g) Objectives need to be evaluated at regular intervals for ensuring its relevance. (h) Write behavioral objectives only for higher level behaviors to avoid triviality and (i) Use SMART attributes-objectives should be specific, measurable, attainable, relevant and time bound.

## The SMART Attributes

Learning objectives should have the following SMART attributes.
- **Specific:** Concise, well defined statement of what students will be able to do.
- **Measurable:** The goals suggest how students will be assessed. Objectives should describe what students will be able to do by the end of a learning activity.
- **Attainable:** Students should be able to do what is envisaged by the objectives, within the allotted time and available resources.
- **Relevant:** Educational objectives should have a direct relationship with the aims of learning, in other words educational objectives should be based on the needs of the learner. To make the objective relevant, skills or knowledge described in the objective should match course or program content.
- **Time-bound:** A learning objective should include a specific time frame by which it will be completed or when students should be able to attain knowledge or demonstrate skills.

## SETTING LEARNER-FRIENDLY OBJECTIVES FOR TEACHING NURSING

Following measures will help in setting learner-friendly objectives.
- **Setting learning objectives that are specific but not restrictive:** Specific learning objectives provide direction for learning. Students know the purpose of acquiring a skill or information. But there is no need to restrict further learning even though objective is specific. For example, when the specific objective is to acquire skill of taking body temperature accurately, there is no restriction in learning the pattern of body temperature in diseases like malaria and typhoid.
- **Communicate the learning objective to learners:** Before every teaching session teacher need to communicate learning objectives to learners. This will help learners in the learning process. If possible inform previous day regarding next day's lesson along with objectives. This will help students to come more prepared for class.
- **Prepare realistic objectives for clinical teaching:** It is essential to prepare realistic objectives for clinical teaching in order to motivate learners. While preparing objectives for clinical teaching, teacher need to consider knowledge and skill of students in addition to clinical facilities rather than blindly following textbooks.
- **Connect learning objectives to previous and future learning:** This is essential for the continuity of learning. For example, while teaching interpretation of ECG, objectives need to focus on normal function of heart taught earlier as well as further learning of variations of ECG during disease process.
- **Help students in setting personal learning objectives:** Each student is unique and differs in the ability to learn. Hence, in addition to setting learning objectives for the whole class teacher need to help students in setting personal learning objectives.

## STRENGTHS OF BEHAVIORAL OBJECTIVES

Morrison and Ridley clearly described the strengths and weaknesses of behavioral objectives. The strengths of behavioral objectives are (a) They are performance based, measurable and observable. (b) They are easily communicated to teachers and students. (c) They facilitate organization by specifying goals and outcomes. (d) They clarify thinking and planning and resolve ambiguities. (e) They are 'teacher-proof' and clear to anxious teachers. (f) They are highly prescriptive. (g) They make clear assessment and evaluation criteria. (h) They specify behaviors.

## WEAKNESSES OF BEHAVIORAL OBJECTIVES

The weaknesses of behavioral objectives are: (a) They are highly instrumental, regarding education as instrumentally rather than intrinsically worthwhile. (b) They render students and teachers passive recipients of curricula rather than participants in a process of negotiation. (c) They only cover the trivial, concrete and observable aspects of education, thereby neglecting long-term, unobservable, unmeasurable deeper-seated aims and elements. (d) Education becomes technicist, tending toward low level training rather than higher level thinking. (e) Because they are 'teacher-proof' they build out teachers' autonomy. (f) They lead to predictability rather than open-endedness, discovery, serendipity, creativity and spontaneity. (g) The process of education is overtaken by outcome dependence. (h) They replace the significance of understanding with an emphasis on behavior. (i) Epistemologically they mistake the nature of knowledge, seeing it as products and facts, supporting a rationalist rather than an empirical view of knowledge. (j) They mistakenly 'parcel up' and atomize knowledge.

## SUMMARY

Educational objectives are those desired changes in behavior as a result of specific teaching-learning activity or specific teacher-learner activities. Behavior is what the student should know or able to do after the teaching-learning activity. Educational objectives can be classified in different ways like general or institutional objective, intermediate or departmental objective, instructional or specific objective, central objective, contributory objective and indirect or concomitant objective. Bloom's taxonomy of educational objectives classifies objectives into cognitive, affective and psychomotor domains with subdivisions.

Educational objectives should be relevant, feasible and achievable, measurable, unequivocal, observable and logical. Objectives are stated in four different forms, namely teacher-centered, subject matter-centered, learner-centered and behavior-centered. Behavior-centered way of stating objective is the most preferred way to state objectives. Components of a behavioral objective include conditions of performance, student behavior and performance criteria or standard. Knowledge regarding the strengths and weaknesses of behavioral objectives will assist the nurse educator in framing objectives in a realistic way suitable to the aims of nursing education.

## MULTIPLE CHOICE QUESTIONS

1. **Educational objectives mainly focuses on change in:**
    a. Behavior
    b. Skill
    c. Knowledge
    d. Attitude
2. **Instructional objectives are formulated by:**
    a. Institution
    b. Individual teacher
    c. Apex bodies
    d. Department teacher

3. **Objective for each lesson is known as:**
   a. Central objective
   b. Intermediate objective
   c. General objective
   d. Specific objective
4. **Cognitive domain is related to:**
   a. Knowledge
   b. Attitude
   c. Values
   d. Skills
5. **Affective domain is related to:**
   a. Skill
   b. Attitude
   c. Knowledge
   d. Values
6. **Psychomotor domain is related to:**
   a. Skill
   b. Attitude
   c. Knowledge
   d. Values
7. **A relevant objective is based on:**
   a. Needs of learner
   b. Level of learner
   c. All of the above
   d. None of the above
8. **"Perception" is a level of:**
   a. Cognitive domain
   b. Affective domain
   c. Psychomotor domain
   d. None of the above
9. **Receiving is a level of:**
   a. Cognitive domain
   b. Affective domain
   c. Psychomotor domain
   d. None of the above
10. **Comprehension is a level of:**
    a. Cognitive domain
    b. Affective domain
    c. Psychomotor domain
    d. None of the above

## ANSWER KEY

| | | | | | |
|---|---|---|---|---|---|
| 1. a | 2. b | 3. a | 4. a | 5. c | 6. a |
| 7. a | 8. c | 9. b | 10. a | | |

# CHAPTER 4

# Curriculum

## LEARNING OBJECTIVES

**After completing this chapter, reader will be able to:**

- Define curriculum.
- Define nursing curriculum.
- Explain the modern concept of curriculum.
- Describe the models of curriculum.
- Identify the components of nursing curriculum.
- Explain the nature of curriculum.
- Recognize the criteria for a desirable curriculum.
- List down the types of curriculum.
- Realize the levels of curriculum planning.
- Explain the principles of the organization of curriculum.
- Explain the principles of curriculum development.
- Identify the factors influencing the development of nursing curriculum.
- Describe the steps in curriculum development.
- Prepare rotation plan.
- Prepare course plan.
- Prepare unit plan.
- Prepare lesson plan.
- Distinguish between syllabus and curriculum.
- Explain core curriculum.
- Explain the process of curriculum revision.

Education aims the behavior modification of learners. Behavior modification is achieved through a series of activities. Curriculum is concerned with guiding the teachers and students in the educative process. Since a detailed discussion of curriculum is difficult within the limits of this book, our discussion is limited to some important aspects of nursing curriculum.

## MEANING AND DEFINITION

The term curriculum is derived from the Latin word *"currere"* which means 'run'. Thus, curriculum is a runway for attaining the goals of education. Curriculum may be considered as the blueprint of an educational program. It is the base of education on which the teaching-learning process is planned and implemented. It nearly resembles a 'cake' in which carefully selected experiences are blended together little by little, stirred by the hand of an expert teacher and slowly baked in the oven of experience, allowing each ingredient to complement and permeate the others. The quality of the final product depends not only on the quality of the ingredients and the sequence in which they are combined, but equally in the blending process itself and the 'setting' of the oven.

According to Cunningham, "Curriculum is a tool in the hands of an artist to mold his material, according to his ideals in his studio". In this definition, artist is the teacher, material is the student, ideals are the objectives and studio is the educational institute.

Alberty regards curriculum as "the sum total of student activities which the school sponsors for the purpose of achieving its objectives."

As per Florence Nightingale International Foundation, "Curriculum is a systematic arrangement of the sum total of selected experiences planned by a school for a defined group of students to attain the aims of a particular educational program."

Nursing curriculum is the learning opportunities (subject matter) and the learning activities (clinical experiences and practices) that the faculty plans and implement in various settings for a particular group of students, for a specified period of time in order to attain the objectives.

## MODERN CONCEPT OF CURRICULUM

In the past, life was very simple and the needs of the society were also not very complicated and numerous. So only a few subjects in the curriculum began to be considered as synonymous with academic subjects of instruction. Now, of course, when education is viewed as a dynamic process, the old concept of curriculum cannot be accepted. The courses of study are only a part of the curriculum. The experiences of pupils gained at school and in the community under the guidance of teachers are also included in the curriculum. Modern curriculum encompasses all the meaningful and desirable activities outside the school provided that these are planned, organized and used educationally. As such, curriculum is something more than textbooks, more than the subject matter and even more than the course of study. The secondary education commission has also pointed out as "according to the best modern educational thought, curriculum does not mean only the academic subjects traditionally taught in the school, but it includes the totality of the experiences that a pupil receives through the manifold activities that go on in the school—in the classroom, library, laboratory, playgrounds and in the numerous informal contacts between teachers and pupils. In this case, the whole life of the school becomes the curriculum which can touch the life of the students at all points and help in the development of a balanced personality." The acknowledgement of the fact that experience is the best teacher has helped to formulate a result-oriented curriculum.

## MODELS OF CURRICULUM

Models of curriculum help to understand the nature of curriculum. Some of the useful curriculum models are discussed below in a very brief manner.

### Behavioral Objective (Product) Model

This model was developed by Ralph Tyler (1950). He was one of the most influential of the early curriculum theorists and has arguably developed a considerable and lasting influence on present-day thinking about the nature and function of the curriculum. His theories reflect very much the need to organize and the utility of purpose and concern for an end product of quality and practical application. He views curriculum objectively and in terms of its function and clearly includes teaching and learning as integral parts of it. For him, the function of the curriculum is to set forth the order and scope of what has to be taught so that learning may be enhanced. He identifies four fundamental questions to be answered in the process of developing a curriculum, such as: (a) What educational purposes should the school seek to attain, i.e., objectives? (b) How can learning experiences be selected that are likely to be useful in attaining these objectives? (c) How can learning experiences be organized for effective instruction? and (d) How can the effectiveness of learning experiences be evaluated? This notion of rational curriculum planning led to the development of the generic model of curriculum which consists of four main components namely objectives, content, method and evaluation.

Hence this model give importance to the achievement of objectives by the student. Thus, this is an output model. Tyler stressed the importance of stating objectives in terms of student behavior. By the beginning of 1980, behavioral objectives were almost universally implemented in both classroom and clinical settings by the nurse educators.

## Stenhouse's Process Model

Lawrence Stenhouse (1975) formulated the process model. This is an input model, i.e., emphasis is on learning experience or the process of education. He believed that it was possible to organize curriculum without having to specify in advance the expected behavioral change in students. According to him, the content of curriculum can be selected on the basis that it is worthwhile in itself and not merely as the means to achieve behavioral objective. Similarly, teaching methods and learning experiences can be selected in terms of the worthwhileness as learning activities. Teacher's role is to appraise the student's work, with emphasis in developing self-appraisal quality among students. In this model, the teacher's commitment to professional development is vital. Teachers need to see themselves as learners rather than as experts and to be continually striving to improve their performance and judgment.

## Lawton's Cultural Analysis Model

Lawton's model (1983) was a reaction against what he saw as the dangers of the behavioral objectives models. This model proposes a curriculum planned on the technique of cultural analysis. Culture is defined as the whole way of life of society and the purpose of education is to make available to the next generation what we regard as the most important aspects of culture. Cultural analysis is the process by which a selection is made from the culture and in terms of curriculum planning.

## Beattie's Fourfold Model

Beattie (1987) suggests that there are four fundamental approaches in relation to the task of planning a curriculum for nursing. They are:

- **The curriculum as a map of key subjects:** This approach consists of mapping out the key subjects in nursing curriculum.
- **The curriculum as a schedule of basic skills:** This approach emphasis the explicit specification of basic skills of nursing practice.
- **The curriculum as a portfolio of meaningful personal experiences:** This approach places the students at the center of things by organizing the curriculum around their interests and experiences.
- **The curriculum as an agenda of important cultural issues:** This approach avoids giving detailed subject matter, focusing instead on controversial issues and political dilemmas in nursing and health care.

## COMPONENTS OF CURRICULUM

As curriculum is the total learning experience intended to bring out behavioral modification of learners, it is difficult to list down precisely the whole components of a curriculum. As there exists lot of approaches to curriculum development, it is difficult to predict all components of a curriculum. But a curriculum should definitely include the following components or elements:

1. A framework of assumptions about the learner and society such as learners' needs, development stage, ability, aptitudes, motivation, interests and values as well as societal needs and resources available in society.

2. The statement of aims and objectives of educational program. Objectives are statements that describe the end-points or described outcomes of the curriculum, a unit, a lesson plan or learning activity.
3. Content or subject-matter with selection of what is to be taught and learnt, scope of the subject–matter and its organization like courses, units, lessons.
4. Modes of instruction which deals with the process of teaching–learning and includes methodology of teaching, learning experiences both within the institution and outside, learning environment, teaching materials and learning materials.
5. Evaluation methods and techniques for ascertaining attainment of objectives.
6. Guidelines for conducting online classes if institution is closed for a certain period due to unexpected reasons like coronavirus disease-2019 (COVID-19) pandemic in 2020.
7. Guidelines for conducting online assessment if institution is closed for a certain period due to unexpected reasons like COVID-19 pandemic in 2020.
8. Guidelines for dividing content into topics that can be preferably taught by online mode and direct student-teacher interaction. Nowadays, online teaching is equally important as traditional classroom teaching. One reason to conduct teaching-learning activities through online is the unexpected closing down of educational institution for a long period due to pandemic outbreak like COVID-19. Another reason is to promote social distancing by reducing classroom teaching hours in order to prevent community spread during a pandemic outbreak like COVID-19. In other words, future education is based on blended or hybrid learning. Blended or hybrid learning is a combination of online teaching and traditional classroom methods.
9. Another component is curriculum timing. Curriculum specifies period required for completing the educational program. It also specifies time required for completing each course and every unit in a course. This specification of time frame is called curriculum timing. For example, in MSc nursing program, educational psychology is a course and in educational psychology "characteristics of adolescence" is a unit.

## COMPONENTS OF NURSING CURRICULUM

Curriculum invariably contains:
 a. The statement of philosophy of the educational program.
 b. The statement of the objectives of educational program.
 c. Total duration of the educational program.
 d. Detailed course plan for each course (for example, mental health nursing is a course in the nursing educational program. See course planning) which spells out the placement of the course, subject matter, allotted time in terms of theory and practical hours, learning experiences like areas of clinical posting and class by nurse educators or other professionals, teaching and learning methods, etc.
 e. Program of evaluation, such as type of examinations, various grades according to the results, percentage meant for internal assessment in the university examinations, etc.

The basic purpose of nursing education is to prepare the students to render comprehensive nursing care and health guidance to individuals and families based on nursing process. For such a preparation, the nursing curriculum draws its components from various branches of knowledge like medicine, behavioral sciences and natural sciences in addition to the professional nursing areas subjects like fundamentals of nursing, midwifery, community health nursing, etc.

## NATURE OF CURRICULUM

- **Curriculum as objectives:** By way of objectives, curriculum guides the process of behavioral modification among students. According to Tyler, any statement of the objectives of the school should be a statement of changes to take place in students.
- **Curriculum as subject matter:** Curriculum offers socially valued knowledge, skills and attitudes to students through a variety of arrangements during the time they are at school, college or university.
- **Curriculum as student experience:** Curriculum is all the learning which is planned and guided by the school whether it is carried on in groups or individually, inside or outside the school.
- **Curriculum as opportunities for students:** A curriculum is all the educational opportunities encountered by students as a direct result of their involvement with an educational institution.

The nature of curriculum resembles that of education and its nature, therefore can be summarized as follows: (a) Is dynamic and flexible in meeting the constantly changing demands of the society. (b) Has a societal orientation. (c) Is oriented to life situation. (d) Has a positive attitude toward the needs of the learners. (e) Has a blending of ideal and realistic approaches. (f) Is dependent on the philosophy and objectives of the respective educational program. (g) Is influenced by technological and scientific advancements.

## NATURE OF NURSING CURRICULUM

In addition to the above said features, nursing curriculum is (a) Health-oriented. (b) Flexible to meet the changing health needs of the society. (c) Influenced by the developments in other healthcare professions. (d) Influenced by transnational trends in nursing education and nursing service. (e) Influenced by the policy decisions based on national health policy.

## CRITERIA FOR A DESIRABLE CURRICULUM

Since the curriculum includes the sum total of all activities, it must possess certain criteria to bring about the necessary changes in behavior. The criteria are:

- The curriculum should describe the theory form, i.e., subject in the real form of community needs.
- Curriculum should cope with the knowledge explosion and scientific advancements.
- Curriculum should use all the teaching personnel in the most efficient and economic way.
- Curriculum should use the logical, precise and effective technology which are currently available in the same as well in the allied discipline.
- The curriculum should be consistent with the theoretical framework of all the subjects included in it.
- The curriculum should enable the student to do active practice.
- The curriculum should provide facilities for testing the learned behavior in reality for the students.
- The curriculum should be as such to produce graduates who are capable of being creative for the next 15-20 years at least.
- A curriculum which is planned should spend a reasonable length of time in order to accomplish the goals.
- The curriculum should be enriched with the activities for professional and personal growth of the learners.

In short, nursing curriculum should be learner centric, patient centric, competency based, gender sensitive, outcome driven, consideration to co-curricular activities and confirms to global trends in health care and nursing education. It should also promote active learning than rote learning by allotting more time for self-directed learning.

## TYPES OF CURRICULUM

The common types of curriculum can be classified as follows:

### Explicit Curriculum

The explicit, overt or written curriculum is commonly referred as the "curriculum in use". This is the curriculum followed at the institutional or school level. It is the formal curriculum that explains explicit steps and procedures to achieve the aims of educational program. It is also called institutional curriculum.

The explicit curriculum is divided into two components. (a) Educational activities conducted through online method and (b) Educational activities conducted through traditional classroom teaching.

Sometimes due to unexpected reasons it is impossible to conduct all teaching activities through traditional classroom manner. For example, during COVID-19 pandemic classes were conducted through online manner. To make students familiarize with online education, it is advisable to conduct online classes along with traditional classroom teaching instead of following only traditional classroom methods.

### Hidden Curriculum

As the name indicates hidden or implicit curriculum refers to the unintended outcomes occur while implementing explicit curriculum. Hidden curriculum represents the kinds of learning students derive from teacher's attitudes and school environment. This learning can be either conscious or unconscious. For example, when a student is influenced positively by the teacher teaching mathematics, the learner unconsciously develops an interest in learning mathematics. A school's rigid class schedule may make students perceive learning as an inflexible and authoritarian process.

The hidden curriculum conveys both positive and negative messages to learners depending on the teacher's attitude and influence of school environment. Hence, teachers need to be aware about the implications of hidden curriculum while teaching. A great teacher always takes precautions to overcome negative impacts of hidden curriculum while teaching.

### Null Curriculum

The null or absent curriculum is what is not taught. Null curriculum is created when certain aspects of explicit curriculum is excluded either intentionally or unintentionally from the explicit curriculum. Teacher may not teach some ideas due to order from school authorities, lack of knowledge or deeply ingrained assumptions or biases. For example, teacher teaches about war but not peace, we teach about certain select cultures and histories, but not about other cultures. A teacher should implement her null curriculum carefully. By not teaching a subject area, she communicates its irrelevance.

Null curriculum created intentionally by excluding some aspects of explicit curriculum when it is impossible to teach all aspects is called essential curriculum. For example where institutions are closed for a long period due to COVID-19 pandemic institutions opted for essential curriculum.

## Essential Curriculum

The essential curriculum is the curriculum implemented for conducting the educational program when it is impossible to continue with the already written or explicit curriculum due to unforeseen reasons. It is also known as the optional curriculum. For example, when educational institutions remain closed for a longer period due to COVID-19 pandemic institutions opted essential curriculum or optional curriculum to conduct classes. Salient features of the essential curriculum are:

- New strategies are formulated to achieve the aims of educational program.
- The very essential content of curriculum is retained by removing not so essential content. "Must to be taught" topics are given preference than "likely to be taught" topics.
- It is implemented only for a single academic year.
- Highly disruptive in nature. Significantly alters the concepts of teaching, learning, discipline and role of teachers and learners. For example, institutions so far banned mobile phones in campus are now conducting online classes through mobile phones.
- Heavily depend on information and communication technology. Digital platforms like zoom, Google classroom are widely used to conduct classes.
- Equal importance to web-based resources and textbooks or teaching materials prepared by teachers.
- Highly flexible when compared to explicit curriculum.

## Societal Curriculum

According to Cortes, "societal curriculum is the massive, ongoing informal curriculum of family, peer groups, neighborhoods, organizations, mass media and other socializing forces that "educate" children". This type of curriculum can now be expanded to include the powerful effects of social media like YouTube, Facebook, etc., and how it actively helps in creating new perspectives.

## Official Curriculum

The official curriculum or the formal curriculum is the curriculum prepared and recommended by apex bodies for conducting educational programs in a region, state or country. Curriculum prepared by universities, state education boards, and regulatory bodies like INC are examples of official curriculum. The main aim of preparing an official curriculum is to bring out uniformity and standardization in conducting an educational program. For example, all nursing colleges need to follow curriculum recommended by INC while conducting nursing programs. Educational institutions develop explicit or written curriculum from the official curriculum prepared by apex bodies.

## Received Curriculum

The "received curriculum" or the "learned curriculum" is what the students actually learn. It is the most important of all curricula. It is the real or actual experience of students. Hence, it is also known as the "actual curriculum". Through assessment, we are really evaluating this curriculum. There is a gap between the official or planned curriculum and the received curriculum. The teacher needs to put more effort to reduce this gap. In short, the knowledge, skills attitude and values the learners attain can be included in the received curriculum.

**Olivia Bevis recommends four types of nursing curricula namely, the legitimate curriculum, illegitimate curriculum, hidden curriculum and the null curriculum for every nursing institute.**

## Legitimate Curriculum

This is the one agreed by the faculty either implicitly or explicitly. Sometimes it is written into plans, sometimes not. But, regardless, it is recognized and acknowledged by faculty and students as 'real' curriculum. It is approved by the accreditation bodies and is the one that generates the learning tasks, episodes, papers and tests with which both students and teachers contend. Currently in nursing this curriculum is generally behavioral objectives driven. In other words, only those items describable in behavioral terms, explicitly chosen by faculty as worthy and correctly formulated into objectives, guide the curriculum by dictating the learning experiences to be chosen and evaluations to be made. This is the curriculum that is acknowledged by the faculty. The normal discourse regarding curriculum refers to this curriculum.

## Illegitimate Curriculum

This is the curriculum that, because of the constraints of the behavioral objective driven curriculum prevalent in nursing, cannot be graded or officially acknowledged or sanctioned because it does not lend itself to descriptors that are behavioral. It is the curriculum that values and teaches, among many other things, caring, compassion, power and its use. This curriculum exists in the behaviorist curriculum and is often taught quite openly because teachers feel a moral obligation to their students to recognize things beyond the explicit. This is the curriculum of insights, patterns, creativity, strategies, inquiry and understanding: a curriculum that is seldom expressed in easily manifested behaviors and it lies within the learners influencing life choices, taste, approaches, values and style.

## Hidden Curriculum

It is the curriculum in which we are unaware of the messages given by the way we teach, the priorities we set, the type of methods we use and the way we interact with students. This is the curriculum of subtle socialization of teaching how to think and feel like nurses. It is the curriculum that covertly communicates priorities, relationships and values. It colors perceptions, independence, initiative, caring, colleagueship and the mores and folkways of being a nurse. It is taught by subtle, out-of-awareness things that pervade the whole educational environment: when classes are scheduled, how much time is given to a subject in relationship to other subjects, how many test items are assigned to a topic, whether or not a test paper is conducted, how the teacher responds to students who openly differ in opinion from the teacher, how students are or are not encouraged to work together and how teachers interact with students. All of these give the value messages to students that shape their learning in this curriculum.

## Null Curriculum

This is the curriculum that exists only in the hearts and mind of educators but seldom exists in reality. This may be because teachers are not taught the art of provoking cognitive dissonance and raising issues and questions that support the general aims of education like critical thinking, enquiry and intellectual development. We speak of critical thinking, enquiry and intellectual development and would like to teach it, but seldom do we raise the questions with students that would require any response beyond the 'rationale' for a nursing decision.

It is the goal of all good professional programs to be educative, to have no null curriculum and no illegitimate curriculum and to reduce the hidden curriculum to the barest minimum.

However, in nursing institutions we have four curricula: The legitimate, the illegitimate, the hidden and the null. These curricula, although they may differ in content, are also different in reality because of the primacy of their agreed-upon acceptability by the faculty and their fit within the approved curricular philosophy regarding learning and the perceived importance of sciences to nursing. In other words, it is not the content that makes them legitimate, illegitimate or hidden, but the degree of value placed upon the content, how overtly that value is spelled out or the implicit messages in the environment and climate of the school.

## NATURE OF TWENTY FIRST CENTURY CURRICULUM

### Blended Curriculum

The curriculum of coming years will be blended in nature. It explains how aims of education can be achieved through online teaching as well as traditional classroom teaching. Blended curriculum is recommended because we cannot depend only on traditional classroom teaching to achieve aims of education if institutions remain closed for a long period due to unexpected reasons like COVID-19. In blended curriculum equal importance is given to online education and traditional classroom teaching.

Blended curriculum clearly classifies topics that can be taught through online and traditional methods. It clearly defines the role of technology, media, learner and teacher in the educative process in this digital age. More reliance on technology never underestimate the role of teachers in the educative process. Blended curriculum recognize the evolving role of teacher in education and thereby the human component in the teaching–learning process.

### Evolving Curriculum

Twenty first century curriculum can be described as an evolving curriculum. This is especially true in the case of institutional curriculum when compared to official curriculum, the institutional curriculum always bear the scope to evolve in a desirable manner. In other words, institutional curriculum should always be an evolving curriculum based on:

- Recent research findings in the cognitive neurosciences
- Twenty first century digital and network tools to access information
- Twenty first century life skills identified by WHO
- Changes in job market
- Promoting collaboration than competition

### Creative Curriculum

Twenty first century curriculum need to promote creativity by encouraging learners to think out of the box or no box manner. Young brain, especially adolescent brain is a gold mine of creativity. Best examples are Bill Gates and Larry Page. If nurture youngsters properly, modern education can create more Bill Gates. Curriculum should not only focus ways necessary to develop reasoned and logical construction of new knowledge in various field of study but also should aggressively cultivate a culture that nurtures creativity in learners. Curriculum should enable learners to come out with creative ideas that are actionable, rational and constructive.

Enabling learners to develop a "high concept" and "high touch" approach to life as explained by Daniel H will help them develop creativity. "High concept" involves the capacity to find relationship between facts and combine various ideas to create something meaningful. "High touch" involves the ability to empathize with others, to understand the importance of human interaction and value humanity in all circumstances. This approach makes life more creative, meaningful and beautiful.

## Coherent Curriculum

By all means twenty first century curriculum needs to be a coherent curriculum. As per the glossary of education reforms coherent curriculum or aligned curriculum refers to an educational program that is (a) Well organized and purposefully designed to facilitate learning, (b) Free of academic gaps and needless repetitions and (c) Aligned across lessons, courses, subject areas and grade levels. In short, in a coherent curriculum there is coherence among all elements involved in educating students, including content, academic expectations, learning standards, assessments, standardized tests, textbooks, assignments, lessons and instructional techniques.

**Curriculum mapping:** It is a processes that enable teachers to build a coherent curriculum. Curriculum mapping involves activities based on the four questions:
1. What do we want our students to know and be able to do?
2. What are we currently teaching?
3. What are the overlaps or repetitions and gaps in the current teaching?
4. What to do to overcome these over laps and gaps.

## Entrepreneurship Curriculum

Entrepreneurship mindset curriculum is a curriculum put forward by Delhi government from classes IX to XII in government schools to build awareness and knowledge of various aspects of entrepreneurship among students. Twenty first century curriculum need to incorporate certain aspects of this curriculum to promote entrepreneurship among youngsters. The objectives of the curriculum are: (a) develop key attributes such as critical thinking, confidence and creativity, (b) develop foundational abilities like problem solving, communication and collaboration, (c) develop entrepreneurial abilities like recognizing opportunities, taking risks and bouncing back from failure, (d) to enable students to dream big and pursue their dreams, (e) be happy and joyful and be lifelong learners.

According to State Council of Educational Research and Training (SCERT), this curriculum will inspire students through various entrepreneurial stories case studies and many mindfulness activities and approaches. It focuses on imparting the personality and character traits of successful entrepreneurs other than business aspects of entrepreneurship.

## Curriculum for Excellence

The curriculum for excellence has been developed in Scotland to help young people and children attain the attributes, skills and knowledge necessary to equip them for today's life. By incorporating certain aspects of this curriculum all schools can convert curriculum to curriculum for excellence. The purpose of curriculum for excellence is to help young people become confident as individuals, successful as learners, responsible citizens and also effective contributors to society as a whole.

The four "contexts for learning" included in the curriculum for excellence are: (a) curriculum subjects and areas, (b) the life and ethos of school, (c) interdisciplinary learning opportunities and (d) opportunities for personal achievement.

## RESPONSIBILITY OF CURRICULUM DEVELOPMENT

The construction of nursing curriculum is the responsibility of the faculty of the nursing institute, but the minimum requirement which are prescribed by statutory bodies like nursing council or university in the name of syllabus (see syllabus) has to be followed by all institutes. Since the needs of students as well as the needs of the society vary from place to place, individual nursing institute can adopt as much as is required from the minimum prescribed syllabus in order to achieve the educational objectives. Knowledge regarding the changing health needs of the society, developments in the field of general education, scientific and technological advancements, changes in the healthcare delivery system, advancements in the medicine and allied fields will assist the faculty in the process of curriculum development. The curriculum of nursing education is formulated by *curriculum committee*. Nowadays, whole faculty members are included in the curriculum committee. Curriculum will be developed by this committee on the basis of several discussions. Every faculty member is given a chance to bring out their logical and valuable suggestions related to curriculum. After discussing these suggestions, the valid ones are considered while developing the curriculum.

## LEVELS OF CURRICULUM PLANNING

According to Goodland, there exists three levels of curriculum planning, namely societal curriculum, institutional curriculum and instructional curriculum.

- **Societal curriculum:** This is the curriculum planned for a specific population of students by experts outside the educational institution and who are legally appointed. In nursing education, the societal level curriculum is planned by different statutory bodies like Indian Nursing Council, National League of Nursing Education, etc. Giving adequate consideration to societal curriculum will help in achieving the much needed uniformity and standardization of nursing education.
- **Institutional curriculum:** This is the curriculum which is prepared by the faculty of the institute for a particular group of students for a definite period of time. Institutional curriculum is synonymous with the actual type of curriculum.
- **Instructional curriculum:** As the name indicates, this is the curriculum prepared by the individual teacher at the instructional level.

## ELEMENTS IN PLANNING A CURRICULUM

Curriculum planning ranges from deciding the overall goals of curriculum to lesson planning as shown in **Figure 4.1.** The salient features of course planning, unit planning and lesson planning are explained at the end of this chapter.

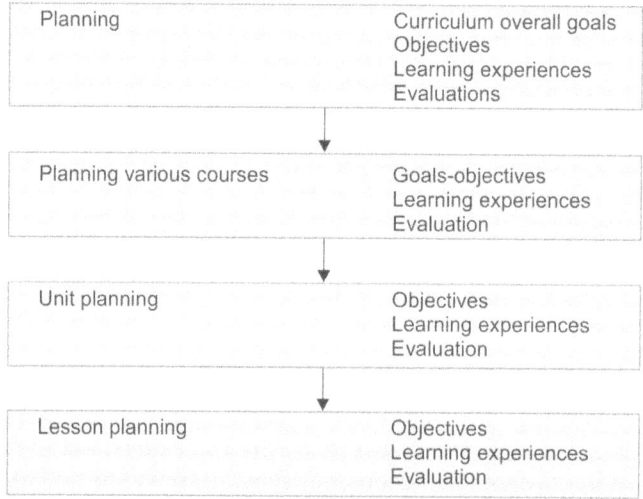

**Fig. 4.1:** Elements in planning a curriculum.

# ORGANIZATION OF CURRICULUM

Organization of curriculum is the systematic arrangement of the learning activities by applying the principle of sequence, continuity, correlation and integration. The following principles have to be observed while organizing the curriculum:

a. An ideal curriculum should be neither too flexible nor too rigid—an appreciable amount of flexibility has to be maintained.
b. Curriculum should be planned and organized in an integrated form in order to maintain wholeness.
c. Curriculum should consider the needs, especially the psychological needs of the students.
d. Curriculum should be organized on the basis of desirable attitudes, abilities and skills, including social, moral, intellectual and aesthetical values of life.
e. Curriculum has to be organized effectively, efficiently, logically and should allow the precise use of educational technology.
f. Curriculum should take into account the knowledge explosion and scientific advancements.
g. Curriculum should be organized in such a way that it should provide appropriate learning experiences required for attaining mastery in relevant areas of knowledge.
h. Democratic approach and leadership styles have to be followed while organizing the curriculum.
i. Opinions of experts from other disciplines should be given due consideration while organizing the curriculum.

# CURRICULUM DEVELOPMENT

The curriculum is what happens, what actually takes place among teachers and students, so that learning occurs. Even though curriculum cannot be entirely preplanned and prescribed, to a great extent a curriculum that satisfies the needs of the students as well as the society can be developed.

# STEPS IN DEVELOPING OFFICIAL CURRICULUM

The steps involved in the development of an official curriculum can be explained as follows:

1. **Constituting a curriculum development team:** A curriculum development team is constituted by including experts from the concerned fields, usually a well experienced and qualified curriculum developer is appointed as the chairman of the curriculum development team. Role and functions of each member is explained in detail.
2. **Conducting situational analysis and needs assessment:** According to Benson Sitwe, situational analysis is the process of examining factors that exist (situation) in the society or environment where the curriculum is going to be implemented. Kaufman defined needs assessment as "a formal analysis that documents gaps between current results and the desired results". He further defined a need is a gap between what is and what should be. Need assessment mainly aims arranging needs in priority of order and selection of the most important needs. Once analyzed the information, it is then used to set appropriate goals and objectives in curriculum development.
   The importance of situational analysis and needs assessment is that they will help in identifying the needs of society as well as the abilities of the learner. This will further help in the formulation of curriculum objectives, content, selection of learning and teaching activities. In other words, situational analysis and needs assessment guide educationists in meeting the needs and expectations of the society.

3. **Statement of educational objectives:** Intended outcomes or education objectives states what the learner will be able to do as a result of successfully completing the educational program or participating in the curricular activities. This step involves (a) defining intended outcomes, (b) determining the components of the intended outcomes (condition, performance and standard), (c) example of intended outcomes and an overview of learning behavior.
4. **Selection of content or subject matter:** Content or subject matter helps in the attainment of educational objectives. It will assist learners to attain knowledge, skills, attitudes and values for achieving behavior modification. Kenner proposes the following criteria for selecting content:
   - *Validity*: The content of the curriculum is valid if it helps in the attainment of already stated educational objectives. In other words, content promotes the cognitive, affective and psychomotor development of learners. Validity is also about the authenticity, relevance and significance of the content.
   Content become significant when it is useful in solving the problems of the society. Culture sensitivity of content also contributes to validity. When learners belongs to different cultural background and races then the content must be cultural sensitive.
   - *Interest:* Content should arouse interest among students. Students learn best if the subject matter is meaningful to them. Only a learner centered curriculum can arouse interest among students and the best way to create a learner centered curriculum is to make the content meaningful to learners.
   - *Learnability:* Content should be appropriate to the level of learners and should be within their experience. Content need to be organized in a way to maximize the learning capacity of students.
   - *Self-sufficiency*: Content should enable learners to attain self-sufficiency in the most beneficial manner. Teachers need to devise most appropriate ways for achieving this criteria.
   - *Utility*: The knowledge, skills, attitudes and values attained through mastering content should be useful for now and in future.
   - *Consistent with social realities*: Content should address properly the needs of the society and abilities of the learner. Content must be acceptable to the culture and the belief system of the people.
5. **Selection of learning experiences:** Learning experience refers to any interaction between teachers and learners or learners and the environment with an intention to modify their behavior by attaining appropriate knowledge, skills, attitudes and values. Learning experiences include planned teaching activities by the teacher as well as other activities performed by the learners themselves for attaining educational objectives. The criteria for selecting learning experience should be based on the principles of learning. Kenner recommends following criteria for selecting appropriate learning experience. They are:
   - *Validity*: Learning experience is valid when it is based on already stated educational objectives. The learning experience should try to involve cognitive, affective and psychomotor domains of objective in a holistic manner.
   - *Variety*: Learning experience need to provide a variety of learning experiences rather than a few type of experiences. Varied learning experience satisfies the need of learners with different interests and abilities of learning.
   - *Arouse interest*: Learning experiences need to arouse interest among learners. This will result in proactive learning among learners.

- *Relevance to life*: Learning experiences must be relevant to real life situations in the school and in the society. This will help learners understand the problems of society and find solutions for problems.
- *Suitability*: Learning experience must not be too simple or complex but rather be suitable for the level of the learners and appropriate to the concerned content.
- *Comprehensive*: Learning experience must cover all the stated objectives in lesson; it must range from the simplest learning experience to the most complex, covering all the domains of learning.
- *Base for further learning*: A learning experience should provide strong base for further learning. In other words, learning experiences should result in multiple learning.

6. **Organization of learning experiences and integration of learning experiences with content or subject matter:** This step involves (a) division of content into courses and units with specific time frame for completion. For example, in MSc nursing program educational psychology is a course and adolescent health is a unit in the course of educational psychology course, (b) division of content into areas which can be preferably taught through online teaching and traditional teaching methods. On the post-COVID period it is better to divide content in this manner so that teachers and students can familiarize with online classes if the school is forced to close down for long periods like the COVID-19 pandemic lockdown, (c) selection of teaching methods for each units in a course and (d) selection of reference materials like textbooks, web resources, etc. for each course.

Content and learning experience can be organized in two relationship bases namely **vertical and horizontal relationship**. Vertical organization is the arrangement of learning experience and content over a time sequence from simple to complex manner. For example, simple topics of medical nursing is taught during second year and more complex are taught during third year classes. Horizontal organization occurs, when the learning in one subject enhances knowledge skill and attitude in another subject within the same class. For example, knowledge acquired in pharmacology helps in learning medical nursing.

Kenner recommends following criteria in organizing learning experience and content they are:

- *Continuity*: It is the recurring emphasis on the learners' experiences on a particular element or kinds of activities until mastery in achieved. For example, a first year student get familiarized with physical examination in the beginning and attains mastery by completing second year.
- *Sequence*: it is also related to continuity as well as progressively moving from the lower to the higher level of knowledge and from simple to complex. Each experience reinforces and extends the previous one. Curriculum ensures sequence by arranging experiences based on chronological order or logical order and sometimes from simple to complex order. For example, a learner attains proficiency in English language after completing schooling.
- *Integration*: It refers to the relationship among learning experiences which brings about a unified view regarding knowledge. For example, knowledge in pharmacology helps in learning medical nursing.

7. **Selection of assessment strategies:** This step involves selection of assessment methods for each course in the educational program. Assessment strategies include assessment for learning or formative assessment and assessment of learning or summative assessment. Class tests and unit tests are examples of formative assessment. Final year examination conducted by school or university for promoting to higher level is an example of summative evaluation.

8. **Preparation of draft curriculum.**
9. **Publishing curriculum** in the website for seeking opinion of public as well as stakeholders.
10. **Finalizing curriculum** by including suggestions from public if required.
11. **Implementing curriculum.**
12. **Evaluating curriculum.**
13. **Revising curriculum.**

## PRINCIPLES OF CURRICULUM DEVELOPMENT

Aggarwal describes curriculum as a tool in the hands of the teachers for giving training to students in the art of living together in the community. It is a tool which considerably helps to inculcate those standards of moral action which are essential for successful living in society and for getting true satisfaction out of life. It is, therefore, very essential that the curriculum should be based on sound principles. Aggarwal suggests the following principles for developing a fruitful curriculum.

- **Conservative principle:** It has been stated that nations live in the present, on the past and for the future. This means that the present, the past, and the future needs of the community should be taken into consideration. The past is a great guide for the present as it helps us decide what has been useful to those who have lived before and what will be useful to those who are living now. Thus, the function of the school is to preserve and transmit the traditions, knowledge, experience and way of life to the present generation. This principle will be of help only when we carefully select as to what things of the past are likely to help us in the present. All the things of the past may not suit us. It is, therefore, essential that we should select only those subjects and activities which are required by the present generation.
- **Forward-looking principle:** Children of today are the citizens of tomorrow. Therefore, their education should be such as it enables them to be progressive minded persons. Education should give them a foundation of knowledge that will enable them to adjust with the environment.
- **Creative principle:** In the curriculum, those activities should be included which enable the child to exercise his creative and constructive powers.
- **Principle of totality form:** The total learning experience and total learning opportunity may have to be well planned as a whole curriculum and the teaching-learning activity needed for the entire period of time has to be considered while developing the curriculum.
- **Activity principle:** The curriculum should be developed in terms of activity and experience rather than of knowledge to be acquired and facts to be stored. Growth and learning takes place only where there is activity 'Experience' rather than 'instruction' is required to meet the needs of the various stages of growth.
- **Principle of preparation for life:** This is the most important principle in the development of curriculum. Curriculum must include those activities which enable the child to fulfill his responsibilities when he becomes an adult.
- **Principle of connecting to life:** The curriculum which is planned and developed for a particular educational program should provide worthwhile life experiences; in other words, subjects included in curriculum should be linked with some of the actual life situations.
- **Child-centered curriculum:** While developing the curriculum due consideration should be given to the students age, their educational level, needs and individual difference. Curriculum should be a student-oriented one rather than teaching-oriented. It should be adapted to the grade of the students and to their mental and physical development. The experiences provided should be within the comprehension of the students.

- **Principle of integration and correlation:** While developing the curriculum, each year's course should be built on what has been done in previous years and at the same time should serve as basis for subsequent learning. Different courses of the educational program should not be considered as watertight compartments. The wholeness may have to be achieved through the principle of correlation and integration.
- **Principle of comprehensiveness and balance:** The curriculum should be framed in such a way as every aspect of life, like economic relationships, social activities, occupations, etc., is given due emphasis.
- **Principle of loyalties:** The curriculum should be planned in such a manner that it teaches a true sense of loyalty to the family, the school, the country and the international community at large.
- **Principle of variety and flexibility:** While constructing curriculum, variety should be provided in terms of learning and teaching activities. Curriculum should not be too rigid so that appropriate modifications can be done as and when needed.
- **Principle of connecting to community needs:** Curriculum development should address the community needs. The lifestyle of the people, cultural background, aspirations of the people and needs of the community should be considered while constructing the curriculum.
- **Principle of connecting with social life:** Curriculum has to maintain a relation with social life. Sociology has to be given due recognition so that students can be prepared in such a way that they will be able to lead a well adjusted life in the democratic society.
- **Training for leisure:** In the curriculum development, there should be some provision for the cocurricular activities, relaxation, library utilization and electives according to choice. While developing the curriculum, the whole allotted time of curriculum should not be fixed exclusively for teaching and learning activity.
- **Principle of core or common subjects:** There are certain broad areas of knowledge, skill and appreciation with which all the children must be made conversant and these should find a place in the curriculum.
- **Principle of all-round development of body, mind and spirit:** All kinds of experiences should be provided to the students so that they may develop their all powers.
- **Principle of democracy, secularism and socialism:** Curriculum should be such as it trains the child to imbibe ideals and values of a democratic, secular and socialist state.
- **Principle of dignity of labor:** Curriculum should make provision for socially useful productive work. Curriculum should help the students to develop a positive attitude toward all kinds of jobs in addition to the white-collar ones.
- **Principle of character building:** Curriculum should provide those activities and experiences which promote human and social values. Well planned cocurricular activities will help the students develop these values.

## PRINCIPLES RELATED TO THE DEVELOPMENT OF NURSING CURRICULUM

In addition to the above mentioned principles, below mentioned ones should be kept in mind while developing nursing curriculum.
- Nursing curriculum should equip the students with the essential knowledge, skills and attitude so that they can fulfill their duties and responsibilities during the upcoming professional life.
- The expected results of the curriculum should be made clear to the students as well as the teacher. Since the modern nurse educator is considered as a facilitator of learning this principle deserves special attention.

- Curriculum development should consider the community needs with special emphasis to the health needs, lifestyle and cultural background of people, health services available and changes in the health pattern of the community.
- As nursing students are living under the influence of media and modern lifestyles, special measures has to be formulated in the curriculum for inculcating right attitude in them.
- Posting to the concerned clinical area should be preceded by adequate coverage of the related theory. Curriculum should offer adequate teaching-learning activities in the classroom, clinical area and community settings.
- Curriculum development has to consider the guidelines laid down by the statutory bodies like nursing council, universities, examination boards and the like.
- Curriculum development should give due importance to high-tech high-touch approach in the nursing care. This will help maintain the human component of nursing in the midst of technological advancements in patient care.
- Curriculum should allow a participatory approach in the teaching-learning process where students are mainly responsible for their learning and teacher assumes the role of a facilitator of learning.
- The learning environment should closely resemble the life situation where the nurses will perform on being qualified from the educational program.

## FACTORS INFLUENCING CURRICULUM DEVELOPMENT IN NURSING EDUCATION

The major factors which influence curriculum development are: (a) philosophy of nursing education, (b) educational psychology, (c) society, (d) student, (e) knowledge explosion and scientific advancements, (f) technological advancements in patient care, (g) educational technology, (h) transnational career opportunities and (i) resources.

- **Philosophy of nursing education:** The purpose of nursing education is to bring about desirable behavioral changes in nursing students so as to enable them to render comprehensive nursing care. The determination of desired changes in behavior is being written down in the form of educational objectives. The objectives can be formulated only on the basis of the philosophy of education. Hence philosophy is regarded as a major factor influencing the curriculum development. As said elsewhere, philosophy of education also determines the selection of students, recruitment of staff, teaching-learning activities and evaluation system.
- **Educational psychology:** Educational psychology furnishes necessary information required for the selection of appropriate teaching-learning activities. Principles of learning and principles of teaching are derived mainly from educational psychology. Educational psychology provides information and principles which serve to help in the selection, organization and evaluation of learning experience in the curriculum.
- **Society:** Educational institutions are social institutions which exists within the society. Hence, the needs of the society may have to be considered while developing curriculum. Nursing education is considered as a social institution related to health. So, we have to give due consideration to the health needs of the society while developing the nursing curriculum. Due to emerging and reemerging diseases the societal pressure on healthcare professions is mounting. Adequate knowledge regarding the nature of the society and its health needs are essential to develop a viable nursing curriculum. This will enable nursing education to produce competent nursing professionals who are capable of confronting the challenges faced by the society in the area of health care in a successful yet cost-effective manner.

* **Student:** Since the modern education is student centered, nursing education has to address the needs of the students in a more humanitarian way without neglecting the patient's rights. Majority of the students joining for nursing educational programs are in their late adolescence and provision for guidance and counselling in the curriculum will help solve many of their problems, either related to learning nursing or personal life. As nursing students are living under the constant influence of media and modern lifestyles, curriculum has to formulate special measures to inculcate proper attitude in them. Curriculum should also give importance to high-tech high-touch approach in nursing care so that students can maintain the human component of nursing without undermining the advantages of the technological advancements in patient care. Curriculum should allow a participatory approach in teaching-learning process where students are mainly responsible for their learning and teacher assumes the role of a facilitator of learning. It should not impose unnecessary restrictions on nursing students by citing the age old traditions. It is high-time to remove unwanted restrictions and to consider nursing students as just like any other health professional students. Through a perfect blending of student needs and patient needs we can develop a student friendly nursing curriculum. Curriculum should also prepare the students to lead a balanced life in the future by fulfilling other roles in addition to that of a professional nurse such as a family member, a responsible citizen, etc. In short, curriculum has to prepare the student as a good human being who possesses the qualities of a professional nurse. This will make them more sensitive to the health needs of the people and enable them to render care as empathetic care givers. Thus, nursing curriculum aims the total development of students.
* **Knowledge explosion and scientific advancements:** In modern world, knowledge is regarded as power and the success of professional life is determined by the type and quantity of knowledge one possess. Since a profession is defined as a dynamic integration of various faculties of knowledge, nursing curriculum has to address the knowledge explosion properly. Nowadays, enormous quantity of knowledge is generated through research and other activities. Due to the developments in the information technology, knowledge is available at the fingertip of students. Curriculum should guide the students properly to select the much needed information from the jungle of information. As nurse educators cannot give all the knowledge required for the students, curriculum has to propose innovative measures for motivating the students "to hunt for the knowledge." For delivering comprehensive care nurses have to possess knowledge from various disciplines along with the nursing expertise. Hence, while developing curriculum, pooling of essential knowledge from various disciplines are to be considered. Curriculum should motivate students to learn the recent scientific advancements related to patient care.
* **Technological advancements in patient care:** Technological advancements are assisting the nurse to save the life of the patient in a more reliable manner, at the same time it is eating away the human component of nursing. In a society which value technology we cannot ignore the advantages of technological advancements in patient care. We have to preserve the human component of nursing without undermining the merits of technological advancements. Giving emphasis to the high-tech high-touch approach in nursing care throughout the nursing curriculum will help us reach a consensus between human component and technological advancements.
* **Educational technology:** Curriculum should utilize educational technology to the maximum extent possible. Effective use of educational technology will help develop new teaching-learning methods and improve the student friendly nature of the existing ones.

❖ **Transnational career opportunities:** This factor is not influencing the nursing education universally. The influence of this factor is evident in the nursing curriculum of developing countries from where many nurses are seeking jobs abroad for better prospectus. Since the fate of nursing education in these countries is determined by the abroad career opportunities, this factor deserves special attention. The dominance of English and geriatric nursing in our curriculum exemplifies the influence of this factor. As more nations are curbing the restrictions imposed on healthcare professionals, transnational career opportunities will continue to influence our curriculum development at least for the coming 20 years.

❖ **Resources:** The development of a viable curriculum depends upon the availability of tangible and intangible resources. Tangible resources are teachers, textbooks, physical facilities, etc. Intangible resources are the resources within ourselves like motivation, attitude, interests, intelligence, etc.

## ASPECTS OF CURRICULUM DEVELOPMENT

According to Bevis critical points that need to be identified and decided on in curriculum development are:

❖ A determination of the desired characteristics of the graduates of the program.
❖ The identification and structure of knowledge that is critical to nursing practice.
❖ The understanding of the culture of nursing as it relates to roles, ethics and acceptable practice parameters.
❖ An explanation of nursing's role in society in general and health care in particular.
❖ An identification of curriculum, content that will foster nursing's contribution to society.
❖ The identification and organization of healthcare problems that graduates will be dealing with both present and future.
❖ Identification of teaching and learning strategies that will foster critical thinking, inquiry and the ability to meet one's learning needs.
❖ The ability to assist students in developing to context (both within and outside of nursing) in which to understand the discipline of nursing.

## STEPS IN CURRICULUM DEVELOPMENT IN NURSING EDUCATION

According to Ralph Tyler, there are four main steps or tasks in curriculum development. They are as follows **(Fig. 4.2):** (1) Formulation of educational objectives. (2) Selection of learning experiences. (3) Effective and efficient organization of learning experience. (4) Evaluation of the curriculum.

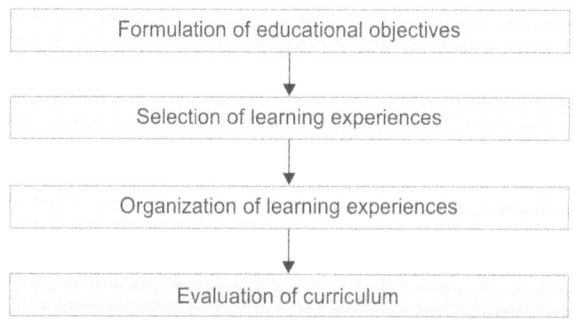

**Fig. 4.2:** Steps in curriculum development in nursing education.

# FORMULATION OF EDUCATIONAL OBJECTIVES

Educational objectives are the statements of those desired changes in behavior as a result of specific teaching-learning activity or specific teacher-learner activity. (*see* Chapter 3: Educational Objectives)

## Data Required for Formulating Educational Objectives

The following information will help formulate educational objectives in an effective manner:
a. Philosophical statement of the institute.
b. Social and health needs of the society.
c. Needs of the students.
d. Resources available in the society.
e. Entry criteria or level of students.
f. Specifications of positions to be held by the students on the completion of the program like staff nurse, nursing tutor, etc.
g. Minimum requirements in terms of clinical and other facilities prescribed by the statutory bodies like nursing council, universities, etc.
h. Future trends in nursing.
i. Criteria to be fulfilled in order to appear for internationally reputed qualifying examinations like CGFNS, MOH examinations, etc.

## Criteria for the Selection and Statement of Objectives

*Following criteria will help to state the objectives in a meaningful way:*
a. Objectives have to be stated in terms of desired changes in behavior and the area of subject matter through which behavior is to operate.
b. Objective should be stated in the form which makes them most helpful in selecting the learning experiences and guiding the teaching activity.
c. The desired changes in behavior should be in consistent with the accepted educational objective.
d. The objectives for the specific subjects or the units or lesson should have a direct contribution to the attainment of overall objective of the curriculum.
e. The objectives should be attainable and practicable in the specific teaching-learning situation.
f. Objectives selected should be worthwhile, contributing both to the social needs and social changes.
g. Objectives should consider the needs, ability and level of students.
h. The objectives of each course, unit, topic and lesson should contribute to the continued and total development of students.
i. The objectives selected should serve as a motivating factor for teachers as well as students.
j. Objectives should be easily accepted and understood by the teacher and learner.
k. Objectives have to be stated by making it possible to maintain continuity, sequence, correlation and integration of learning activity.
l. Objectives should be cooperatively planned and developed by all teachers and by the teacher and student whenever and wherever possible.
m. Objectives have to be so worded that each statement contains only a single objective.
n. Objectives should not be too detailed—detailing of objective will permit wide flexibility in teaching and learning. Hence, the objective should be simple and concise in nature.
o. While developing and formulating the objectives, the scheme of evaluation may have to be planned and developed.

## Steps in the Formulation of Educational Objectives

According to Ralf Tyler, there are nine essential tasks or steps in the formulation of educational objectives. They are as follows **(Fig. 4.3)**: (1) Identify the needs of the learner. (2) Identify the needs of the society. (3) Study the suggestions of the expert. (4) Formulate the philosophy. (5) State the objectives inferred or gathered from various sources in a proper way. (6) Formulate a theory of learning. (7) Screen the objectives through educational philosophy and educational psychology and select the appropriate ones. Screening of objectives through educational philosophy will help select objectives in relation to human values and thereby contribute to the total development of the student. Screening through educational psychology helps determine the methods of teaching, principles of teaching, methods of learning and the like. (8) Define the objectives clearly in terms of content. (9) State the educational objectives in terms of behavioral outcomes or change.

## SELECTION OF LEARNING EXPERIENCES

Learning experience is defined as deliberately planned experiences in selected situations where students actively participate, interact and which result in desirable changes of behavior in the students. In nursing education, selection of learning experience is concerned with the decision about the content of subject matter and clinical, community and laboratory practice. Thus, selection of learning situations together with corresponding learning activities will comprise the learning experiences. When these are in relation to the selection of subject matter, i.e., different theoretical courses of study, these will form the theoretical learning experiences. When learning experiences are selected in terms of community and clinical nursing practice and laboratory work these will constitute practical learning experience. In short, learning experiences are those experiences which make appropriate responses among students as indicated in the objectives.

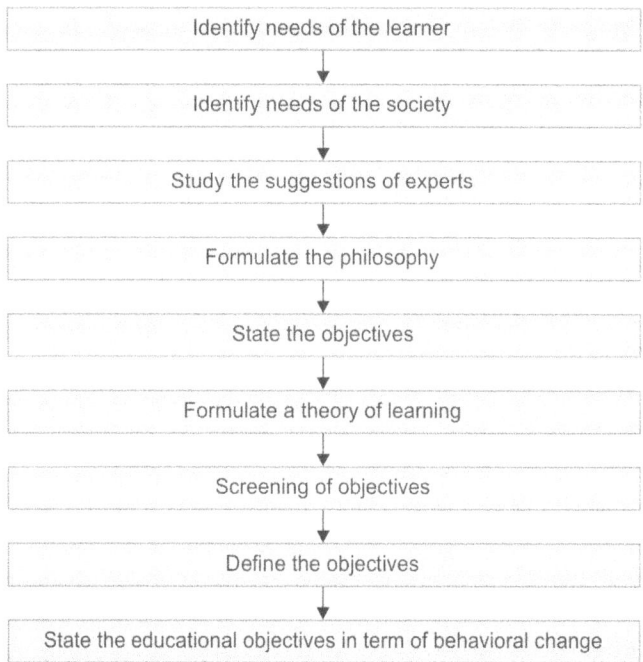

**Fig. 4.3:** Steps in formulation of educational objectives.

## Principles to be Followed in the Selection of Learning Experiences

1. All learning needs should be in relation to the selected objectives.
2. Learning activities should be in relation to those real life situations where the students are expected to practice after being qualified.
3. Selection should be in a manner that there is an effective integration between theory and practice.
4. Reactions sought must be within the range of possibility for the students concerned.
5. The same learning experience will result in several outcomes and several learning experiences may bring out the same outcome.
6. Learning experiences should be selected in such a way that learners are constantly motivated.
7. Learning experiences should be planned and organized in such a way that the student gets meaning out of each experience and the student should see the relationship between past and present experiences and focus on the future needs.
8. Learning is enhanced by utilizing a wide variety of teaching-learning methods.
9. Students will learn effectively, if the experiences are satisfactory to them.
10. Learning experience should consider the students' ability to undergo the desired changes in behavior.
11. Learning experiences selected should not be beyond the particular stage of development of the students.
12. Learning experiences selected should be according to the needs of the students and every student should be given similar learning experiences.
13. Learning experiences selected should provide same or equal chances for all students.

## Characteristics of Good Learning Experience

Characteristics of good learning experience are: (a) Learning experience should allow the student to learn by doing. (b) Learning experience should create motivation and interest among students. (c) Learning experience should be challenging to students. (d) Learning experiences should satisfy the needs of the time. (e) Learning experiences selected should bring out multiple outcomes in students. (f) Learning experiences should help students acquire needed knowledge, skill and attitude. (g) Learning experiences should be helpful in hunting or gathering information. (h) All learning experiences which are planned and selected should be helpful to the student in attaining the educational objectives.

## Criteria for the Selection of Learning Experiences

Following criteria will help in selecting the appropriate learning experiences:

1. Learning experience selected should be consistent with the philosophy of the institute and lead to the achievement of the objectives of the program.
2. Learning experiences should be varied and flexible enough. This can be achieved by keeping in mind the learners abilities to undergo the desired change of behavior and not going beyond their particular stage of development.
3. Learning experiences should be so selected that it will give the student an opportunity to practice the kind of behavior implied in the objective. It should provide sufficient opportunity for self-activity so that the transfer of knowledge remembered, skill acquired and desirable attitudes become habitual.

4. Learning experiences should provide opportunity for the development of independent thinking and decision making, sound judgment, intellectual resourcefulness, self-discipline and sound integrity of purpose.
5. Learning experiences should be adapted to the needs of the students so that they can obtain satisfaction from behaving in the manner implied in the objective.
6. Learning experience are arranged in a manner that provides continuity, correlation and integration of theory and practice and clinical learning experience.
7. Learning experiences are planned and evaluated cooperatively by the teacher and the student. The various experiences provided will be effective, interesting and useful if the evaluation can be cooperatively planned by the teacher and the student.
8 Learning experiences are selected and arranged to give appropriate emphasis and weightage according to the relative importance of the various learning experiences and contents.

## Constraints in the Selection of Learning Experiences

According to Halstead J, constraints in choosing and implementing learning experiences may arise from faculty, student, time and resources (**Table 4.1**). Even though it is difficult to eliminate all constraints, careful assessment of each source of constraint help avoid shortenings.

## ORGANIZATION OF LEARNING EXPERIENCES

Organization of learning experiences has to be done carefully, systematically and sequentially. According to Tyler, primary aim of organization of learning experiences in the curriculum is to bring and relate various learning experiences together to produce the maximum cumulative effect in order to give a unified view of the whole so that the educational objectives are achieved. *Continuity, sequence and integration* has to be followed while organizing the learning experiences. Continuity is achieved through building each experience one after another. Sequence refers to building of learning experience one over the other more deeply and broadly. Integration is relating learning experience in such a way that the learner gets a unified view of whole learning.

**TABLE 4.1:** Constraints in selection of learning experiences.

| Source | Constraint |
|---|---|
| Faculty | • Faculty/student ratio<br>• Lack of experience<br>• Lack of knowledge<br>• Lack of understanding of students knowledge |
| Students | • Distractions<br>• Inability to use technology<br>• Lack of prerequisite knowledge and skills<br>• Stress/anxiety<br>• Student-faculty ration too large |
| Time | • Inadequate for activity<br>• Inadequate for debriefing |
| Resources | • Copyright restrictions<br>• Inadequate clinical facility<br>• Inadequate classroom facility<br>• Inadequate funds<br>• Inadequate AV aids |

Learning experiences have to be *vertically and horizontally* organized. In vertical organization, the learning experiences planned for the entire curriculum have to be arranged in such a way that the learning progresses week by week, month by month, semester to semester and year to year and two important criteria of continuity and sequence are maintained. In horizontal organization, all the learning experiences have to be related in all areas of students' experience so that the learning takes place in different times and are automatically related to learning of another situation or subject. In horizontal organization, learning becomes more wider and deeper and criteria of integration becomes possible.

## Principles to be Followed While Organizing Learning Experiences

a. Learning experiences have to be so organized that succeeding experiences build upon those which preceded.
b. Learning experience in one area and other areas should be related to each other.
c. Learning experience should utilize the allotted time in a cost-effective manner.
d. Learning experiences should be organized in broad areas in order to facilitate relating the learning experience in allied areas.
e. Broad principles of education has to be applied and emphasized.
f. Provide ample opportunities for the student to concentrate and relate the various activities in different areas of learning so that the required ability and skills are easily attained.
g. Provide opportunity to concentrate on one or more electives.
h. In organizing nursing educational program, the curriculum may have to be organized in terms of broad subject matter areas like humanities, behavioral sciences, biological sciences and nursing sciences.
i. Organization of learning experiences in the curriculum should be neither too flexible nor too rigid.
j. Clinical experience and assignments should be valued on the basis of experiences provided to students.
k. Learning experiences have to be organized in such a way that the student is able to practice professional nursing for the next few years.

## Elements of Organizing the Learning Experiences

Elements to be considered while organizing the learning experiences are: (a) Grouping learning experiences under subject headings. (b) Preparation of master plan for curriculum. (c) Placement of learning experiences in the total curriculum. (d) Preparation of the correlation chart. (e) Organization of clinical experience. (f) Types of teaching system have to be followed.

## Grouping Learning under Subject Headings

After selecting the learning experiences, we have to organize them with an intention to provide optimum experience to the students. The practice of grouping learning experience under subject headings is the most preferred method of organizing the learning experiences. In nursing educational programs, subject matter can be grouped into humanities, behavioral sciences, nursing sciences, medicine and the like.

## Preparation of Master Plan for Curriculum

Preparation of master plan will guide the teachers in the placement of subject matter and clinical experience. This will give a clear picture as to how, in which year and in what stage is the subject matter going to be taught and the relevant clinical experiences to be offered. Master plan should be prepared in accordance with the requirements prescribed by the statutory bodies like Indian Nursing Council and universities. The master plan should also spell out the hours of planned instructions and required hours of clinical experience per week or per month of the year. Invariably, the master plan explains the following: (a) Total duration of the program, for example, three years for diploma program and four years for graduate program. (b) Explanation of different courses of study with special reference to theory and practicals, for example, theory and practical experience meant for medical surgical nursing, mental health nursing, etc. (c) Total allotted hours in terms of theory and practical for each course. Course plan of each course with details like total units, hours and objectives for each unit. Guidelines for providing practical experiences, master rotation plan, etc. Specific mention about the core content of the curriculum, i.e., the most important content in each course, for example, the nursing process approach of giving patient care is emphasized in all courses. (d) Teaching-learning methods. (e) Scheme of evaluation. (f) Details of student activities like cocurricular activities, health check-up, vacation, etc.

### Placement of Learning Experiences in the Total Curriculum

All elements of the curriculum should be related to one another. The learning experiences should be so organized that they continuously reinforce each other and broaden and deepen the understanding and skills of the learner. Following the principle of sequence, integration and correlation will help organize the learning experience in an effective manner.

### Preparation of Correlation Chart

Preparation of correlation chart will help identify the extent of correlation achieved in the total curriculum in relation to the different courses of study and the various subjects and clinical experience offered in the program.

### Organization of Clinical Experience

Clinical experience is the vital element in the curriculum of any nursing educational program. How well the students develop nursing expertise will be determined by the volume and quality of clinical experience they receive. Students achieve speed and accuracy in carrying out the nursing procedures only through a well planned and organized clinical experience. Considering the importance of clinical experience, a separate session is devoted for it in the coming pages.

### Teaching System

Teaching of various subjects can be organized in different ways like *complete block or teaching block system, partial block system and study day system.* In the teaching block, the classroom teaching and clinical postings are divided into specific blocks. Certain blocks are devoted for theoretical instruction while some other blocks are meant for specific clinical experience. In partial block system, the theoretical instruction as well as the clinical experience go hand in hand. The student may attend the classes in the afternoon and go for postings in the morning or vice versa depending when the experience would be varied and rich in accordance with the fulfillment of objectives. In study day system, one day or more per week is completely kept for taking classes and the other days students will be in the clinical areas. Usually a combination of these systems is followed. Teaching block is preferred in the beginning of academic year, especially in the case of first year students. Since all students cannot be withdrawn from the clinics for teaching block at a time, academic year of senior students usually starts with partial block. For first year students, partial block begins after a few weeks of full day postings in the clinical area.

# ORGANIZATION OF CLINICAL EXPERIENCE

Organization of clinical experience in the curriculum is done on the basis of the syllabus and regulations laid down by the statutory bodies like Indian Nursing Council and universities. Organization of clinical experience is the responsibility of the faculty. Clinical experience related to each course should be planned according to the objectives so that students will get enough opportunities for developing the desired nursing skills and attitude. Preparing a *clinical rotation plan* will help in providing clinical experience to the students in an effective manner. Clinical rotation plan is the statement which explains the order of the clinical posting of various groups of nursing students belonging to different classes in relevant clinical areas and community health settings as per the requirements laid down by the statutory bodies. A well planned clinical rotation plan will help students to gain maximum experience from the clinical area and community settings. Thus, clinical rotation plan will contribute toward the attainment of overall objectives of the nursing educational program.

## Factors Influencing the Clinical Rotation Plan

Multiple factors influence the planning of clinical rotation plan. They are: (a) Requirement stated by the statutory bodies like Indian Nursing Council and universities. (b) The objectives of the course, for example, while planning clinical rotation plan for mental health nursing, objectives of the mental health nursing course should be considered. (c) Only a limited number of students can be posted in a particular clinical area, especially in critical care areas. Hence the number of students should be taken into account while preparing the clinical rotation plan. (d) Infrastructure of various clinical areas. This factor is particularly important in institutions which conduct more than one program. (e) Duration of experience in each area. (f) Nurse educators available for supervision.

## Principles of Developing Clinical Rotation Plan

Principles related to the development of clinical rotation plan will help accomplish the objectives of the clinical postings in a more effective manner. The principles are: (a) The clinical rotation plan must be developed in accordance with the master plan of the curriculum. Theoretical instructions should precede as closely as possible the clinical experience. (b) The rotation plan must be made in advance with the cooperation of all the faculty members involved in the clinical teaching. (c) Maxims of teaching should be followed while selecting areas of experience. (d) Principle of continuity, sequence and integration should be followed to the maximum extent possible. (e) Enough teaching staff should be made available in the clinical areas for giving proper instructions to the students. (f) Seeking suggestions of the nursing staff working in the clinical areas will ensure their cooperation. Moreover, giving adequate weightage to the suggestions of nursing staff will help post the students in such a way that they will get enough exposure to the patient care activities rather than spending time in the name of clinical experience. (g) First 3-year students should receive maximum supervision and attention. (h) All students should get enough experience as per the clinical rotation plan. If any student misses experience in an area due to unavoidable reasons, provision should be there to compensate the same. Students should be motivated to continue in the clinical areas more than the prescribed hours required for attending the university or board examinations. (i) All assignments related to the clinical area should be finished before the completion of the postings, especially when the students are posted in institutions other than the parent institution. (j) Overcrowding in the clinical area with different groups of students is not advisable.

## Types of Rotation Plan

Rotation plan can be mainly classified into *master rotation plan and individual rotation plan*. Master rotation plan is an overall plan of rotation of all students in a particular educational institution showing the entire teaching-learning activities and related events during an academic year like details of theoretical instruction, duration and areas of clinical instruction, particulars of community health nursing postings, period of vacation, study leave for university examinations, examination week, etc. Usually, master rotation plans of all batches are prepared as a combined chart for getting a unified view regarding the placement of students on various occasions. This will help avoid duplication and the resulting confusion.

Individual rotation plan is made to make sure that each student in a particular block posting undergoes experience in each area. For example, in a four-week period of operation theatre posting where the student needs to gain experience from different theaters like gastroenterology, orthopedics, etc. an individual rotation plan can be made for each student by indicating different areas of posting during this period in order to ensure adequate experience.

## EVALUATION OF THE CURRICULUM

Evaluation of nursing curriculum has become a major concern of nurse educators in recent years. Curriculum evaluation involves an assessment of the philosophy of the institution, program goals of the institution, nursing content taught in each course, course objectives, teaching-learning methods, course evaluation methods and the relationship of non-nursing courses to the overall plan of study.

Student participation can also be elicited in curriculum evaluation. Evaluation of a curriculum should be efficient and effective, characteristics which can be enhanced by advanced planning. Spreading evaluation throughout the year will lighten the load. One way to assure efficiency is a plan with specific timetables and inexpensive non-time consuming evaluative tools that cover variables in a particular program. Evaluation that burdens the already busy faculty or students will be regarded as unwelcome or will be ignored and tools must be practical to administer and analyze.

In curriculum evaluation, the evaluation of five M's are done, They are: (a) Men—whether curriculum has been organized and implemented properly by the faculty members and other personnel involved. (b) Money—whether money meant for curriculum development is utilized properly. (c) Materials—evaluation of textbooks, literature and the like used for the development and implementation of curriculum. (d) Methods—whether teaching-learning methods which are planned in the curriculum are appropriate. (e) Minutes—whether adequate time is given for theory and practical in each course like medical-surgical nursing, mental health nursing, etc.

### Principles of Curriculum Evaluation

Principles of curriculum evaluation are: (a) Evaluation of curriculum should consist of finding out to what extent the objectives are being achieved. (b) Objectives for evaluation should be in terms of behavior or the reactions to be measured and also in terms of content which is being planned through which the behavior is to operate. (c) Plan of evaluation should be comprehensive enough to measure adequately the behaviors which are considered important or significant. (d) Techniques and methods used in evaluation should be on the basis of specific behaviors expected and measured. (e) Satisfactory evaluation program should include a variety of evaluation tools or instruments. (f) The decision on whether the student has had adequate experience in a given area should be in terms of excellence of performance and not in terms of time spent. (g) Records of clinical practice should reflect the objectives of practice and give evidence of the extent to which students have achieved the objectives.

## SYLLABUS AND CURRICULUM

Curriculum is a systematic arrangement of the sum total of selected experience planned by a school for a defined group of students to attain the aims of a particular educational program. There is a considerable difference between the syllabus and the finished curriculum. The syllabus was given by the statutory body like Indian Nursing Council and it is the responsibility of the nursing faculty to interpret the syllabus and create a curriculum. Thus, syllabus is a list of the content of a course or a collection of courses which may or may not be in logical order. A syllabus generally lists a series of topics which should be covered and which may form the basis of examination questions.

## CORE CURRICULUM

According to Fredgreaves, core curriculum means the central area of concern, the central theme or thread which provides the 'main route' for the students through the curriculum or part of it. It can also mean the areas of curriculum which are compulsory, rather than electives or special options. Nursing process approach of giving nursing care can be regarded as the core curriculum in any nursing educational program.

## CURRICULUM FOR EXCELLENCE IN NURSING EDUCATION

Curriculum for excellence in nursing education is intended to achieve professional as well as soft skills essential for leading a successful life as a nurse. It prepares nursing students to explore more possibilities in addition to service and education sector. For example, curriculum for excellence in nursing enables a graduate nurse to reach in coveted positions like Indian administrative service. Curriculum for excellence in nursing education focuses on the following aspects.

1. **Benchmarks or content standards:** Benchmarks or content standards in curriculum for excellence in nursing education explains what learners need to know and do to achieve a particular level or standard across all curriculum areas. This is very important. According to Wilson, these standards should be clear, detailed and complete; reasonable in scope; rigorous and scientifically correct; and they should be built around a conceptual frameworks that reflects sound model of student learning. They should also describe example of performance expectations for learners in clear and specific terms so that all concerned will know what is expected from students.

   Clearly stating educational objectives covering cognitive, affective and psychomotor domains is essential for determining benchmarks. Lack of knowledge about benchmarks can create problems to students. For example, evaluating university answer paper of anatomy by a person not familiar with nursing curriculum may result in high failure rate.

2. **Experience and outcomes*:* Experiences and outcomes are a set of clear and concise statements about students learning and progress in each curriculum area. They are essential to plan learning and assess progress. This aspect of curriculum focus on outcome based teaching-learning process and evaluation. It also highlights the need of providing adequate facilities for simulation and clinical experience.

3. **Recent developments in cognitive neurosciences:** Cognitive neuroscience is the study based on mind and brain research aimed at understanding the psychological, computational

and neuro scientific bases of cognition. Nursing curriculum need to incorporate recent developments in cognitive neurosciences. This is essential for developing more student friendly teaching-learning methods.
4. **Relevance:** Curriculum for excellence in nursing education needs to consider the relevance of contents of curricular areas with special consideration to nursing procedures. Many nursing procedures are outdated with the advancements of technology in health care. This aspect also highlights the need of recommending appropriate teaching methods in nursing education.
5. **Developments in educational technology:** Curriculum needs to consider developments in educational technology for devising appropriate methods of teaching. Since GNM program is phasing out, educational technology will help to develop appropriate programs for diploma holders to acquire equivalency with degree program.
6. **Recent trends in healthcare delivery system:** Trends in health care definitely influence nursing education. Hence, nursing curriculum needs to address trends in healthcare system.
7. **Research orientation:** Curriculum focuses on inculcating a positive attitude toward research among students. Research orientation not only aims high end research but also motivate students to think about the "why" and "how" related to nursing process and nursing procedures.
8. **Challenges:** Curriculum effectively deals with challenges facing by nursing education and nursing service. Challenges can be confronted effectively by adopting learner friendly teaching methods with adequate consideration to patient safety.

## CONCEPT OF HAPPINESS CURRICULUM AND NURSING EDUCATION

Happiness curriculum is a form of value based learning developed mainly for school children. The idea was to focus on students EQ (Emotional Quotient) and SIG (Social Intelligence Quotient) which are not given much attention like IQ (Intelligence Quotient). Happiness curriculum is focused on helping children manage their life better. It motivates students to view world more positively and holistically.

As nursing is a caring profession, integrating aspects of happiness curriculum helps to improve life of nursing students. Inculcating values along with higher level of competence assist students to build a successful career by becoming a good human being. A higher level of social intelligence quotient helps nursing students to become more empathetic and responsible. When become more empathetic and responsible they concentrate more on studies than attracted by social media.

Nursing education is the most value based professional education in the modern world. By adopting few more measures to enhance EQ and SIQ of students as well as teachers we can integrate the concept of happiness curriculum into nursing curriculum. A happiness curriculum transfers all nursing college from mere professional colleges to a centre of excellence capable of bringing out good human beings with qualities of a competent professional nurse.

## CURRICULUM REVISION/CHANGING THE CURRICULUM

Curriculum revision means making the curriculum different in some way, to give it a new position or direction. This often means alteration to its philosophy by way of its aims and objectives, reviewing the content included, revising its methods and rethinking its evaluating procedures.

## Approaches to Curriculum Revision

The three main approaches to curriculum revision are *addition, deletion and organization*. In *addition*, new elements are added to the existing curriculum. In deletion, some elements are deleted to modify the curriculum. In reorganization, nothing is added or deleted but only restructuring of the existing curriculum is done. The basis for any major curriculum revision is significantly to improve the existing curriculum. Before any changes can be initiated, therefore, a complete analysis is required of the existing curriculum to identify its strengths and weaknesses and areas of compatibility with the new ideology. This analysis is usually carried out using data acquired through the normal formative and summative evaluation of the old curriculum. From this data, the assessment of future needs can be made along with a determination of what needs to be changed and the selection of possible solutions to problems and the means by which the necessary changes can be achieved.

## Stages of Curriculum Revision

Fredgreaves describes the following seven stages in revising a nursing curriculum.

**Stage 1:** If a curriculum development and evaluation committee does not exist, one should be formed to act as coordinating group for implementing the planned curriculum changes.

**Stage 2:** Appraise the existing nursing and educational practices which are representative of the currently operating curriculum. Study carefully the existing curriculum and identify its strengths and weaknesses by considering its overall intentions and purposes, including the basic values and beliefs which are currently part of the institute's philosophy. Consider the extent to which the curriculum is offering educational and training experience for the students.

**Stage 3:** Make a detailed study of the existing curriculum content to see whether it is still relevant and appropriate to meet a knowledge base adequate for the changing role of the professional nurse. This will mean giving consideration to whether the skills, attitudes and knowledge to be learned are still worthwhile and whether the present developing conceptual frameworks of nursing knowledge are sufficiently represented in the curriculum.

**Stage 4:** Establish criteria for decisions about what needs to go into the curriculum and what needs to come out and how the curriculum materials and methods might be changed.

**Stage 5:** This involves the design and writing of the new curriculum changes and these may include the revised philosophy and aims of the curriculum including the new intentions and purposes. It also includes the revised objectives and the reformed content along with any new teaching-learning approaches. Some of the existing evaluation procedures would need adjustments to fall in line with new content and methodology.

**Stage 6:** Within this stage the actual implementation of changes is put into action. Implementing the changes successfully involves having knowledge of the change and the securing of the participation of those people necessary to enable the implementation. Teachers, students and other concerned people need to be well informed with respect to the changes that are to take place.

**Stage 7:** Following the implementation of the new changes it is important to evaluate the effects of those changes and it is with evaluation that this final stage is concerned. Evaluation is directed at the identification and collection of data and its analysis, in order for the effects of changes to be measured and appropriate decisions and judgments made.

## COURSE OUTLINE PLANNING

Any nursing educational program is a combination of various courses like medical surgical nursing, mental health nursing, etc. These courses are placed in an intertwined manner in order to attain the objectives of the educational program. The two levels of course planning are: (a) At the level of the course itself, i.e., organizing both content and learning experiences within the course. (b) Planning in relation to the total program. This level is concerned with the placement of the course in the program and its relationship to other courses. A course is a combination of various but interrelated units (see Unit Planning).

### Principles of Course Planning

The principles of course planning are: (a) State the objectives in behavioral terms. (b) Follow principles meant for selecting the content of a course. (c) Establish sequence. This can be achieved by following the maxims of teaching. (d) Ensure logical and psychological continuity. This principle focuses on the needs of the students without undermining the standard of profession. By way of considering the level of students, organizing the course in a student centered manner, recognizing individual differences, providing a variety of learning approaches including problem solving and problem-based learning logical and psychological continuity can be achieved. This principle also helps divide the course content into student friendly units, promote comprehension and to avoid overlapping and repetition. (e) Principle of integration. Course planning should facilitate horizontal as well as vertical integration so that students can easily transfer the learning acquired in one situation to another area. (f) The courses should give adequate weightage to the core curriculum content. For example, all courses should enrich the students' ability to render nursing care by employing the nursing process approach. (g) Unity curriculum. This principle proposes merging of closely related subjects to form a particular course in order to avoid repetition and overlapping. For example, maternity nursing and gynecological nursing can be merged together and considered as a course. (h) Select learning approaches that are acceptable to all faculty members like problem solving and problem-based learning. (i) Flexibility in selecting teaching-learning methods. Teacher should have enough freedom to select the appropriate teaching-learning method. However, teacher should try to make the teaching-learning method a student centered one irrespective of its merits and demerits. (j) Provide variety in modes of learning. Provision for innovative modes of learning like assignments, group discussions, independent study modules, problem solving approaches, etc., will promote better learning.

### Principles for Selecting the Course Content

Principles for selecting the course content are: (a) Content should contribute to the achievement of the objectives of the particular nursing educational program. (b) It should be appropriate to the level of that group of students to whom it is to be taught. (c) Content should have community orientation. (d) It must be sensitive to the changing health needs as well as the aspirations of the students. (e) It should be experience based. (f) Content should have transcultural perspective. (g) It should provide functional relationship with allied disciplines or professions. (h) It must be wide and comprehensive. (i) It should provide for continuing learning. (j) Content should contribute to the personal as well as professional development of the students.

### Elements of a Course Plan

Essential elements of a course plan are: (a) Course description. (b) Behavioral objectives. (c) Placement of the course by specifying the level of learners, for example, placement of anatomy is stated as first year leading to BSc Nursing (Basic) degree. (d) Explain the time allotted. If clinical experience is needed, specify the time meant for theory and practical experience. (e) In case of courses associated with field experience like community health nursing, details of the field experience. (f) Organize the content into unit wise or lesson plan wise. (g) Details of the resource materials and teaching-learning methods to be followed. (h) Details of learning activities for students. (i) Details of formative and summative evaluation, ratio between internal assessment and university examination, etc. (j) References for teachers and students (see the course outline in your university syllabus for example of a course outline.)

## UNIT PLANNING

Hanna, Hageman and Potler state that "a unit can be defined as purposeful learning experience focused upon behavior of the learner and enable him to adjust to a life situation more effectively." Jorolimek defines unit "as a means of organizing materials for instructional purposes which utilizes significant subject matter content, involves pupils in learning activities through active participation intellectually and physically and modifies the pupil's behavior to the extent that he is able to cope with new problems and situations more competently". From the above definitions, it is evident that a unit consists of a comprehensive series of related and meaningful activities, so developed to achieve the purpose and educational objectives by providing significant educational experiences that would result in appropriate behavioral changes in the learners. A unit is a combination of various but interrelated lessons (*see* Lesson Planning). Depending upon the number of lessons, a unit may be small, taking only few hours to teach or it may be large covering weeks or even months of teaching. For example, Unit on history of nursing takes only few hours to teach, whereas unit on medicine administration may take at least two months to finish.

### Characteristics of a Good Unit

The characteristics of a good unit are: (a) Organize various learning activities or experiences around a central problem or purpose. For example, the unit on cardiovascular system enables the student to care patients with cardiac problems. (b) Unit should be suitable to the needs, capabilities and interests of the students. (c) Provision for a variety of learning experiences like clinical postings, theory classes, field trips, etc. (d) Contribute to the development of students by providing new experiences. (e) As far as possible interrelated topics should be included in a unit. (f) It should deal with a sizable topic so that the length of the unit can be kept within the limits. This will also help sustain the interest of students. (g) It should emerge out of the students' past experiences and should lead to broader interests. It should lead to an integrated learning experience and contribute to the continuity of the student's learning. (h) It should provide opportunities for creative experience. (i) It should allow the utilization of various resources like textbooks, journals, etc.

### Elements of a Unit Plan

Elements of a unit plan include: (a) Selection and statement of objectives. (b) Selection of content. (c) Organization of content. (d) Deciding upon the time allotment. (e) Selection of teaching and learning activities. (f) Determining the teacher expertise depending upon the nature of the unit, certain units are taught by nurse educators, doctors or other professionals. (g) Selection of methods of evaluation. (h) Selection of reference.

### Types of Units

Categorized according to use, there are two general types of units, namely resource units and teaching units.

**Resource unit:** The resource unit is a teacher's guide to planning and action. It is in fact a blueprint of suggestions and resources for developing a theme, problem or topic. A resource unit invariably contains the following elements: (a) Statement of objectives. (b) Problem or topic. (c) An approach or initiation. (d) Content or subject matter basic to the area of study. (e) Direct and related experiences. (f) Evaluation of learning. (g) A collection of instructional resources.

**Teaching unit:** The term 'teaching unit' is used to describe the development of unit for teaching in the classroom. Also referred to as the unit in action, the teaching unit focuses on implementation of the learning activities. In the teaching unit, the areas of learning and the sequences in which they are presented may or may not be prescribed. Always, however the needs, the maturity level and the background experiences of the students set the boundaries of the teaching unit and determine its direction.

Thus, a resource unit contains an organized collection of teaching ideas and suggestions build around a large topic of significance and the teaching unit contains definite plans for teaching a specific group of students under a given set of circumstance. In this way, the resource unit can serve as a reserve from which the teacher may draw ideas, suggestions and teaching aids when she plans a teaching unit to implement. It is in many ways, the heart of effective teaching.

### Principles of Unit Planning

Following principles need to be considered while preparing unit plan.
1. Ultimate focus of unit planning is to enhance teaching–learning process by ensuring sequence and selection of contents.
2. Unit planning provides a holistic view regarding teaching–learning process.
3. Unit planning helps in designing a systematic, sequential, continuous and integrated arrangement of contents in the best possible manner.
4. Unit planning gives adequate emphasis to all important aspects of the course or competencies under consideration.
5. Unit planning ensures opportunity to correlate theory with practice in order to achieve competency in nursing practice.
6. Unit planning provides freedom to teachers for finding the best approaches to achieve aims of teaching-learning process.
7. Unit planning encourages unit wise evaluation for ensuring learning progress.

### Steps in Unit Planning

According to Sandra de Young unit planning involves two major processes, namely sequencing and selection. The main focus of unit planning is to ensure effective learning by learners. Steps involved in the unit planning can be summarized as follows:
   a. Estimate the whole course content/set of competencies to be achieved by the learners for the year.
   b. Estimate the teaching time available to the teachers.
   c. Arrange the given course content/set of competencies in a teaching–learning sequence
   d. Identify inter-linked aspects of course content/competencies
   e. Distribute the whole course content/competencies into units by considering the followings:
      i. A unit should not be too small or too lengthy.
      ii. It should have some element of commonness within its components.

    iii. It should be such that its completion develops a sense of accomplishment to both the teacher and the learners.
  f. For each unit, further breaking up of teaching lessons would be required
  g. For each lesson within the unit decide about the appropriate teaching methods, teaching aids, learner activities and evaluation procedure.
  h. Present units in a tabular form which may be considered to be unit plan.

# LESSON PLANNING

A teaching unit generally contains a number of lessons. Careful planning of lessons is essential for experienced as well as beginner teachers. Experienced teachers use loosely structured lesson plans, whereas beginners use highly structured lesson plans. Lesson planning, in fact is fundamental to effective teaching.

## Meaning and Definition

Lesson plan is a plan prepared by a teacher to teach a lesson in an organized manner. It is a plan of action and calls for an understanding on the teacher's part, about the students, knowledge and expertise about the topic being taught and her ability to use effective methods.

## Purposes of Lesson Planning

Careful lesson planning is the foundation of good teaching. It performs the following functions.
- It demands adequate consideration of goals and objectives, the selection of subject matter, the selection of teaching-learning methods, the planning of activities and the planning of evaluation devices.
- It keeps the teacher on the track, ensures steady progress and a definite outcome of teaching and learning procedures.
- It helps the teacher in effective teaching. The teacher looks ahead and plans a series of activities with an intention to modify students' attitudes, habits and abilities in the desirable directions.
- It prevents waste. It helps the teacher to carry out the teaching activity in a systematic and orderly fashion. It encourages proper organization of subject matter. It prevents haphazard teaching through eliminating disorder and other ills of thoughtless teaching.
- It provides confidence and self-reliance to the teacher. It can ensure that the teacher does not 'dry up' or forget a vital point. A teacher can enter the class and carry out the teaching activity without anxiety.
- It serves as a check on unplanned curriculum. It provides a framework to carry out the teaching at a suitable rate. The hierarchy of lessons becomes well-knit and interconnected. Continuity is assured in the educative process. Needless repetition is avoided.

According to Lester, "A lesson plan is actually a plan of action. It, therefore, includes the working philosophy of the teacher, her knowledge of philosophy, her information about and understanding of her pupils, her comprehension of the objectives of education, her knowledge of the material to be taught and her ability to utilize effective method".

Thus, lesson plan is the title given to a statement of the achievements to be realized and the specific means by which these are to be attained as a result of the activities engaged during the period of 45 minutes or one hour. It points out what has already been done, in what direction the pupils should be guided further and helped and what work is to be taken up immediately. Lesson plan is the teacher's mental and emotional visualization of the classroom experience as she plan it to implement. It is in many ways, the heart of effective teaching.

## Criteria of Lesson Planning

SK Mangal recommends below mentioned criteria for effective lesson planning.
- An effective lesson planning have a written form.
- It must have instructional objectives properly expressed in behavioral terms.
- Proper mentioning of AV aids.
- Proper mentioning about prerequisite knowledge and skill of students.
- Explanation about the method of introduction of the topic.
- The subject matter should be properly selected, organized and presented in the planning.
- Teaching methods and AV aids should be selected and used judiciously.
- Promote active participation of learner in the teaching learning process.
- An effective lesson plan considers the age of student, ability of student. Previous knowledge of student, duration of period, learning environment and resources available at the time of conduct of class.
- Specifically mention the measure of fixation of the contents taught through the lesson in the form of recapitulation, review, etc.
- It should mention the type of black board work or summary, etc., to be developed during the conduct of class.
- It should cater to the individual difference of the students.
- It should follow the principle of correlation and integration in the presentation of subject matter.

## Principles of Lesson Planning

The following principles will help in the preparation of a good lesson plan.
a. The teacher should prepare a careful but flexible plan. The lesson plan is to be *used as a guide rather than as a rule of thumb* to be obeyed blindly. The teacher should have the courage to depart from it according to the needs of the students.
b. The teacher must have mastery of an adequate training in the topic from which the subject matter has been selected for a certain lesson.
c. The teacher must be fully conversant with new methods and techniques of *teaching nursing*.
d. The teacher must know his students thoroughly and organize the materials in a *psychological* rather than merely a *logical* fashion.
e. The teacher must ensure active student participation.
f. Since monotony is a defect, different teaching-learning methods have to be employed while teaching instead of adhering to a single method.

## Steps in Lesson Planning

For teaching nursing effectively, the teacher has to proceed in a systematic manner. For this purpose, some steps have to be followed while preparing the lesson plan. There is no universally accepted step in planning a lesson. The following steps may help in preparing a lesson plan.
1. **Planning:** This step is concerned with the formulation of objectives, selection of the content, organization of the content, selection of teaching-learning methods, selection of audiovisual aids, etc.
2. **Preparation or introduction:** This brief stage is concerned with introducing the lesson to the students in an interesting manner and thereby preparing them to receive new knowledge. Different methods and techniques can be used to prepare the students. Awareness regarding the previous knowledge of the students is essential for the successful implementation of this stage of lesson planning.

3. **Presentation:** During the presentation stage teacher and students actively engage in the teaching–learning process. The objective of the lesson is largely attained during this stage. The teacher employs appropriate teaching–learning methods with the help of various teaching aids. A teacher has to employ multitude of teaching skills to make this stage a successful one (see teaching skills). During this stage nurse educator has to give importance for generalization and application. Through generalization students develop an ability to generalize the learned information. For example, while teaching the importance of maintaining intake output chart, teacher has to motivate the students to recognize conditions which required intake output monitoring from their clinical experiences. Teacher has to teach the theory with a practical orientation so that students can easily apply the learned lessons in various health care settings.
4. **Recapitulation or closing stage:** This is the last step of the lesson and concerned with planned repetition, giving assignments, evaluating pupils progress and diagnosing pupil learning difficulties and taking remedial measures.

## Proforma for a Lesson Plan

Just like the steps of lesson plan, there is no universally accepted proforma for lesson plan. Experienced teachers use a loosely structured lesson plan **(Fig. 4.4)**, while beginner teachers use a highly structured plan as shown in **Figure 4.5**.

### Lesson Plan

Name of teacher  Class
Subject  No. of students
Unit  Date and time
Topic of lesson  Duration
Previous knowledge of students  Venue
Methods of teaching
Resources
Central objective
Specific objectives

| Time | Specific objective | Content | Teacher-learner activity |
|---|---|---|---|
| | | | |

Assignment
References
Remarks

**Fig. 4.4:** Loosely structured lesson plan.

## Lesson Plan

| | |
|---|---|
| Name of teacher | Class |
| Subject | No. of students |
| Unit | Date and time |
| Topic of lesson | Duration |
| Previous knowledge of students | Venue |
| Methods of teaching | |
| Resources | |
| Central objective | |
| Specific objectives | |

| Time | Specific objective | Content | Teacher activity | Students activity | AV aids | Evaluation |
|---|---|---|---|---|---|---|
| | | | | | | |

Recapitulation:
Assignment:
References:
Remarks

**Fig. 4.5:** Highly structured lesson plan.

## SUMMARY

Curriculum is considered as the blueprint of an educational program. Nursing curriculum is the learning opportunities and the learning activities that the faculty plans and implement in various settings for a particular group of students, for a specified period of time in order to attain the objectives. Modern curriculum encompasses all the meaningful and desirable activities taking place inside and outside the school. The behavioral objective model, Stenhouse's process model, Lawton's cultural analysis model and Beattie's fourfold model are some of the useful curriculum models. Olivia Bevis recommends four types of nursing curricula, namely legitimate curriculum, illegitimate curriculum, hidden curriculum and the null curriculum. The curriculum of nursing education is formulated by curriculum committee. According to Goodland, there exists three levels of curriculum planning namely societal curriculum, institutional curriculum and instructional curriculum. Principles of curriculum development will guide in developing a curriculum that satisfies the needs of the students as well as the society. Major factors which influence curriculum development in nursing education are philosophy, educational psychology, society, student, knowledge explosion and scientific advancements, technological advancements in patient care, educational technology, transnational career opportunities and resources. Steps in curriculum development include formulation of educational objectives, selection of learning experiences, effective and efficient organization of learning experiences and evaluation of the curriculum. Teaching of various subjects can be organized in different ways like complete block or teaching block system, partial block system and study day system. Rotation plan can be mainly classified into master rotation plan and individual rotation plan.

There is a considerable difference between the syllabus and the finished curriculum. Core curriculum represents the central area of concern in the curriculum. Curriculum revision is concerned with making the curriculum different in some way to give it a new position or direction. Three approaches to curriculum revision are addition, deletion and reorganization.

Any nursing educational program is a combination of various courses. A course is a combination of different units. According to the use, units can be classified as resource unit and teaching unit. A unit is made up of various lessons. Essential steps in making the lesson plan are planning, introduction, preparation and recapitulation.

## MULTIPLE CHOICE QUESTIONS

1. **Societal curriculum is planned at:**
   a. Institutional level
   b. Teacher level
   c. National level
   d. None of the above

2. **Instructional curriculum is planned at:**
   a. Teacher level
   b. Institutional level
   c. National level
   d. None of the above

3. **Central concern of curriculum is called:**
   a. Core curriculum
   b. Institutional curriculum
   c. Instructional curriculum
   d. Societal curriculum

4. **Social intelligence quotient is more related to**
   a. Hidden curriculum
   b. 21st century curriculum
   c. Null curriculum
   d. Happiness curriculum

5. **Emotional intelligence is more related to:**
   a. Hidden curriculum
   b. 21st century curriculum
   c. Null curriculum
   d. Happiness curriculum

6. **Conducting situational analysis and needs assessment is a part of:**
   a. Curriculum development
   b. Unit planning
   c. Lesson planning
   d. Curriculum revision

7. **Conservative principle is related to:**
   a. Curriculum development
   b. Course planning
   c. Unit planning
   d. Lesson planning

8. **Reorganization is an approach to:**
   a. Curriculum development
   b. Curriculum revision
   c. Curriculum planning
   d. Lesson planning
9. **Recapitulation is a step in:**
   a. Curriculum planning
   b. Unit planning
   c. Lesson planning
   d. Course planning
10. **Giving assignment is a part of:**
    a. Curriculum planning
    b. Unit planning
    c. Lesson planning
    d. Course planning

### ANSWER KEY

| 1. c | 2. a | 3. a | 4. b | 5. d | 6. a |
| 7. a | 8. b | 9. c | 10. c | | |

# CHAPTER 5

# Learning

## LEARNING OBJECTIVES

After completing this chapter, reader will be able to:

- Define learning.
- Explain key concepts of learning.
- Describe characteristics of learning
- Identify factors influencing learning.
- List down principles of learning.
- Explain nature of learning.
- Explain learning theories.
- List down barriers to learning.
- Appreciate relationship between first principles thinking and learning.
- List down types of learning.
- Explain approaches to learning.
- Explain active learning strategies
- Identify determinants of learning.
- List down types of learners.
- Explain characteristics of present-day learners.
- Identify relationship between emotional intelligence and learning.
- Explain relationship between emotions and learning.
- Identify impact of motivation on learning.
- Explain influence of environment on learning.
- Definition of learning nursing
- Explain principles of learning nursing.
- Explain process of remembering and forgetting.

Learning is essential to replenish knowledge. In the light of knowledge explosion, it is assumed that a student gains one-fourth knowledge directly from the teacher, another one-fourth through his own effort, next one-fourth from experiences and the remaining one-fourth will remain unfilled not only during the student period but also throughout the life. Even though the last one-fourth will remain unfilled, the student has to fill it as much as possible by his or her own effort. From the above said facts, it is clear that the students have to play a dominant role in the learning process, whereas role of the teacher is limited to a facilitator or stage setter. A good teacher is always aware about this designated role of students and prepare them to take up their responsibilities in order to ensure fruitful learning. Knowledge regarding some facts or truths about learning will help the teacher prepare the students to handle their responsibilities in an admirable way. As you have already learned much about the general aspects of learning from your educational psychology classes, our discussion is limited to the factors favoring learning, especially the learning of nursing science.

## DEFINITION

- According to GA Kimble, "Learning is a relatively permanent change in behavioral potentiality that occurs as a result of reinforced practice".
  Let us see the details of Kimble's definition. First, learning is indicated by a change in behavior, in other words, the results of learning must always be translated into measureable behavior. After learning, learners do something that they did not do before learning took place. Second, this behavioral change is relatively permanent, that is, it is neither transitory

nor fixed. Third, the change in behavior need not occur immediately following the learning experience. Fourth, the change in behavior results from experience or practice. Fifth, the experience or practice must be reinforced that is only those responses that lead to reinforcement will be learned.
- According to Paivio, "Learning is the process of acquiring new or modifying existing attitude, knowledge, behavior, skills values and preferences". This definition highlights the comprehensive nature of learning. Learning is a continuous process and knowledge gaining through experience is an integral part of learning.

## KEY CONCEPTS OF MODERN LEARNING

R Vanessa put forward the following key concepts of learning.
- **Learning is dynamic and changes over time:** Learning is a skill that we are all born with and develop over time. When we are first born, we learn from our body's natural reflexes. Our eyes, ear, arms and such react and we learn from that. Then as we grow learning becomes more complex. This concept underlines the importance of understanding human growth and development for understanding learning needs of students.
- **Learning is both cognitive and emotional:** Combination of logical thinking skills and emotional skills leads to creativity. Understanding the connection between emotion and cognition helps to reduce stress while learning. There is no thinking without feeling and no feeling without thinking. This concept highlights the importance to affective domain along with cognitive and psychomotor domains (*see* Chapter 3: Educational Objectives).
- **Learning is context dependent:** Students will learn better in certain situations with certain support. This concept highlights the need of good environment in promoting learning.
- **Learning is interactive:** Learning is a social enterprise that happens in association with a variety of active factors in the learning environment including teacher, parents, apps, peers, textbooks, and so on.

## CHARACTERISTICS OF LEARNING

The characteristics of learning are:
- Learning is a process which can be inferred from the behavioral change of the individual.
- The change in behavior need not occur immediately following the learning experience.
- Learning is relatively a permanent change in behavior.
- The change in behavior from learning is distinct from changes due to maturation, motivation, etc.
- Learning is to be differentiated from instinctive behaviors.
- Learning is influenced by experience and practice.

**SK Mangal describes characteristics of learning as follows:**
- **Learning is a lifelong process:** Learning is a continuous process. Learning occurs throughout life. Learning can be formal or informal and it may be direct or indirect. When a learner learns, he develops knowledge, skills, habits, attitudes and aptitudes.
- **Learning is change in behavior:** The result of the learning process can be measured as behavioral changes. This change can be in any form. It can be desirable or undesirable. But in desirable form, these changes should occur in a positive direction. In true sense, learning is a change in desirable manner.
- **Learning is a universal process:** Learning is a universal process. It can happen everywhere. Learning is a process for all living creatures. Human beings across all cultures learn as it is a lifelong process.

- **Learning is purposeful and goal oriented:** Learning always has a purpose. It is goal oriented because a teacher always has learning objectives in mind while teaching. If we don't have any aim or goal, then the process of learning will not bring any change in behavior. Through the process of learning, we can move towards predetermined learning goals.
- **Learning is a process of progress and development:** Learning can occur in any direction. These directions can be desirable or undesirable. Learning aims development in a desirable direction. Learning should try to bring progressive changes in the behavior of the learner always.
- **Learning is the systematic organization of experiences:** The basis of learning is the acquisition of new experiences. Change in behavior occurs as a result of new experience.
- **Learning occurs due to activity and interaction with environment:** Interaction with the environment is very essential for the learning process. The more the children interact with their environment, the more they learn. The absence of activity and interaction hampers the quality of learning. Experiences gain from these interactions bring out changes in the behavior of learner.
- **Learning helps in achieving teaching objectives:** Process of learning helps in achieving the objectives of teaching. With learning, we expect a change in the behavior of individuals. This changes happens with the development of knowledge, insight, interests, skills and attitude, so for achieving teaching objectives, the learning process plays an important role.
- **Learning is the fundamental process of life:** Without learning the progress of an individual is not possible. It acts as the basis for the progress of society and civilization.
- **Learning is the relationship between stimulus and response:** Learning is generally a relationship between stimulus and response. A person is considered as a learned person if he reacts according to the task to be learned. Through learning, a person learns to react appropriately to the stimulus associated with the situation of life.
- **Learning is transferable:** The learning acquired in one situation can be transferred to some other situation. The learner should be careful not to let previously gained knowledge interfere in acquiring new knowledge and experiences.

## FACTORS INFLUENCING LEARNING

Based on modern concepts of learning and theories, like dynamic skill theory, factors influencing learning can be classified under three categories namely learner, curriculum and environment (**Fig. 5.1**).
- **Learner:** Learner's age, health status, readiness for learning, motivation level, ability, maturation, previous experience, genetic inheritance, etc., affect the learning process.
- **Curriculum:** Quality of learning tools like books, other instructional materials, selection and organization of learning experiences, methodology of teaching, teacher–student interaction, etc., influence the learning.
- **Environment:** Learning is a context-dependent process. Hence, environment influences the learning process, physical environment of school and home influence learning. Learner's friends, family, culture and society also influences learning in a big way.

## PRINCIPLES OF LEARNING

Based on above-discussed concepts and definition of learning, we can derive the following principles.
- **Learning is an evolutionary process:** Learning is a skill that we are all born with and develop over time. When we are born, we learn from our body's natural reflexes, our eyes,

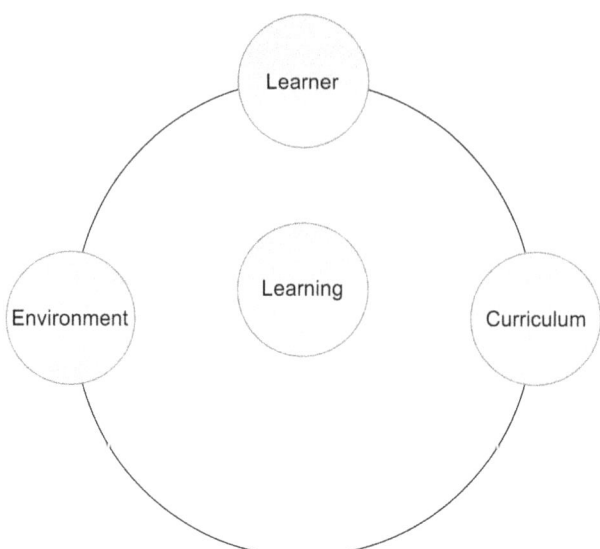

**Fig. 5.1:** Factors influencing learning.

ears, arms and such react and we learn from that. Then, as we grow, learning becomes more complex. This principle is based on life span development of mankind.

- **Learning is a consequence of experience:** Learning is the process of acquiring new or modifying existing knowledge, behavior, skills, values or preference. More skills and knowledge can be acquired only through repeated experience.
- **Learning is a collaborative as well as cooperative social process:** Learning is not competitive as we think. It occurs as a result of collaborative and cooperative process. Learning is a social enterprise that happens in association with a variety of active factors in the learning environment including teachers, parents, peers, textbooks, apps and so on.
- **Effective learning is initiated by the learner:** Intrinsic motivation is essential for effective learning. Intrinsic motivation is the process that leads us to do meaningful things. It involves factors such as self-determination, curiosity, focused attention and hard work. Students with greater intrinsic motivation become successful learners.
- **The process of learning is emotional as well as intellectual:** Learning involves emotions and thinking skills. Combination of logical thinking and emotional skills helps in retention of learned contents.
- **Learning is highly unique and individual:** Each individual has his own style of learning. This principle highlights the need of considering each learner as a unique individual with his own learning needs and abilities.
- **Providing meaningful feedback enhances learning:** Teachers need to clearly communicate what is expected from learners and how they are progressing. Continuous and meaningful feedback is essential for attaining aims of learning.
- **Learners are the center of learning process:** Learning activities should focus on growth and development of learner. This helps learners to participate actively in the learning process.

# NATURE OF LEARNING

Henry P Smith describes nature of learning as follows:

- **Learning brings behavioral changes:** Whatever the direction of the changes may be, learning has to bring progressive changes in the behavior of an individual. This behavioral modification helps him to adjust with his situations.
- **Learning is adaptation or adjustment:** Learning leads to behavior modification and this behavior modification enables individuals to adjust or adapt with his environment. Thus, learning is also described as a process of progressive adjustment to ever-changing conditions, which one encounters.
- **Behavior change must be based on some form of practice, experience or training:** Any change in behavior due to diseases or physical changes does not constitute learning. This change may not be evident until a situation arises in which the new behavior can occur.
- **Reinforcement:** The practice or experience must be reinforced in order for learning to occur. If reinforcement does not accompany the practice or experience, the behavior will eventually disappear.
- **Learning is continuous:** It denotes the lifelong nature of learning. Every day new situations are faced and the individual modifies his behavior to deal with the situations. Learning occurs from birth to death.
- **Learning as growth and development:** Any activity can be called learning as far as it develops an individual. Learning helps a learner to achieve a vision for life and thereby give direction to his efforts.
- **Learning is dynamic and changes over time:** Learning is a skill that we are all born with and develop over time.
- **Learning is both cognitive and emotional:** Combination of logical thinking skills and emotional skills leads to creativity. Understanding the relationship between cognition and emotion enhances learning process.
- **Learning is context dependent:** Students will learn better in certain situations with certain supports. Thus, good environment always promotes learning.
- **Learning is interactive:** Learning is a social enterprise that happens in association with a variety of active factors in the learning environment including teacher, parents, peers, textbooks, apps and so on.

# LEARNING THEORIES

Learning theories try to explain how we learn and teach. As learning is a complex process, one theory alone cannot explain learning. Behaviorism, cognitivism, constructivism, humanistic, connectivism and experiential are the most important learning theories. Other notable theories include the Maslow's hierarchy of needs, elaboration theory, ADDIE (Analyse, Design, Develop, Implement and Evaluate) and Bloom's taxonomy. Let us discuss some important learning theories.

## Behaviorism

John B Watson founded 'Behaviorism' in 1913. It is one of the three primary learning theories. Ivan Pavlov and BF Skinner also contributed much to the development of behaviorism. The primary goal of behaviorism is to form a relationship between a stimulus and a response. According to behaviorism, "learning is a relatively permanent change in behavior brought about as a result of experience or practice". Thus, learning is confirmed through observable behavioral change. Behaviorism is based on the observation that all behaviors are learned through interaction with environment. This theory states that behaviors are learned from the environment and innate or inherited factors have very little influence on behavior. The stimulus-response sequence is a key element of understanding behaviorism or in simple words; according to behaviorism, learning takes place because of the result of stimulus-response sequence. Behaviorism studies learner's observable and measurable behaviors that are repeated until they occur voluntarily.

### Types of Behavioral Learning Theories

Three types of behavioral learning theories are contiguity, classical conditioning and operant conditioning.

1. Contiguity theory is based on the work of ER Guthria. It proposes that any stimulus and response connected in time and/or space will tend to be associated or repeated. For example, a student scoring high marks on a test after trying a new learning technique makes an association between the stimulus and response of scoring high marks.
2. Classical conditioning theory developed by Ivan Pavlov was studying the digestive system of dogs and became interested with his observation that dogs deprived of food began to salivate when one of their associates walked into the room. He began to investigate this phenomenon and established the laws of classical conditioning. Skinner renamed this type of learning as "respondent conditioning" since in this type of learning, individual is responding to stimulus from the environment. In classroom learning classical conditioning is seen primarily in the conditioning of emotional behavior. Activities in the classroom that make students' happy, sad, angry, etc., become associated with stimuli that gain their attention and elicit response.
3. Operant conditioning is the study of the impact of consequences of behavior. Operant conditioning is concerned about the voluntary behaviors of humans. As per operant conditioning actions that are followed by reinforcement will be strengthened and more likely to repeat in the future. Whereas actions that result in punishment or undesirable consequences will be weakened and less likely to repeat. In classroom learnings, operant conditioning highlights the importance of providing proper feedback and positive reinforcement.

### Key Features of Behaviorism and Learning

- Behaviorism equates learning with behaviors that can be observed and measured. Behaviorism helps in learning by creating measurable learning outcomes and guiding learners in mastering a set of predictable skills or behaviors.
- Reinforcement is essential for successful learning.
- Strong emphasis on the stimulus, the response and the relationship between them.
- Recommends learning activities that promote positive feeling among students.
- Suggests a rewarding system that can reinforce positive academic performance.
- Suggests spaced repetition for retaining information during learning.
- Small progressively sequenced tasks ensure that students remain focused during the learning process.
- Negative reinforcement for an undesirable response promotes learning.

## Cognitivism

Cognitivism is a learning theory that focuses on the process involved in learning rather than on the observed behavior. As opposed to behaviorists cognitivists do not require an outward exhibition of learning, but focus more on the internal process and connections that take place during learning. The learner is considered as an information processor. Knowledge can be seen as schema or symbolic mental constructions and learning is defined as change in a learner's schemata. Some important classroom principles from cognitive psychology include meaningful learning, organization and elaboration. According to cognitivists, learning takes place not because of stimulus-response sequence or for rewards. Cognitivists believe that learning takes place because of some inner abilities of learner rather than stimulus-response sequence. Cognitivists also believe that thinking process has a dominant role in learning. The learners according to cognitivism are active participants in the learning process.

Cognitive theory developed as a reaction to behaviorism. Jean Piaget contributed much to the development of cognitivism. He believed knowledge is something that is actively constructed by learners based on their existing cognitive structures. Cognitivism focuses more on the thought process behind the behavior than the observable behavior. Cognitive learning is centered on the mental process by which the learner receives, interprets, stores and retrieves information. According to cognitivism, learners act on beliefs, thoughts, knowledge, attitudes, feelings as well as understanding about their cognitive abilities when interpreting information. Thus, cognitivism is more concerned with knowledge, memory, thinking and problem-solving skills.

## *Key Features of Cognitivism and Learning*

- Learning is a process of organizing information into conceptualized models.
- Teaching should be organized, sequenced and presented in a manner that is understandable and meaningful to the learner.
- Retention and recall is important to build schema in the brain.
- Learning materials need to be prepared in a way to enhance memory of learners.

Teachers must provide tools that help learner's brain in processing information.

## Constructivism

Like cognitivism, constructivism sees learning as an active mental process. Constructivism is the theory that says learners construct knowledge rather than just passively take in information. According to constructivism, learners build or construct knowledge based on social or situational experiences. This allows learners to gain information and to test it through social interactions. Constructivism focuses on the process of assimilation and accommodation. Assimilation refers to the process of taking new information and fitting into a pre-existing knowledge or schema. Accommodation refers to using newly acquired information to revise and redevelop an existing schema.

## Humanistic Theory

Humanistic theory postulates that learning is influenced by motivations, potential and free will. Humanistic theory puts forward the term "self-actualization". It does not recognize a change in behavior as evidence of learning. Learning occurs when learners utilize their potential through observations and accumulated experiences rather than didactic teaching, humanists believe role models are the best teachers.

## Experiential Theory

Experiential theory sees learning as a four-step process that includes concrete experiences, reflective observation, abstract conceptualism and active experimentation. Here, experience leads to reflection, then conceptualization, then testing, which involves new experiences.

It is seen as a self-sustaining cycle with each of the four steps required for learning. Kolb is proponent of experiential theory. Kolb says emotions, prior learning and style of processing are involved in the learning process. As such there are four learning styles. Some learners prefer doing; others prefer watching or observation. Some prefer reading and reflecting. Others prefer a gut-level response followed by experimenting. This theory proposes multi-modality teaching. Experiential teachers use hands-on learning, reflections, reading, watching slides or PowerPoint presentation, lectures, field trips and other methods to accommodate all their students' learning styles.

### Connectivism

Connectivism is one of the newest educational learning theories. It focuses on the idea that people learn and grow when they form connections. This can be connections with each other or connections with their roles and responsibilities in their lives. Hobbies, goals and individuals all can be connections that influence learning.

Teachers can utilize connectivism to help student in learning by encouraging them to make connections with things that excite them. Teachers can use digital media to make good, positive connections to learning. A good teacher–student relationship will motivate learners to learn better. Good relationships with colleagues help teachers to become competent and professional.

## BARRIERS TO LEARNING

Any factor that interferes with actively engaging in learning process can be defined as a barrier to learning. Following are the most widely recognized barriers to learning.

- **Health and emotional problems:** Health problems are the most commonly found barriers to learning. With advances in medical sciences, many of the health problems effecting learning can be easily diagnosed and treated properly. Emotional issues related to learning problems can be managed through providing adequate guidance and support to students.
- **Family problems:** Problems in the family can affect the learning of children. Nowadays, this problem is solved through family counselling centers.
- **Financial issues:** To a certain extent financial issues can interfere with the learning process. By seeking financial help from government and voluntary agencies, financial issues can be solved to a great extent.
- **Lack of adequate teacher and parental support:** Children need adequate support from teachers and parents for effective learning. Each child is unique in abilities and interests. Teachers and parents need to consider this and provide adequate support to children in the learning process.
- **Lack of purpose/interest or attitude:** Without proper purpose, learning is difficult. By arousing interest in learning by properly explaining the need of learning for a successful life helps in overcoming this issue.
- **Lack of adequate student support and guidance program (SSGP):** Student Support and Guidance Program is essential for finding out the learning problems among children and finding appropriate solutions. Lack of adequate SSGP in educational institutions can adversely affect the learning process of students.
- **Environmental issues:** Environment can influence the learning process in a great manner. A hostile environment adversely affects learning process. Hence, providing conductive environment that promotes-learning is important to facilitate learning.
- **Lack of focused attention:** Lack of focused attention can lead to learning problems. Focused attention maximizes concentration for learning.

- **Lack of time management/planning:** Lack of time management or planning is a barrier to learning, especially in higher studies. Lack of planning adversely affects in achieving objectives of learning. By seeking assistance from parents, teachers and peers this barrier can be managed easily.
- **Overuse of social media:** Spending more time to social media is one of the learning barriers of modern times. Irrational use of social media can lead to many health and psychological issues that can adversely affect learning process. The rule "DISCONNECT AND LEARN MORE" will help to overcome this barrier.
- **Failure to embrace boredom:** Boredom is a part of learning process. Embracing boredom is essential for achieving learning aims. We need to be comfortable being bored, for achieving aims of learning.

## FIRST PRINCIPLES THINKING AND LEARNING

First principles thinking is basically the practice of actively questioning every assumption you think you 'know' about a given problem or scenario-and then creating new knowledge and solutions. In other words, by following first principles of thinking you begin learning by understanding the basic concept of a topic under discussion or learning content. For example, when teacher and classmates tell you learning mathematics is difficult, instead of blindly believing their words you have to question their assumptions to find out the reason of difficulty in learning mathematics and through finding answer to your questions you can find easy solution for learning mathematics.

Essentially, first principles thinking will help you develop a unique worldview to innovate and solve difficult problems in a unique manner. Elon Musk recommends 3 simple steps to develop first principles thinking ability in life. They are: (a) Step 1: Identify and define your current assumptions: For example, you think that it is difficult to find enough time to learn all subjects in a time-bound manner. (b) Step 2: Breakdown the problem into its fundamental principles. For, example, adopting first principles thinking, you have to read the whole syllabus, then divide the content based on your perspective into difficult, not so difficult and easy to learn. Instead of blindly following suggestions of others your powerful questions determine the reality about the subject matter. (c) Step 3: Create solutions from basic knowledge gained through analysis: once you identified and broken down your problems or assumptions into their most basic truths, you can begin to create a new insightful solution from scratch, for example, once you divide the subject matter into different segments, you can devote more time to difficult topics than simple ones and thereby able to learn whole subject matter in a time-bound manner.

## TYPES OF LEARNING

Gagne (1970) described the below mentioned eight types of learning.

### Signal Learning

This is the simplest and first level of learning. The person develops a general diffuse reaction to a stimulus. For instance, nursing students become anxious whenever they hear the term university examination because they are experiencing anxiety while appearing for university examination. Because of this association, the term university examination has become the signal that elicits the response, namely anxiety.

### Stimulus-response Learning

Stimulus-response learning involves developing a voluntary response to a specific stimuli or combination of stimuli. If there is doubt in the position of the Ryle's tube, the nursing student is taught to check the position by aspirating for stomach content before resorting to further steps. The clinical instructor may demonstrate and reinforce this measure in the clinical area. Subsequently, whenever this doubt arises, the student responds automatically by aspirating for stomach contents with a syringe. This automatic reaction of aspirating stomach contents with the syringe when a doubt regarding the position of Ryle's tube arises is an example of stimulus-response learning.

## Chaining

Chaining is the acquisition of a series of related conditioned responses or stimulus-response connections. If the doubt regarding the position of Ryle's tube is not cleared even after aspirating for stomach contents, the student is taught to place the distal end of the Ryle's tube into a bowl of water and look for bubbles or inject 5 mL of air and auscultate for it in the stomach area as the second step. This second step becomes another automatic response in a chain of responses.

## Verbal Association

Verbal association is a type of chaining which is very useful in learning medical terminologies. A student who knows that the word 'thermal' refers to temperature can easily learn the new term 'hypothermia' and its definition given by the teacher. This is because the student recognized that the syllable 'therm' connects the two words and finds it easier to learn the new term due to a previous association.

## Discrimination Learning

A considerable amount can be learned through forming large number of stimulus-response or verbal chains. When more chains are learned, the tendency to forget previous chains will increase, so in order to learn and retain large number of chains the student should be able to discriminate among them. This process of discriminating chains with an intention to retain more important chains is called discrimination learning. Nursing student has to learn any number of drugs and it is impossible to keep in mind the full details of a particular drug, so she has to follow discrimination learning to retain the more important aspects. For example, while learning about Ibuprofen, a nonsteroidal anti-inflammatory drug, she has to discriminate the nursing care implications to be followed before, during and after administration of Ibuprofen such as don't administer in an empty stomach or to patients who have been suffering from asthma or renal problems from the chemical structure and other details. This discrimination will help her to retain whatever is essential for a safe nursing practice.

## Concept Learning

Concept learning is learning how to classify stimuli into groups represented by a common concept. Students enter nursing institute with a great deal of experience with concept learning. They have learned so many concepts like smaller, bigger, same and different. Even then they have to learn newer concepts in the nursing curriculum. They learn a concept such as asepsis, first hearing what the word means, then having it pointed out to them in a variety of situations ranging from handwashing to sterile technique in the operating room. It may take a long time, but they will learn to identify the concept of asepsis in new situations and will be able to put the concept into use.

## Rule Learning

A rule can be considered a chain of concepts or a relationship between concepts. A nursing student learns that to prevent a decubitus ulcer the patient must be turned or if there is an open wound, sterile technique must be used. It is possible that a student may learn these statements simply as verbal chains and not understand or be able to apply the concepts. This happens, for example, when students memorize their notes for an examination but do not understand their application. True rule learning involves knowing each concept and being able to put relationships between concepts into use, so the nurse educator has to ensure that true learning is taking place.

## Problem-based Learning

Problem-based learning (PBL) has its origin in medicine and is very much useful for teaching nursing also. PBL is a way of designing and presenting courses that use problems in professional practice or real life as the stimulus for student learning. Regrettably, many teachers immediately claim that they have used this method for years because they incorrectly equate the problem-solving activities of their course with PBL. This kind of teaching is not PBL at all. PBL is a way of seeing the curriculum as being focused on key problems that arise in professional practice and which requires student activity-independently or in cooperative groups to learn from the problems. Students work through the problems, under greater or lesser degrees of guidance from teachers, defining what they do not know and what they need to know in order to understand (not necessarily just to solve) the problem. The justification for this is firmly based on modern theories of learning which have found that knowledge is remembered and recalled more effectively if learning is based on the context in which it is going to be used in the future.

Thus, if basic knowledge is structured around representations of situations or cases likely to be encountered in professional practice in the future, it is more likely to be remembered. Problem-based learning is also integrative, with the need to understand relevant aspects of several disciplines being readily apparent in each case that is presented.

Savoie and Hughes (1994) recommend the following actions for providing problem-based learning experiences to the students: (a) Identify a problem suitable for the students (see selection of the problems). (b) Connect the problem with the professional practice so that it presents authentic opportunities. (c) Organize the subject matter around the problem. (d) Give students responsibility for defining their learning experience and to understand the problem. (e) Encourage collaboration by creating learning teams. (f) Expect all students to demonstrate the results of their learning through a product or performance.

## Selection of the Problems

This is one of the most important considerations while providing problem-based learning. The problems must be of the kind that will be faced by the students after they graduate, but they must also be both broad enough and specific enough to engage students in learning activities that match the curriculum objectives. Problems should not be answerable by simple responses. In general, they should be professional problems that will require students to go through the following process: (a) Analyze the problem. (b) Identify the knowledge required to understand and solve the problem. (c) Obtain agreement on the independent learning tasks to be performed. (d) Obtain agreement on when the learning tasks will have been achieved. (e) Carry out further cycles of the process, if necessary.

# APPROACHES TO LEARNING

Main approaches to learning are simulation-based learning, scenario-based learning, blended learning, reflective learning, observational learning and experiential learning.

## Simulation-based Learning

Simulation is a generic term that refers to an artificial representation of a real world situation to teach students. Simulation-based nursing education is defined as any educational activity that utilizes simulation to replicate clinical scenarios. (*see* Chapter 6: Teaching-Learning Methods) There are mainly three types of simulations namely simulation exercise, simulation game and role-playing. Zly classifies the simulations available for nursing in the following manner:

- Simple models or mannequins.
- Simulated/standardized patients.
- Computer screen-based clinical case simulators.
- Realistic high-tech procedural simulators (task trainers)
- Virtual reality.
- Realistic, high-tech interactive patient simulators.

Simulation-based learning allows the acquisition of clinical skills through deliberate practice rather than mere repetition of procedures. Simulation tools serve as an alternative to real patients. A student can make mistakes and learn from them without the fear of harming the patient. Simulation-based learning has been found to enhance clinical competence at the undergraduate and postgraduate levels.

Simulation-based learning helps to acquire clinical skills or competencies including communication skills, history taking, professional attitudes, awareness of ethical basis of healthcare, physical examination, procedural skills, clinical laboratory skills, diagnostic skills, therapeutic skills, resuscitation skills, critical thinking, clinical reasoning, problem-solving, teamwork, organization skills, management skills and information technology skills.

Increasing concern for the quality of patient care and safety and changing trends in health care favors simulation based learning. Deliberate practice is essential to achieve desired learning outcomes. According to Lssenberg, "Deliberate practice involves: (a) repetitive performance of intended cognitive or psychomotor skills in focused domain, along with (b) rigorous skills assessment that provides learner's specific, informative feedback that results in increasingly better performance in a controlled setting". From evidence it is found that simulation based learning is best way for providing deliberate practice.

Even though there are merits for simulation based learning it should be considered only as an adjuvant and not a replacement for learning with real patients. Simulation is not intended to replace the need for learning in the clinical environment, so it is important to integrate simulation training with clinical practice to achieve desired learning outcomes.

## Scenario-based Learning

Scenario-based learning (SBL) uses interactive scenarios to support learning strategies such as problem-based learning or case-based learning. For example, teacher creates a home-like situation in community health nursing lab for allowing students to solve problems related to geriatric care. It normally allows students to solve a problem which they are required to solve. In the process, students must apply their subject knowledge and critical thinking and problem-solving skills in a safe, real world context. SBL usually provides immediate feedback to students regarding their performance. Scenario-based learning may be conducted as a single session or as part of larger assignment. When conducted as a part of larger assignment, students later complete the scenario and then provide a written or oral self-assessment on the process.

SBL can be used in a wide range of contexts but usually to simulate real world practice, providing opportunities which may be difficult for students to experience within the limitations of real-life situations. SBL can be also used as part of either formative or summative assessment. SBL enhances decision-making and critical thinking abilities of students.

Steps in creating scenario-based learning can be summarized as follows:
- **Identify the learning outcomes:** It is important to identify what your students want to achieve on completion of the scenario and plan activities to achieve the desired outcome.
- **Decide on your format:** Is your scenario going to be delivered in the face-to-face or online environment? What media (Photographs, audio, video) and other resources will you need?
- **Choosing a topic:** Remember to consider using 'critical incidents' and challenging situations while choosing SBL.
- **Identify the trigger event or situation:** This will be the starting point of your scenario. As you create the scenario, identify key areas for feedback and student reflection. Creating a storyboard is an effective way to do this.
- **Peer review your scenario:** Ask colleagues to work through the scenario to ensure that it happens in the way you expect and achieves intended learning outcomes.

Clark's advice to go through the following checklist before deciding SBL approach as the right option:
- Are the learning outcomes based on skills development or problem-solving?
- Is it difficult or unsafe to provide real-world experience of the skills?
- Do your students already have some relevant knowledge to assist decision-making?
- Do you have time and resources to design, develop and test on SBL approach?
- Will the content and skills remain relevant for long enough to justify the development of SBL?

## Blended Learning

"Blended learning is the interdependent combination of face-to-face and online education. It involves combining the best of these two modes of learning in such a way that they complement and supplement each other". Effective blended learning occurs when online and face-to-face modalities are used to their full advantage for optimal interaction and when there is enough opportunity for student-paced and student-directed learning.

In many cases the act of "blending" achieves better student experiences and outcomes and more efficient teaching and course management practice. It involves a proper mix of teaching delivery modes, teaching approaches and learning styles. Advances in technology provide new opportunities for students to learn in diverse environment and for courses to be designed and delivered in a way that enhances the role of teachers in the teaching-learning process.

Advantages of blended learning environment are: (a) It broadens the spaces and opportunities available for learning. (b) It supports course management activities (e.g., communication, assessment submission, evaluation and feedback). (c) Enhance the availability and authenticity of information and resources for students and (d) Engages and motivates students through greater opportunities for interactivity and collaboration.

Blended learning approach can be used to support face-to-face teaching, large group and small group learning, self-directed learning, communication between the teacher and individual students or groups of students, as well as between students themselves. You can "blend" time (e.g. face-to-face with recorded lectures), place (small group tutorial on-campus with online discussion forum; traditional field trip with virtual field trip using websites and online chat with experts) people (video link with guest lecturers or virtual classroom to include both on-campus and off-campus students), resources and activities (textbook with online readings; in-class with online quiz).

## Observational Learning

Most of the initial learning happens through observation. Observational learning is the process of learning by watching the actions or behaviors of others. The targeted behavior is observed, memorized and then mimicked. Also known as shaping and modeling, observational learning is most common in children as they imitate behaviors of adults. While adults observe experts to learn new information, observational learning isn't always intentional, especially in young children. A child may learn to avoid or smoke cigarettes by watching adults. They are continually learning through observation, irrespective of the target behavior is desirable or not.

### Four Processes of Observational Learning

According to Bandura, there are four processes that influence observational learning:

1. **Attention:** To learn, an observer must pay attention to something in the environment. They must notice the model and behavior occurring. Attention level can vary based on the characteristics of the model's degree of likeness or the observer's current mood.
   In humans, it is likely the observer will pay attention to behaviors of models that are high-status, hardworking, intelligent or similar to observer in some way.
2. **Retention:** Simple attention is not enough to learn a new behavior. An observer must also retain or remember the behavior at a later time. To increase chances of retention, the observer must structure the information in an easy to remember format.
3. **Reproduction:** Reproduction is the process where the observer must be able to physically perform the behavior in the real situation. Often, performing a new behavior requires hours of practice to develop the skills.
4. **Motivation:** All learning requires some degree of personal motivation. For observation learning; the observer must be motivated to perform the desired behavior. Sometimes this motivation is intrinsic to the observer. Other times, motivation can come in the form of external enforcement-rewards or punishments promoting observational learning.
   An expert teacher always behaves in a professional manner by showing only desirable behaviors that can be adopted by students in their life. By exhibiting only desirable behaviors, teacher becomes a role model to students. Role modeling is the first and foremost quality of a great teacher. Through role modeling teacher can become a living example for students regarding merits of a good living.

## Experiential Learning: The Future of Learning

Simon Fraser University defines experiential learning as: "the strategic, active engagement of students in opportunities to learn through doing, and reflection on those activities which empower them to apply their theoretical knowledge to practical endeavors in a multitude of settings inside and outside the classroom".

Experiential learning is the preferred method of learning in many universities. Experiential learning focuses on learners reflecting on their experience of doing something, so as to gain conceptual insight as well as practical expertise. Kolb's experiential learning model suggests four stages in this process **(Fig. 5.2)**.

1. Concrete experience—a new experience or situation is encountered, or a reinterpretation of existing experience.
2. Reflective observation of the new experience—of particular importance if any inconsistencies between experience and understanding.

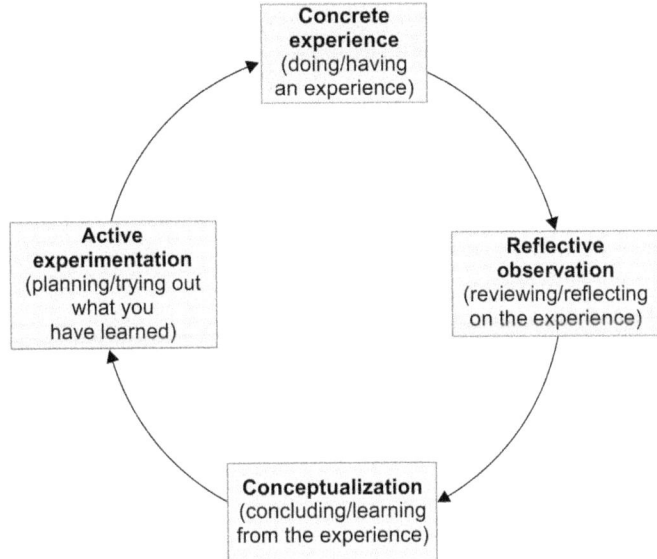

**Fig. 5.2:** Kolb's experiential learning model.

*Source*: Kolb DA. Experiential learning: Experience as the source of learning and development. Englewood Cliff: Prentice Hall; 1984.

3. Abstract conceptualization—reflection gives rise to a new idea, or a modification of an existing abstract concept (the person has learned from their experience).
4. Active experimentation—the learner applies their idea(s) to the world around them to see what happens.

Moon suggests following design models for experiential learning which uses technology to ensure development of knowledge and skills needed for students in this digital age. The design models are:
* Laboratory, mainly simulations, workshop or studio works
* Apprenticeship
* Problem-based learning
* Case-based learning
* Project-based learning
* Inquiry-based learning
* Cooperative (work- or community-based) learning

Rajiv Jayaraman cites following reasons for considering experiential learning as the future of learning.

1. **Accelerates learning:** Repetitive learning or learning by rote has long been replaced by 'Learning by Doing'. Experiential learning methodology uses critical thinking, problem-solving and decision-making to teach a subject. This has become an established method to accelerate learning.
2. **Provides a safe learning environment:** Simulations use real-life scenarios that depict several challenges, which learner eventually face after the course completion. Learning from mistakes in a stimulated environment provides an opportunity to learn in a safe controlled environment.
3. **Bridges the gap between theory and practice:** By moving beyond theory to the realm of "learning by doing" the learner gets a first hand experience of practicing what has been taught. This helps in retaining concepts and ideas.

4. **Produces demonstrable mindset changes:** There are very few learning methods that have a positive impact on the learner's mindset. Experiential learning is one of them. Many things cannot be learned by simple reading only. Experiential learning provides opportunity for "learning by doing".
5. **Increases active participation or engagement of learners:** The high focus on collaboration and learning from each other benefits the learners as it increases engagement in learning. As the learner is involved in problem-solving activity it enhances learning also.
6. **Ensures optimum learning outcomes:** Experiential learning is personal and effective in nature, influencing both feelings and emotions as well as enhancing knowledge and skills. It goes beyond classroom learning and ensures that there is high level of retention, thereby ensuring optimum learning outcomes in comparison to traditional methods of learning.
7. **Enables personalized learning:** Experiential learning methodology enables personalized learning due to its distinct characteristics. By combining technology and teaching methods, experiential methods allow learners to set their own pace of learning.

## Reflective Learning

### What is Reflection?

According to Kinzer, "Reflective thinking is an active, intentional and purposeful process of exploration discovery and learning". Reflection is not just looking back on what happened but to understand what has happened and make use of it; the idea of learning from the past, especially trying not to repeat mistakes happened in the past. Race said that reflection is a process of personalizing and understanding the contents, process and the rationales for what we have learned. Through reflection we relate our personal experience to a wider perspective, which helps us to see the bigger picture. Winitzky viewed reflection as a process to retrieve, apply and analyze knowledge and to relate that knowledge to larger context. Reflection is an active, disciplined and deliberate strategy.

Reflection is active, persistent and careful consideration of any belief or form of knowledge in the light of the grounds that support it and the further conclusions to which it leads. According to Devey, reflection is the kind of thinking that involves in processing an information or subject in the mind and giving it a serious thought.

### Importance of Reflection in Learning

Reflection enables learners to generalize the main ideas, principles and abstract concepts from experience. The process of reflection includes debriefing and reframing to expand students' beliefs and understanding. Reflection also helps learners to create knowledge and generalize practical examples into explicit knowledge. Through reflection students integrate and generalize accepted arguments. Students can also recapitulate actions and learn lessons from their experiences.

Reflection enables students to evaluate, synthesize and understand the examples shared by the teacher. In order to make conscious decisions about the use of information and selecting problem-solving strategies, students need to use appropriate reflective thinking. Reflection can be used to influence students' learning from experience, increase their awareness of their thoughts and actions-increase their recall of experiences, when students do reflections, they repeatedly retrieve the information from memory and this will enhance their retention ability.

Reflection stimulates students to judge their beliefs and make connections between their personal beliefs and knowledge. Developing a reflection means that a student begins to automatically challenge and question why he is doing tasks in a certain way rather than how they were carried out.

Reflection is not just an individual activity. Reflection can also be a collective activity. Joint reflection with peers helps individuals as they refine, develop and enhance learning skills from various perspectives. According to Florence, collaborative reflection can bring different perspectives when we have discussion with others, when others view things differently, ask question or challenge our assumptions.

Reflective learners develop their ability to learn by understanding themselves as learners. They are concerned with the process as well as the products of their learning and strategies essential to become life-long learners. Skilled reflection deepens understanding and permits students to apply their knowledge in new contexts. Thus, reflective learners are self-regulated and life-long learners. According to David White Bread, children developing self-regulatory abilities predict academic outcomes and emotional wellbeing more powerfully than other aspects of children's development.

Reflection helps students to develop a deeper understanding of what they are learning through making new connections and relating different ideas.

## Reflective Student: Learning How to Learn

Reflection is essential to become an engaged, self-regulated and lifelong learner. Reflection is an active, disciplined and deliberate strategy. According to Watkins, "Effectiveness as a learner depends on the ability to be versatile as a learner. To have a rich view of learning and learning orientation which is in turn linked to the ability to plan, monitor and review one's learning". Meta-cognition (thinking about thinking) is a general term used to describe when learners plan, monitor, evaluate and subsequently make changes to their learning behaviors. Another term developed by Watkins to describe the very specific idea of reflecting on and regulating learning, is "meta learning".

According to Cambridge University, reflective learners are not only strategic in their thinking but are able to reflect upon their thinking-in- progress, using their strategies and revising them as appropriate. They thrive in the unfamiliar or unknown, actively learn from failure or setbacks and have developed a considerable degree of resilience and determination.

In Watkin's words learning to learn is concerned with developing the capacity to accurately reflect on one's learning and deliberately apply this understanding to learning in the future. Thus, this involves making learning an object of learning'. In short, a reflective learner adopts a number of learning habits, strategies and process incorporating metacognitive knowledge and regulation including:

- Self-awareness of how I am learning and how effective my learning is.
- Identifying and overcoming barriers to learning.
- Questioning assumptions.
- Delaying gratification, sticking to a task, enjoying challenges and difficulties.
- Organizing learning effectively.
- Being willing and able for help, understanding when one's own resources are limited.
- Learning from mistakes and setbacks.
- Trying new strategies.

## How to Support Reflective Learning?

In Robert's words, "Reflection without connection to study material will not result in learning. Reflecting on the professional level is important. However, it is also necessary to reflect on private matters since through reflecting on private matters and sharing each other's personal experiences, learners will find more connections and a sense of safety and belonging. It will also provide each other with social support in the process.

To support reflection, teachers can help learners externalize their tacit mental activities by prompting them to reflect on what they have done before, during or after an event. Teachers can also promote reflection by critically assessing assignments of students through fruitful discussions. The purpose of discussion is to improve the ability of learners to reach to a higher level of reflection, increases their self-awareness in their work and convert their implicit knowledge to explicit.

To make reflection useful to students' academic performance, reflection "should be implemented in a well-structured, intentional manner with focus on learning outcomes or objectives throughout the educational program.

## ACTIVE LEARNING STRATEGIES

Most commonly followed active learning strategies are team-based learning, journaling and problem-solving learning.

### Team-based Learning

Team-based learning (TBL) is defined as "an active learning and small group instructional strategy that provides students with opportunities to apply conceptual knowledge through a sequence of activities that includes individual work, team work and immediate feedback". TBL was originally designed by Larry Michaelsen.

### Key Components of TBL

- **Carefully formed and managed teams:** Students should be assigned to teams using a transparent process to ensure there are no pre-existing friendship groups-based teams and to ensure each team has a diverse mix of students. Teachers motivate teams to "stay together for as long as possible" to enhance team dynamics, trust and diversity of resources within the group, continuity of learning and cohesiveness of teams.
- **Frequent and timely feedback:** Providing immediate feedback is an important aspect of TBL. It ensures that students are provided with an understanding of their level of content knowledge. Feedback fosters critical thinking, knowledge acquisition, retention and team development.
- **Problem-solving:** During problem-solving activities, teams are required to use their collective knowledge, reasoning, ethical views, skills and values to solve complex problems. Participation in the problem-solving activities encourages learning and team development through the use of challenging cases.
- **Peer evaluation:** In TBL, students contribute to the grades of other students through provision of quantitative and qualitative feedback.

### Journaling

According to key Burke, "Journal writing results in more reflection and encourages students to take charge of their learning and their feelings". Journaling help students make connections between what is really important to them, the curriculum and the world. Journaling helps students to express themselves. It also gives students time to organize their thoughts and prepare responses, which give confidence to participate in classroom discussion.

Another important aspect of journaling is its contribution to the physical and mental development of students. Journaling helps to introspect and adopt a healthy lifestyle.

By encouraging students to do daily journaling, giving direction, reviewing students' work and encouraging self-evaluation teacher can promote journaling among students.

## Problem-solving

Problem-solving is the highest level of learning. To solve problems, the learner must have a clear idea of the problem or of the goal being sought and must be able to recall previously learned rules that relate to the situation. The next step is a thinking process in which the learner combines the recalled rules to form a new, higher order rule that is then available for use in similar situations in the future. Therefore, a problem once solved, theoretically will never be a problem again. The person will have only to recall the solution upon encountering that problem or a similar one.

Another way of viewing problem-solving is a process of formulating and testing hypotheses. The student, confronted with the problem, begins to formulate hypotheses, a process analogous to combining recalled rules to form a higher order rule. Tentative solutions are mentally or actually planned and tested to see if they work, then modified as necessary.

An example of how nursing students use problem-solving in the process of learning might be helpful at this point. Suppose a learner is planning care for a patient who has been stabilized after a myocardial infarction but is still on strict bed rest. As the instructor, you ask the learner how he or she is going to prevent muscle weakness in this patient yet also prevent strain on the heart. The problem has now been identified. The learner will recall rules that relate to exercise, muscle tone and strength and will remember that passive isotonic exercise puts the least demands on the circulatory system, making it relatively safe for the stabilized myocardial infarction patient to maintain some muscle strength. The learner will then test the solution in actual practice. The learner has now learned a solution to this exact problem and related problems and will probably be able to recall the solution in future situations. If the learner had simply been told the solution, problem-solving learning would not have taken place; the learner might not have understood the concepts involved and might not retain the information.

Bigge differentiates between "understanding level" teaching and "memory level" teaching. He states that "if understanding level teaching is successful, students will know, in addition to the facts, the principles by which the facts are related; memory level teaching tends to ignore principles, or at best handles them on such a superficial level that they have little meaning". If students are to understand and retain information and have insight into problems, most of their nursing education should be at the rule learning, problem-solving and understanding levels. Moreover, the WHO also recommends problem-solving type of learning in nursing.

Teacher has to play an important role in problem-solving learning. First, teacher can help the student to define the problem and the goal. Teacher can simply state the problem or help the student put it into words by verbal coaching. Teacher should be fairly certain at this point that the student has already learned the concepts and rules that will be needed to solve the problem. In the second step, teacher should help the student to recall the necessary rules by means of questions, suggestions, or demonstration. Students are learning a large number of rules and concepts in a short period of time and probably need help to select the rules that may apply to the problem situation.

## DETERMINANTS OF LEARNING

Haggard classifies determinants of learning as follows:
1. Learning needs—what learner needs and want to learn.
2. Readiness to learn—when the learner is receptive to learning.

3. Learning styles—how the learner best learns or in simple words learner's knowledge of how to learn

## Learning Needs

According to Healthcare Education Association, "Learning needs are defined as gaps in knowledge that exist between a desired level of performance and the actual level of performance". In other words, a learning need is the gap between what a learner knows and what learner needs or want to know. Such gaps may arise because of lack of knowledge, attitude or skill.

Of the three determinants of learning, teachers must identify learning needs first so that they can develop an instructional plan to rectify any deficits in the cognitive, affective or psychomotor domains. Once the teacher discovers what needs to be taught, he can determine when and how learning outcomes can be achieved in a better manner. Often learners are not aware of what they do not know or want to know. So it is the duty of the teacher to help learners in identifying, clarifying and prioritizing their needs and interests. Once this information is collected, teacher can plan effective ways to achieve learning outcomes.

Learning needs can be categorized into **mandatory needs, desirable needs and possible or nice-to-know needs.** Mandatory needs must be learned for attaining competency. For example, a nursing student must know how to do cardiopulmonary resuscitation or a BEd student must know how to take class effectively using a lesson plan. Desirable needs are related to the overall ability to perform duties with responsibility. For example, health-care workers and teachers need to update their knowledge by attending in-service programs or by self-effort. Possible needs are information that is nice to know but not essential or required or situations in which the learning need is not directly related to daily activities. For example, a teacher need not be an expert in all teaching methods because she is not using all teaching methods on a daily basis.

## Readiness to Learn

Once the teacher has identified learning needs, the next step is to determine the learner's readiness to receive information. Readiness to learn can be defined as the time when the learner demonstrates an interest in learning the information necessary to maintain optimal health or to attain competency or qualification for a job. Readiness to learn occurs when the learner is receptive, willing and able to participate in the learning process. It is the responsibility of the teacher to identify exactly when learners are ready to learn, what they need or want to learn and how to make learners adapt to learning situation.

According to Lichtenthal, there are four types of readiness to learn—**physical readiness, emotional readiness, experiential readiness and knowledge readiness.** These four types of readiness are commonly referred by an acronym "PEEK". Five major components of physical readiness are measures of ability, complexity of task, environmental effects, health status and gender because they affect the degree or extent to which learning will occur.

Learners must be emotionally ready to learn. Like physical readiness, emotional readiness includes several factors that need to be considered. These factors include anxiety level, support system, motivation, risk taking behavior, mindset and developmental stage.

Experiential readiness involves level of aspiration, past coping or adjusting mechanisms, cultural background, locus of control and orientation. Knowledge readiness includes present knowledge base, cognitive ability, learning disabilities and learning styles.

## Learning Style

Recent research findings not supporting the old belief that learning styles are the best way to learn for a student. Even then, learning styles help a teacher recognize the preferred way in which a student processes and retains information. Even though there are many models related to learning styles, the VARK model is among the most widely used since it sufficiently addresses learner diversity and needs.

The VARK model stands for four learning styles namely **visual, auditory, reading/writing and kinesthetic.** Not all learners follow exactly single style. Learners use different styles single or together depending on the subject matter and activity.

**Visual learners** like to see and observe the things that they are learning about. Visual learners like to use pictures, diagrams and written directions to acquire and process information. This learning style has also been known as 'spatial'. Students who are visual or spatial learners might draw, make lists or take notes in order to acquire and process information. Some of the more traditional styles of teaching support visual learners such as white boards or projecting information into a screen. Assignments involving pictures or diagrams also help visual learners. In addition, providing class notes or handouts that students can follow motivate visual learners. It is difficult for visual learners to understand lectures as they need more time to process information that they receive auditory.

**Auditory learners** learn best by listening and relating information to sound. These are students who prefer listening to a lecture or a recording rather than taking written notes. They may also read aloud for understanding information. Auditory learners often repeat what a teacher has said to process the information. Including discussion while teaching can support auditory learners. They want to hear others' opinion and share their own ideas in order to learn and process information. While giving a lecture, asking auditory learners to repeat what they have learned will enhance their learning. Call and response or question and answer processes can also benefit auditory learners. In addition, auditory learners like watching videos about a topic and listening to audiobooks or recordings.

**Reading/writing learners** like to learn using the written word. This may seem like visual learning but reading/writing style learners express themselves through writing. They also enjoy reading articles and writing in diaries or journals. Most of the traditional educational system supports this type of learners. The reading/writing learner learns by researching, reading books and writing. They are happy with writing an essay or with writing projects. More than giving answers vocally they can express themselves well with written words.

**Kinesthetic or tactile learners** learn by experiencing and doing. They like to use their hands and bodies as learning instruments, often acting out events and using their hands when they talk. Students who are particularly good athletes or dancers may be kinesthetic learners because they adapt at following the directions of a game or a dance using their body. Since kinesthetic learners learn through movement, teachers may ask them to act out scenes from a book or use movement in other ways during the learning process. Kinesthetic learner can benefit by walking in place while trying to memorize facts.

## TYPES OF LEARNERS

According to Association for Psychological Science, learners can be classified: as (a) visual learners, (b) auditory or aural learners, (c) kinesthetic or hands on learners and (d) reading and writing learners.

### Visual Learners

Visual learners learn well when they can visualize relationships and ideas. Charts, videos, diagrams and even essays help visual learners to learn well. When teachers teach with the help of appropriate audiovisual aids, visual learners learn in a better manner.

### Auditory Learners

Auditory learners prefer listening for learning rather than reading or seeing visuals. Auditory learners may speak or/and read slowly. Auditory learners learn better through discussion with others. Listening and discussion helps auditory learners to process information, retain information and recollect information than reading or seeing visuals.

### Kinesthetic Learners

Kinesthetic learners are the most hands-on learning type. They learn best by doing and may easily get distracted while attending lectures. Kinesthetic learners learn well when they can participate in activities or solve problems in a hands-on manner. They tend to remember what they do best.

### Reading and Writing Learners

Reading and writing learners are more interested in written words. They prefer to process information by reading and learn better by preparing self- learning materials. Traditional way of imparting knowledge through textbook or lecture notes is more preferred by reading and writing learners.

## CHARACTERISTICS OF PRESENT-DAY LEARNERS

Due to various factors that influence behavior of adolescents, it is difficult to explain all the characteristics of present-day learners in a precise manner. Even then awareness about the general characteristics of learners is essential for setting effective educational objectives or learning outcomes and attaining them. Let us discuss the general characteristics of present-day learners in a brief manner.

- **More depend on technology:** Present-day learners consider technology as an extension of their body. Wider availability of Internet, affordable data plans as well as gadgets enable present-day learners to depend more on technology for attaining learning outcomes. Dominance of online classes due to closure of educational institutions during COVID-19 pandemic also forced learners to depend on technology for meeting learning needs more than ever before.
- **Use a combination of resources for learning:** Present-day learners use a wide variety of resources like social media, learning apps and other learning platforms in addition to textbooks and classes by teachers for gaining knowledge. Easy access to various resources made learning more affordable and convenient when compared to the past.
- **Follow a combination of learning styles:** In a way, learning styles become outdated as students follow a combination of learning styles rather than one style for gaining knowledge with the easy access to information, now they can learn at any time and at any place. 3D animated videos and virtual classrooms enable students to combine various learning styles in an effective manner.
- **Applying first principles thinking in learning:** Many present-day learners knowing or unknowingly follow first principles thinking in learning by trying to find out the basic cause of a problem or relationship between facts. Critical thinking, reasoning, problem-solving

skills and easy access to information enable present-day learners to apply first principles thinking in learning.
* **Enhanced physical literacy:** Present-day learners are more aware about the importance of maintaining physical wellbeing for a better life. They believe physical wellbeing is essential for maintaining and improving cognitive skills. Present-day learners give importance to daily exercise and other habits essential for leading a healthy lifestyle.
* **Adapted to different modes of teaching:** Present-day learners are familiar with offline as well as online mode of teaching. They become more familiar with online teaching during COVID-19 pandemic when institutions were closed for a long period of time. Another reason is the widespread use of learning apps and easy access to massive open online courses (MOOCs) other than traditional classroom learning.
* **Preference to choices more than abilities:** With the introduction of a lot of new generation educational programs, present-day learners opt for programs that may not suit with their abilities. For example, a learner who is interested in maths may opt for health science program considering the high chance of getting a job. In other words, present-day learners select educational programs based on the trends in job market rather than considering their aptitude.
* **Prefer interactive, experiential and collaborative learning:** Present-day learners believe in collaboration than competition. They also prefer learning by doing than merely memorizing the content.
* **Consider teacher as a facilitator and guide:** Present-day learners consider teacher as a facilitator and guide. For them the best teacher is one who inspires them primarily through role modeling. Present-day learners consider teacher as a guide who helps them to become lifelong learners for leading a good life.
* **Aware about their rights and responsibilities:** Present-day learners are very much aware about their rights and responsibilities. They demand safe and positive learning environment. They do not tolerate irrational restrictions that violate their fundamental human rights as learners.
* **Up-skilling through online courses:** Present-day learners prefer to join online courses along with the regular educational program for enhancing skills for a good living. Easy access to massive open online courses (MOOCs) is the main reason for this desirable trend.
* **Demand a combination of teaching methods:** Present-day learners prefer a combination of teaching methods than mere traditional lecture. Hence, teachers need to follow a combination of teaching methods by effectively utilizing resources, especially technology to achieve learning outcomes. As they don't prefer long lectures, teachers need to use video clips, concept charts, short PowerPoint presentations, etc., to engage learners. Easily distracting nature of present-day learners is the main reason for recommending a combination of teaching methods.
* **Aware about the importance of acquiring 21st century life skills:** Present-day learners are aware about the importance of acquiring 21st century life skills like critical thinking, problem-solving, reasoning, creativity, research skills, etc., for leading a balanced life. Hence along with learning they try to acquire these skills in a meaningful manner.
* **Know the need of learning, unlearning and relearning:** Present-day learners are lifelong learners. Hence, they are aware about the importance of learning, unlearning and relearning for updating knowledge and skills.

## EMOTIONAL INTELLIGENCE AND LEARNING

Emotional intelligence or emotional quotient is the ability to understand, manage and express emotions in positive ways, relieve stress in a positive manner, communicate effectively, empathize with others, overcome challenges and resolve conflict. Having emotional intelligence helps students to learn in a better manner. The benefits of having emotional intelligence include:

- **Self-management:** Students are able to control impulsive feelings and behaviors, manage their emotions in healthy ways, take initiative for learning, fulfill their commitments and adapt to changing circumstances.
- **Self-awareness:** Students can recognize their own emotions and how they effect their thoughts and behavior. Students can realize their strengths and weaknesses and have self-confidence.
- **Social awareness:** Students develop more empathy and compassion for others. This will help them to understand the emotions, needs and concerns of other people, understand feelings of others and feel comfortable with others. This will help them to become a good human being.
- **Relationship management:** Students know how to develop and maintain good relationship, communicate assertively and clearly, inspire and influence peers, work well as a team member and manage conflicts.
- **Higher motivation for learning:** Students with adequate emotional intelligence have high intrinsic motivation for learning. They rarely depend on external motivation to initiate learning and achieve learning goals.
- **Stress management:** Students with adequate emotional intelligence manage their stress in a positive manner. They find out positive ways to relieve stress.
- **Better communication and decision-making:** Emotional intelligence helps students to communicate in an assertive and clear manner. It also helps in taking good decisions by choosing best among the alternatives.

Teacher can help students to develop and improve emotional intelligence in the following ways. Unlike intelligence, emotional intelligence can be developed and nurtured through conscious effort.

- Helping students to identify and manage emotions.
- Listening to students' feelings.
- Having empathy towards students
- Teach problem-solving skills
- Becoming a role model to students in both professional and personal life.

## EMOTIONS AND LEARNING

Emotions influence the cognitive process in humans including perception, attention, learning, memory, reasoning and problem-solving. Emotions particularly influence attention and motivation. Attention and motivation are closely related to learning. Thus, emotions influence learning depending on the situations. For example, tests, examinations, homework and assignments create different emotional states like frustration, anxiety and boredom. Even subject matter influence emotions that affect one's ability to learn.

Increasing acceptance of computer-based multimedia educational technologies such as intelligent tutorial systems (ITSs) and massive open online courses (MOOCs) are gradually replacing traditional face-to-face learning environment. This also induces various emotional experiences in learners. Hence, teachers need to consider emotional influences in learning while teaching for maximizing learner engagement and thereby ensuring better learning outcomes situation.

## Characteristics of Emotions

Research conducted by Otto Euler and Mandi shows the following three characteristics of emotions.
1. An emotion is an affective reaction which can be determined and described in a relatively precise manner (for example, enjoyment, anger, pride, sadness, etc.) and can be due to a cause or an incident. Thus, we talk about emotions when talking about a student's enjoyment in learning or a teacher's anger about indiscipline of students.
2. The experience of an emotion is related to situations which are of importance for the individual. If a situation, an event or content is significant for us or if we are influenced by something, emotions are likely to be evoked. Learner will only experience joy, frustration, anxiety, pride or satisfaction if the learning content or the learning process is relevant to them.
3. Emotions also create an increased self-awareness. Emotions are very difficult to avoid. They are mainly expressed towards others but rarely towards oneself.

## Components of Emotion

In Schutz's opinion, emotions can be explained as 'ways of being' and as 'holistic episodes that include physiological, psychological and behavioral aspects. Emotions are interrelated with cognitions, motivation and actions of an individual. Emotions can be expressed and observed. Emotions are also felt in the body. According to Scherer and Izard, emotions have five components as described below.
1. The affective component is the subjective, individual experience of a person (e. g. feelings of anxiety during a presentation in front of a large audience).
2. The cognitive component represents all thoughts in relation to the emotion (e. g. Thinking about the consequences of possible failure or success).
3. The expressive component represents all the possibilities for expressing an emotion (e. g. A tensed face).
4. The motivational component addresses the impulses for action, stimulated or inhibited by the emotion (e. g., Working on easy tasks before doing the difficult tasks)
5. And finally, the physiological component includes the physiological reactions associated with an emotion (e. g., increased heart beat).

## Impact of Emotions in Learning

According Charis Drew, emotions impact learning in the following four ways.
1. **Motivational impact:** Positive emotions can help students engage with learning longer because they stay motivated. Emotions during learning also influence students feeling towards learning. Absenteeism is less among students with positive emotions. Students with positive emotions learn proactively and this will be very good for them in the long run. In short, students with positive emotions learn because of an internal drive to learn and this internal drive is called intrinsic motivation. Learners with negative emotions need external factors called extrinsic motivation for learning. Using extrinsic motivation is an inferior way to learn and would likely lead to poorer results in the long run.
2. **Psychological impact:** Positive emotions make learners feel better about learning. Learner with positive attitude towards learning takes responsibility of their own learning. This self-directed learning leads to increased effort. Increased efforts naturally results in better learning outcomes. Better learning outcomes in turn further motivate learners for putting more effort in learning. In short, positive emotions ensure success in life through life-long learning.

3. **Social impact:** Positive emotions improve collaboration among learners. When learners feel good about learning, they are more likely to obey instructions of teachers and contribute their own ideas and thoughts in group discussions. In other words learners who feel good with their learning will interact more socially with teachers and other learners.
4. **Cognitive impact:** Moderate levels of negative emotions like stress or anxiety is necessary for learning difficult concepts. This concept is called Kort's emotional learning spiral which states that learners go through a necessary pattern of emotions to learn something new. According to Kort, there are four stages in emotional learning spiral.
   a. In stage 1, learners feel great about the idea of learning a new concept. But when learners are confused with challenging information, they move to stage 2.
   b. In stage 2, learners start feeling confused and anxious. The new information is challenging and difficult to understand.
   c. In stage 3, learners enter into a state of frustration. Learners start thinking to get new answers to difficult questions. Here learners do not feel very positive emotions at all. Even though there are no positive emotions, it is a necessary stage of cognitive development essential for learning new information or things. This third stage motivates us to unlearn and relearn by questioning our old beliefs and thoughts.
   d. In stage 4, learners feel emotions like determination and hopefulness because they are understanding a new concept.

## MOTIVATION AND LEARNING

According to Kendra Cherry, motivation is the process that initiates, guides and maintains-goal-oriented behavior. Motivation and learning are closely related. If the motivation for learning is high student's learning outcomes are also high. Motivation involves biological, emotional, social and cognitive forces that activate behavior.

### Components of Motivation

There are three major components of motivation: activation, persistence and intensity.
1. Activation involves the decision to initiate behavior such as taking admission for a BSc nursing program.
2. Persistence is the continued effort toward a goal even though obstacles may exist. An example of persistence is joining for MSc nursing program after BSc nursing program although it requires significant investment of time, energy and resources.
3. Intensity enhances the concentration and hard work of a student to achieve the goal of learning. For example, one student might learn without much effort, while another student will study regularly, participates in discussions and takes advantage of research opportunities outside of class. The first student lacks intensity while the second pursues his educational goals with grater intensity.

### Types of Motivation

Most common types of motivation associated with learning are **extrinsic motivation and intrinsic motivation.** Extrinsic motivation is that arises from outside of the learner. It depends on external factors. It is doing something to gain a reward or avoid adverse reactions. For example, a learner studying for an examination to get good grade or stopping unwanted behavior to avoid punishment.

Intrinsic motivation is that arising from within the learner. It refers to learner's personal interests, satisfaction and enjoyment. Intrinsic motivation is guided by factors within the learner. This could be a passion for the subject, curiosity, love of challenges and more. In learning, intrinsic motivation is more desirable as it is linked to (a) Increased results, (b) Increased interest in learning, (c) A greater number of successfully accomplished goals and (d) More autonomy.

## Enhancing Intrinsic Motivation of Learners

In his self-determination theory, Thomas Callahan identifies three drives of intrinsic motivation: **autonomy in learning, relatedness and competence.** These core principles provide a useful framework for teachers in creating a learning environment that enhances intrinsic motivation among students. Christina Hinton explains these core principles in the following manner.

### Autonomy in Learning

When students have a sense of control over their learning, their intrinsic motivation improves and they are likely to do hard work to complete difficult academic tasks and they learn to assimilate or process information at a deeper level. To support students' autonomy teachers can encourage them to set their own learning objectives, contribute to course material and use learning techniques that are suitable for them.

One key way to support autonomy is to give students choices. Hinton suggests following examples: (a) instead of assigning students a specific book to read, allow students to select from a list of books to read, and (b) Rather than having all students write an essay, offer them the opportunity to demonstrate their understanding through digital and other media.

### Relatedness

Relatedness refers to the desire to feel connected to and cared by others. Research shows that social isolation and loneliness are linked to student anxiety, lower intellectual achievement, diminish self-control and poor health. But when students feel a sense of belonging, they experience more meaningful relationship, higher self-esteem, better academic performance and improved wellbeing. Group projects help students to feel connected to one another. Good interpersonal relationship between teacher and students also boosts relatedness. Good relationship with teacher creates a comfortable learning environment in which students feel free to ask questions and discuss ideas.

### Competence

Students need to be challenged by school work and know that expectations are high but they also need a sense of competence—a feeling that they are capable to meet these challenges and standards. Once students feel themselves as competent in learning subject matter, they develop more intrinsic learning motives even when facing obstacles. Hinton recommends following ways to develop competence among students: (a) Introduce activities that are optionally challenging, (b) Provide noncritical feedback, along with information on how to improve learning, (c) Encourage students to follow effective learning strategies, and (d) Show students how to learn so that they can demonstrate competence.

## Factors Affect Students' Motivation

According to Victor Silva, motivation has a very positive impact on performance of students and learning outcomes. According to her motivation is the state that can initiate and maintain students' attention, curiosity and desirable behavior essential for attaining learning outcomes. Motivation has a variety of effects on students' behavior, preferences and results. She suggested eight following factors that influence students' motivation in learning.

1. **Class and curriculum structure:** When students sense or see that classes follow a structure and the curriculum and teaching materials have been prepared beforehand, it provides them with a greater sense of security. The feeling of security is one of our basic needs. When that is provided in a learning environment, it allows students to fully focus on the learning. To help students feel more secure, teachers need to plan classes and curriculum. All learning materials that will be used in class should be prepared in advance. Teacher also needs to formulate educational objectives of a course or class at the beginning of the academic year or semester.
2. **Teacher behavior and personality:** If a student has a negative emotion such as fear or disliking towards their teacher, that can negatively affect their attitude toward the subject as a whole. If a teacher shows a preference towards certain students or uses derogatory and humiliating language, that can lower their motivation for learning.
   On the other hand, kindness, optimism, positive feedback and encouragement can positively affect students' motivation to learn.
3. **Teaching methods:** Students are more likely to retain their motivation in learning if teachers use different teaching methods. This creates interest and prevents students from getting distracted and bored. Students in a single class are likely to have different styles of learning and learning needs. Thus, a teacher is more likely to meet these needs by using different teaching methods. In some cases, allowing participation in extracurricular activities or support from a teacher can help students to achieve their learning goals.
4. **Parental habits and involvement:** A few parental habits can indirectly affect the motivation of learners, especially intrinsic motivation. These include: (a) Showing interest in the child's learning material, (b) Inquiring about their day, (c) Active listening, (d) Helping with specifications or skills taught at school, (e) Attending parent meetings, (f) Encouraging children to complete homework or study for a test and (g) Another habit that improves motivation is reading. Reading to and with small children helps them develop literacy faster than talking does.
5. **Family issues and instability:** Same as lack of security in the classroom, the lack of security at home can negatively impact motivation in learning. Children who live with both parents, on average, get better grades than children who don't. Family conflicts and disruption can result in poor academic performance. As a result, in certain situations, additional support may be needed from school to help students with their issues.
6. **Peer relationships:** As children grow older, the influence peers have upon them increases as well. Therefore, problems and conflicts with peers can make students feel less secure about their social status among peers, increase their stress levels and lower motivation in learning. Checking conflicts, bullying and other peer issues can prevent serious problems.
7. **Learning environment:** School environment or school climate is another factor that affects motivation in learning. School environment refers to different norms and regulations that determine the overall climate of the school. Positive school environment makes students feel safe and secure, meets their basic needs such as daily meals and provides an optimal environment for them to build healthy social relationships.
   Too many classes and rigid learning environment can also lower motivation in learning. Adding humor while taking classes can help to ease the learning atmosphere and improve motivation and learning outcomes. Allowing enough time for play and rest also improves motivation in learning.
8. **Assessment:** While standardized assessment increases the standard of attainment, it can negatively influence students' motivation in learning, especially at a younger age. Students may lose motivation if tests are continuously too challenging. This does not provide a

sense of achievement and lowers motivation in learning over time. Thus, it is important for teachers to experiment with and apply different assessment methods which would be able to address the different learning needs of students.

## ENVIRONMENT AND LEARNING

Like any other human activity, learning is also influenced by the environment. Learning environment encompasses the physical, psychological, social and cultural aspects of the learning context. The learning context may be home, educational institution, online resources or outside environment.

Educators believe that learning environment has both a direct and indirect influence on student learning, including their engagement in learning, their motivation to learn and their sense of wellbeing, belonging and personal safety. How adults, especially teachers and parents and how students interact with one another may also be considered as important aspects of a learning environment. Phrases such as "positive learning environment" or "negative learning environment" are commonly used in reference to the social and emotional dimensions of learning context.

## Characteristics of Positive Learning Environment

While considering the impact of environment on learning teacher needs to consider four factors, such as (a) The increased presence of personal, networked devices (for example laptops and mobile phones) in the classroom, (b) Increased access to information through web and the subsequent transition of teachers role from disseminator of information to facilitator of learning, (c) Increasing importance of virtual learning environment and (d) Encouraging collaboration more than competition among students for achieving better learning outcomes.

Sheifer believes that a positive learning environment is one in which students feel a sense of belonging, trust others, feel encouraged to ask questions and promote curiosity, critical thinking and creativity. Such an environment provides relevant content, motivation for hard work, clear learning goals, appropriate feedback, proper assessment, opportunities to build social skills and strategies to develop ways of effective learning.

## Creating a Safe and Positive Learning Environment

Effective teachers create a positive learning environment by clearly stating teacher expectations, maximizing instruction time, encouraging students to become proactive in learning, offer guidance and support to manage stress, assuming responsibility of students learning and above all considering each student as unique individual. Considering each student as unique individual is essential for addressing needs of individual students in a better manner. Following factors are essential for creating a safe and positive learning environment.

* **Good relationship with students:** The most important aspect in a safe and positive learning environment is the relationship between a teacher and his or her students. When the students understand that their teacher cares about them and wants them to do well, students feel comfortable in the class. To build these kinds of relationship the teacher should take initiative to understand each student's strengths and interests as well as their struggles and frustrations. Teacher needs to act as a positive model for learning by celebrating achievement and supporting students to overcome shortcomings.
* **Promoting collaboration among students rather than competition:** Promoting collaboration among students is another necessary aspect of creating a positive learning environment. Students need to understand what they have in common with their classmates. It is the duty of the teacher to create collaboration among students so that each one can

know another's differences. One advantage of collaboration in classroom is that students become accountable for their own learning by creating a good classroom environment.

- **Fostering motivation among students:** Another important responsibility of a teacher is to develop a learning environment where students' feel motivated to do the right things and help one another. It is important for teachers to give emphasis on intrinsic motivation to keep student interests and pursue their own learning goals. In addition, extrinsic motivation helps students understand expectations of teacher and this will in turn enhance intrinsic motivation. These kinds of motivations include praise, positive reinforcement and reward for exceptional behavior.
- **Better classroom management:** Better classroom management is essential to create a safe and positive learning environment. Students cannot learn effectively in an environment where the teacher has no control. When teachers' classroom management plan is fair, consistent and organized, the students understand what to expect and make wise choices and take responsibility for their actions.
- **Establishing a supportive learning culture:** This aspect is similar to the second aspect we discussed earlier. Each member of the class should have the feeling of connectedness. They must feel that they are contributing to the overall environment while being a bigger and important part of a support learning culture. For this, a proper support system or mentorship program should be developed that would provide students the required assistance when needed.
- **Addressing learner's needs:** Just like adults, learners also have some psychological needs like order and security, love and belonging, competence and personal power, and freedom and even fun. It is important to meet these needs and to help learners progress and be taught with a positive attitude. Any learning environment, where instructors consider these intrinsic needs, learners tend to be happier and engage more in the teaching-learning process.
- **Appropriate feedback:** Feedback is the great way to guide students in the right direction to achieve learning goals. Feedback is important for learners as it helps them to understand their progress in learning and make appropriate changes if needed. It helps students recognize their weak areas while improving the strengths. A feedback informs the learners where they are missing the mark and what is needed to be done. A feedback is not only a key to motivate the learner but this timely and consistent feedback ensures an interactive learning environment.
- **Celebrate achievement of learners:** In addition to feedback and appreciation another way to establish a positive and effective learning environment is to celebrate the learner's success. When learner's achievements are recognized and shared by teachers and classmates, it creates sense of achievement and fosters healthy learning behavior.
- **Provide safety:** A good learning environment offers a safe platform for learners. For learners need to succeed academically, they should feel safe mentally and physically. While most institutions take physical safety measures, not many institutions consider mental safety of the learners. Safety in a learning environment goes beyond physical well-being. In order to maintain a safe learning environment, learners must feel supported, welcomed and respected. Hence, building a positive learning environment is more about maintaining a healthy culture where the expectations are well communicated and learners are fully aware of the code of conduct.
- **Maintain positive relationship with parents of students:** A well-functioning parents-teachers association can contribute much in creating a safe and positive learning environment. Teachers should communicate on a monthly basis with students' parents

for ensuring progress of learners. Involving parents builds up a large amount of trust. And when the parents trust teachers, the chances of the student trusting the teacher increase considerably.

- **Set high expectations:** Setting high teacher expectations about students is very essential for creating a safe and positive learning environment. When teachers expect best from students, they put more effort in learning and try to achieve the goals teachers expecting from them. High expectations always enhance self-confidence of students. This will ultimately lead to a highly motivated environment in the classroom essential for a safe and positive learning environment.
- **Follow high-tech high-touch approach in teaching-learning process:** Although technology is capable of transmitting knowledge, there are many areas which technology cannot replace teacher. For example, no technology can mould the character and creativity of students. Hence, human element in teaching needs to be preserved for creating a safe and positive learning environment.
- **Proper assessment:** Proper assessment of performance of teacher and students is important for creating a positive learning environment. Regular assessment should occur in the classroom to ensure everyone is improving and students are informed and engaged. But all assessment doesn't have to be in the threatening form of a test, assignment or project. Providing timely feedback is an important part of assessment. Adopting a variety of creative assessment methods optimizes learning ability of students.
- **Encouraging leadership and adaptability:** Leadership and responsibility gives students a sense of achievement and accomplishment. It also allows children to understand various leadership styles. Make sure every student has an opportunity to become a leader. They may accept or not accept the challenge of leadership but option of working towards leadership is a valuable life skill.
- **Self-directed learning:** A positive learning environment is one where students develop essential life skills. Promoting life-long learning is a way to inspire students to achieve success in life. Problem-based learning and research projects where students have to hypothesize, explore and discover will enhance critical thinking and problem-solving skills. This will enable students to take responsibility of their own learning.

## DEFINITION OF LEARNING NURSING

Author believes that "Learning nursing is an ongoing behavior modification by way of attaining relevant knowledge, insights, skill and attitude essential for providing meticulous nursing care". This definition has three main components.

1. **Ongoing behavior modification:** Learning occurs as a result of behavior modification. As healthcare science is rapidly changing, nursing students as well as nurses need to learn more by modifying their behavior. This is a continuous process as reskilling is essential to maintain competency in nursing care. Hence, we use the phrase ongoing behavior modification in the definition.
2. **Relevant knowledge, skills and attitude:** Knowledge, skills and attitude need to be updated to make them relevant or valid. Only through relevant knowledge, skill and attitude, one can achieve desired behavioral modification.
3. **Nursing care:** Attaining competency in providing safe and quality nursing care is the output of learning process. Nursing student learns to provide meticulous nursing care in different healthcare settings as a result of learning nursing.

## PRINCIPLES OF LEARNING NURSING

It is hoped that below mentioned principles serve as guidelines for learning nursing. As these principles are self explanatory, no further explanation is needed. In addition to these principles a nurse educator or nursing student can develop her or his own principles of learning nursing for assisting learning process.

- As attitude is caught by students and not taught to them, learning nursing focuses on developing proper attitude towards nursing among students.
- Learning nursing involves continuous modification of behavior by way of acquiring relevant knowledge, skills and attitudes.
- Technology only makes learning easier not better. Hence, teacher-student interaction, especially in clinical area, is important in learning nursing.
- Proactive learning resulting from intrinsic motivation is the most preferred way of learning nursing.
- Deliberate practice is an integral part of learning nursing. It is learning with intense concentration and purpose.
- Learning nursing prepares students for taking up expanding or evolving professional roles in nursing.
- Learning nursing is a lifelong process in accordance with the changes in the healthcare delivery system.
- Learning nursing prepares the student for life by becoming a good human being with qualities of a professional nurse.

## REMEMBERING AND FORGETTING

Factors that affect remembering and forgetting are the attitudes of the student toward the material, the amount of interference from other activities, the degree to which the material is originally learned and the types of learning followed by the student. Students tend to remember information with which they agree and forget that with which they disagree.

Techniques to enhance retention are known as *mnemonics. Acronym and acrostat* are the commonly used mnemonics. Acronym is a term coined by adding the initial letters of words which we have to keep in memory. For example, the acronym for fat-soluble vitamins is adek. Acronym can also be made by correlating the facts to well-known abbreviations. For example, the acronym for water-soluble vitamins is WBC, which is the abbreviation of white blood cells. Acrostat is made by formulating a sentence with words whose initial letters represent the facts. For example, from the sentence— other than lolipop—we can easily recollect the different types of diuretics like osmotic diuretics, thiazide diuretics, loop diuretics and potassium-sparing diuretics. *Please note that mnemonics is only a technique to remember the learned material and not a substitute to effective study habits.*

Effective study habits will enhance retention. Teachers have a responsibility to help students develop better study habits or to refer them to other professionals who can help them. Students need to learn the importance of spaced review versus cramming for an exam, of understanding notes and applying them versus simply reading them and of overlearning through repeated practice.

Teacher can also assist students in retention of learning by planning for certain conditions. First, the teacher should make sure that the material to be covered is at the appropriate level of students. Then, the content should be presented in an organized manner, using a strategy that includes active participation of the student, if possible. If new learning is likely to interfere with already learned material, the teacher should spend extratime reinforcing both old and new concepts to help the student remember both. The teacher should not shy from using repetition to reinforce important material. It is helpful to summarize the content periodically, especially before beginning new content areas. When dealing with skill learning, the teacher should provide adequate time for student practice-supervised practice if possible. Considering the tremendous amount of content that nursing students are asked to learn, anything that teachers can do to enhance retention and prevent forgetting will be worthwhile.

## SUMMARY

Knowledge explosion demands active participation from the students in the learning process, whereas the role of the teacher is limited to a facilitator. Learning aims of higher education like disseminate knowledge, develop the capability to use ideas and information, develop the student's ability to test ideas and evidence, develop the students' ability to generate ideas and evidence and facilitate the personal development of students are also applicable to nursing education. Watson's selected thirteen propositions about learning deals with reinforcement, immediate feedback, threat and punishment, practice, stimulation, motivation, problem-solving, concepts, frustration, peer learning, values and attitudes, situational learning and techniques for learning. It is earnestly hoped that these propositions will assist the nurse educator to achieve the teaching objectives in a better way. Types of learning include stimulus-response learning, chaining, verbal association, discrimination learning, concept learning, rule learning and problem-solving. Even though all these types of learning are common in nursing, problem-solving is the most recommended one. Problem-based learning is a way of designing and presenting courses that uses problems in professional practice or real life as the stimulus for student learning.

There are three approaches to learning namely surface approach, deep approach and strategic approach. Learning psychomotor skills is essential for a successful nursing practice. Skill learning can be divided into two phases namely getting an idea of the movement and fixation/diversification. Nurse educator has to play an important role in promoting skill learning among nursing students. Transfer of learning is the carryover of information from the time and setting in which it was originally learned to new and different situations. Much of what is taught in nursing is transferable. Transfer of learning is classified as negative, positive, lateral and vertical. Applying the tips to maximize transfer will help the teacher to ensure adequate transfer of learning. Knowledge regarding characteristics of an effective learning situation is essential for creating an effective learning situation in the classroom. Successful learners are knowledgeable, self-determined, empathetic and able to develop effective learning strategies.

## MULTIPLE CHOICE QUESTIONS

1. **Artificial representation of a real-world situation to teach students is called:**
   a. Simulation-based learning
   b. Blended learning
   c. Experiential learning
   d. Observational learning
2. **Virtual reality is an example of:**
   a. Simulation learning
   b. Observational learning
   c. Experiential learning
   d. Reflective learning
3. **Which learning involves intentional and purposeful process of exploration discovery and learning?**
   a. Reflective learning
   b. Observational learning
   c. Experiential learning
   d. Blended learning

4. **VARK model is related to:**
   a. Learning style
   b. Types of learners
   c. Memory
   d. None of the above
5. **Hands-on type learners are called:**
   a. Visual learners
   b. Auditory learners
   c. Kinesthetic learners
   d. Reading learners
6. **All thoughts related to emotions are part of:**
   a. Affective component
   b. Cognitive component
   c. Expressive component
   d. Motivational component
7. **Persistence is a component of:**
   a. Motivation
   b. Emotion
   c. Learning
   d. Remembering
8. **Motivation arising from within the learner is called:**
   a. Intrinsic motivation
   b. Extrinsic motivation
   c. None of the above
   d. All of the above
9. **Learning with intense concentration and purpose is called:**
   a. Deliberate practice
   b. Deep learning
   c. Surface learning
   d. Experiential learning
10. **Mnemonics is a technique related to enhance:**
    a. Remembering
    b. Learning
    c. Writing skills
    d. Reading skills

## ANSWER KEY

| 1. a | 2. a | 3. a | 4. a | 5. c | 6. a |
| 7. a | 8. a | 9. a | 10. a | | |

# CHAPTER 6

# Teaching–Learning Methods

## LEARNING OBJECTIVES

After completing this chapter, reader will be able to:

- Explain the meaning of teaching.
- Define teaching.
- Explain teaching as an art as well as a science.
- Explain the principles of teaching.
- Explain the maxims of teaching.
- Explain the marks of good teaching.
- Explain teaching styles.
- Identify characteristics of effective teaching.
- List down the qualities of a good teacher.
- Practice essential teaching skills effectively.
- Recognize the qualities of a good nurse educator.
- Explain the classification of teaching–learning methods.
- Distinguish between teaching strategies and teaching–learning methods.
- List down the guidelines for the selection and practice of teaching–learning methods.
- Practice teaching–learning methods effectively.
- Identify the role of assignments in teaching.
- Define teaching nursing
- Explain principles of teaching nursing
- Define clinical teaching
- Practice clinical teaching methods effectively

Transferring or imparting knowledge is equally important as generating knowledge. Knowledge transferred in a down to earth manner will simplify the learning process and help the students to retain what is taught and to recall learned lessons as and when needed. Fruitful transfer of knowledge can be achieved by employing various student-friendly teaching–learning methods. Student-friendly teaching–learning methods always consider the interests, needs and level of students.

Teaching nursing also involves effective application of different teaching–learning methods, some of which are especially devised to impart knowledge and clinical skills essential for a successful nursing career. Forthcoming discussion aims to cover various aspects of teaching, teaching–learning process and teaching–learning methods.

## MEANING OF TEACHING

Education institutions have two core processes namely: teaching and research. The output of teaching is learning and the output of research is a contribution to knowledge. Teaching is an integral part of education. Special function of teaching is to impart knowledge, develop understanding and skill. Teaching is establishing harmonious relationship between the educator, educant and the curriculum or subject matter. As special skill is required to impart knowledge and to establish the above said relationship, teaching is considered as a skilled occupation. The proverb "to teach is to learn twice" clearly explains the hard-work involved in the teaching activity. Teaching is an activity in which communicating and disseminating information are significant aspects. In broad sense, teaching is the art and science of establishing objectives, selecting and organizing content, organizing teaching aids, designing learning activities and evaluating performance in ways that enable students to learn.

## DEFINITION OF TEACHING

- **Flanders:** "Teaching is an interaction process. Interaction means participation of both teacher and student and both are benefited by this. The interaction takes place for achieving desired objectives." This definition is appreciated for its purpose of teaching and roles designated to the student and teacher. Nowadays, *participatory approach* is widely recognized as a worthwhile way of teaching. In participatory approach, students are allowed to actively participate in the teaching–learning process by keeping an aim or objectives in mind.
- **Burton:** "Teaching is the stimulation, guidance, direction and encouragement of learning." Burton believes that teaching is much more than imparting knowledge and he says that "teaching is a matter of helping the child to respond to his environment in an effective manner. The teacher simplifies the technique, modifies the environment, helps the children to adjust, to strengthen the knowledge and helps them to develop beginning skills, abilities and knowledge." Burton's further explanation for his simply articulated and concised definition motivated educationists to analyze the multiple aspects of teaching other than imparting knowledge.
- **Yoakm and Simpson:** "Teaching is the means whereby the society trains the young in a specific or selected environment to adjust themselves to the world in which they live as quickly as possible." This wisely coined definition conveys the real sense of teaching. Various educational programs ranging from the kindergarten to postdoctoral levels exemplifies this definition. New educational programs emerging out of societal changes and technological advancements and the induction of computer training even from the primary classes justifies this definition. Considering the relevance of this definition in the coming ages, this definition can also be regarded as the "futuristic definition" of teaching.

## TEACHING IS A SCIENCE AS WELL AS AN ART

For effective teaching, teacher has to follow some specific principles based on certain precise knowledge. In this sense, teaching is a science. In order to teach effectively, teacher has to adapt to varied circumstances by using different techniques. There is an element of art in the selection of proper techniques for adaptation. In fact, the art of teaching is being able to choose correct technique at the right time. When we say teaching is an art, authors believe that teaching is not a centpercent tutored art, so in addition to attending teacher training programs, teacher has to develop or cultivate his or her own style of teaching in order to become an efficient teacher.

## TEACHING–LEARNING PROCESS

Even though teaching and learning activities reciprocate each other to a certain extent, effective harmonization of teaching and learning activities are essential to ascertain the fulfilment of desired outcomes. Teaching-learning process is concerned with achieving this harmonization. By definition, teaching-learning process is a means through which the teacher, the learner, the curriculum and other variables are organized in a systematic manner, in order to attain predetermined goals and objectives. Teaching-learning process is aimed at the acquisition of knowledge, skills and attitudes which enable the students to lead a well-adjusted life. Teaching-learning process is basically an interaction between the teacher and learners, which is aimed to bring about behavior modification in learners. This interaction is characterized by a three-way communication. In the initial communication, teacher communicates the relevant information to the learners. After receiving the information, learners process it and communicate their response to the teacher and this is regarded as the second communication. The teacher after interpreting and evaluating the students' response once again communicate to the students, through this third communication, teacher conveys the feedback information. This feedback information helps the students to assess themselves. If a student's response is not good as expected, teacher can motivate the student by giving a positive feedback or reinforcement like "your answer conveys some sense, for a person like you, it is easy to give the exact answer, do not worry, try once more". Through this three-way communication teacher can carry out the teaching activity confidently in the right direction and the students can easily make out their progress in learning.

Even though the human component or human interaction in the teaching–learning activity remains unaffected, the traditional dominance enjoyed by the teacher in the teaching–learning process has come down in the recent years owing to the increased complexity of life, knowledge explosion and creation of new channels of information by the information technology. Nowadays, participatory approach is widely recognized and practiced in the teaching–learning process. In the participatory approach, the student is motivated and equipped to enjoy an active role in the teaching–learning process instead of passively quenching the thirst for knowledge by accepting the spoon-feeding offered by the teachers.

## Elements of Teaching–learning Process

An analysis of the above-discussed teaching–learning process will reveal the following elements.

- **A learner**, whose nervous system, senses and muscles are operating in sequences of patterned activity, which we speak of as behavior.
- **A teacher**, selecting and organizing teaching–learning methods, consciously planning and controlling a situation directed to the achievement of optimum student learning.
- **A series of learning objectives**, related to students' anticipated and desired behavioral changes. As discussed elsewhere, objectives are intended learning outcomes, the level of attainment of which can be observed and measured.
- **A sequence of stimulus-response situations** affecting teacher and learner, resulting in persistent and observable changes in the learner's behavior from which we may infer 'learning'. That learning is directed by the teacher to an enhancement of students' cognitive, affective and psychomotor abilities.
- **Reinforcement of that behavior**. By 'reinforcement' we refer to an activity which increases the likelihood that some event will occur again; it may take the form of a response of the environment, an automatic response of the student or something added to the learning situation by an individual other than the student, for example, an overt expression of approval by the teacher.
- **The monitoring, assessment, and evaluation** of the learner's changes in behavior in relation to the objectives of the teaching–learning process.
- **Appropriate media and technology:** In today's teaching–learning process selection of appropriate media and technology is important.

## PRINCIPLES OF TEACHING

According to J Gullibert, purposes of teaching is to help students: (a) Acquire, retain and be able to use knowledge; (b) Understand, analyze, synthesize and evaluate; (c) Achieve skills; (d) Establish habits; (e) Develop attitudes. Principles of teaching will assist the teacher to achieve these purposes. Moreover, principles of teaching will help the teacher to develop an insight regarding his strengths and weaknesses and provide information on vital elements pertaining to teaching like whom to teach, why to teach, where to teach, what to teach, how to teach and when to teach. Following principles is a combination of psychological principles and general principles of teaching.

- **Principle of motivation:** The best teacher is one who inspires the student. The human mind is like a parachute and it works only when open, so through teaching, teacher should try to unleash the talents of the students by motivating them. Motivation is a combination of recognizing, communicating and participating. Teacher has to recognize students as individuals, encourage their participation while teaching and communicate enthusiasm. Motivation promotes proactive learning and thereby enabling students to achieve success in a systematic way. This principle holds good during the entire nursing educational program, especially during the first year period. Presence of a motivating teacher during the initials days of any nursing educational program will provide an atmosphere of confidence and help students to develop a positive attitude towards patient care.

- **Principle of activity:** Teaching is basically an active process. While teaching, teacher should be alert, smart and follow the most suitable method of teaching. Teacher should also participate in various activities along with the students like discussions or conducting research. Activity generates the drive and drive is essential to achieve more heights in life. Teacher must provide various types of activities, such as assignments or projects to enhance creative skills of students.

  *In nursing foolproof repetition of an activity with a purpose will result in the development of a nursing skill.* Moreover, in nursing theoretical knowledge without the corresponding skill is useless. A nurse educator who is actively involved clinical teaching besides classroom teaching will certainly help the students to attain proficiency in clinical practice.

- **Teacher should arouse interest among students:** Even though we say teaching is sharing of knowledge, knowledge will not flow from one person to another just like money. To make students receptive, teacher has to elicit interest by adopting suitable methods like telling a story, citing an example or by asking questions. For example, when teaching moist heat sterilization, teacher can elicit interest of the students by advising them to take *iddli* for breakfast while travelling not only because *iddli* is a combination of pulses and cereals but also it is prepared in steam, i.e., in moist heat, which is considered as one of the best methods of sterilization.

- **There should be well-defined objectives:** To attain good results, all teaching activities should be based on predetermined objectives. With an objective in mind, it is easy to prepare the content, select suitable method and evaluate the effectiveness of the teaching session. Statement of well-defined objectives in advance will make the teacher more confident and enthusiastic. If you are planning to take a class on lecture method, the following objective will serve the purpose "after attending the class students will acquire knowledge regarding the practice of lecture method, recognize its value as a teaching method and able to practice it effectively by limiting the demerits."

- **Principle of individual difference:** Good teaching always respects the individuality of students. By considering each student as a unique individual, teacher can pay attention to the individual differences and develop strategies to cater the educational needs of the individual student.

- **Principle of creativity:** By applying creativity, teacher can convert a passive teaching-learning situation into an active one. Through creativity teacher can arouse students' natural motivation to learn and this will in turn convert a usually teacher-centered classroom into a more desirable learner-centered classroom.

- **Principle of selection:** Teacher should select the appropriate content, teaching method, teaching situation, media of instruction, AV aids, textbooks and journal articles for teaching a particular subject matter in order to make teaching more meaningful and comprehensible to students. For example, a teacher dealing with pharmacological basis of nursing practice has to give more attention to patient care implications to be followed before, during and after the drug administration rather than the chemical structure or metabolism of the drug.
- **Principle of division:** Particular teaching activity should have definite divisions based on valid reasons. Teacher should be aware about the division and present the content to the students in well organized steps. For example, nursing management of cirrhosis of liver cannot be taught in a single session. Teacher has to divide the content into clear-cut divisions like definition, classification, etiology, pathology, clinical features, investigations, line of management, complications, prognosis and nursing management and teach each division thoroughly before proceeding to the next by giving adequate weightage to the nursing management.
- **Principle of revision and practice:** During a teaching session, teacher has to revise in the middle and in the end. Revising or summarizing the content in the end of a teaching session is called *recapitulation*. In addition to the recapitulation, the teacher has to motivate the students to practice the learned lessons periodically to enhance easy recollection.
- **Principle of correlation:** The function of teaching is to share knowledge, development of understanding and skills. While teaching, teacher has to take care that the transferred knowledge will not remain segregated and as far as possible correlate with the previous or related knowledge. Correlation helps the student to develop a unified view regarding what is taught. Teaching nursing invariably require correlation because to render comprehensive nursing care, one has to correlate different branches of knowledge. For instance, when teaching the doubling of infant's weight by five months and the triplication by one year, teacher has to encourage the students to recollect the dietary requirements during infancy, which they have studied the first year nutritional classes and correlate the nutritional requirements with the weight gaining process.
- **Principle of connecting with life:** Relationship between life and education is proved undoubtfully and teaching is an integral part of education, so all the teaching activities are connected with life. For instance, the maximum attention span of human beings at a stretch is 40–45 minutes and based on this fact, usually a teaching session is planned for 45 minutes. The aim of nursing is the preservation of life with emphasis to quality. Naturally, teaching nursing is connected to the life of the student as well as to the life of the patient. The principle of connecting with life is the reason for giving one day off once in seven days for nursing students in order to recharge their depleted energy levels and teaching students to administer diuretics, preferably in the morning hours to provide an uninterrupted sleep to the patient for maintaining his biological rhythm of life.

## LEARNER-CENTERED PRINCIPLES OF TEACHING

Ambrose, Bridges, Lovett, Dipietro and Norman in their book "How learning works: 7 research-based principles for smart teaching" explain seven learner-centered principles for teaching.

According to them learning is a process that involves change (in knowledge, beliefs, behaviors or attitudes) and it is something students do rather than something that is transmitted to them. Let us discuss the seven principles that is applicable to all teaching settings.

1. **Students prior knowledge can help or hinder learning:** If a student lacks adequate prior knowledge it may not support new knowledge. Furthermore, if prior knowledge is applied in the wrong context, it may lead to students making faulty assumptions or inappropriate

comparisons to other situations. This principle highlights the need of assessing prior knowledge of students by the teacher before teaching.
2. **How students organize knowledge influence how they learn and apply what they know**: This principle focuses on the need of helping students to gain in-depth knowledge through building effective organized knowledge. Faculty should help students to organize knowledge in a more meaningful manner.
3. **Student's motivation generates, directs and sustains what they do to learn:** Student's motivation is essential for successful learning. Teachers can increase or decrease student motivation. Teachers always focus on enhancing student motivation by creating a positive and supportive environment for learning.
4. **To develop mastery, students must acquire component skills, practice integrating them and know when to apply what they have learned:** This principle is concerned with tasks teachers expect students to accomplish. Three elements of mastery of student learning are: (a) acquisition of component skills, (b) practice in integrating these skills, and (c) knowledge of when to apply the skills. Through various activities teachers provide opportunity to attain these elements of mastery in learning.
5. **Goal-directed practice coupled with targeted feedback are important to learning:** This principle underlines the importance of providing feedback to students. Feedback should be targeted to learning goals, timely and frequent. Fundamental purpose of feedback is to keep learners practice moving forward and toward improvement. This principle also emphasize the need of assisting students effort in focusing on what they need to learn (goal) rather than what they already know. When teachers help students to set performance goals at a reasonable and productive level of challenge they also make their own instruction more efficient and focused.
6. **Students' current levels of development interact with the social, emotional and intellectual climate of the classroom and have an impact on learning:** This principle focuses on the relationship between students' level of development and learning outcomes. Students are holistic beings and intellectual, social and emotional climate of classroom influence their learning experiences.
7. **To become self-directed learners, students must learn to assess the demands of the task, evaluate their own knowledge and skills, plan their approach, monitor their progress and adjust their strategies as needed:** This principle focuses on "self-directed learning". Students face challenges in managing their own learning. The skills for achieving "self-directed learning" are: assessing the task at hand; evaluating their strength and weakness; planning appropriate approaches to accomplish tasks; and applying strategies for learning and monitoring performance.

## QUALITIES/MARKS OF GOOD TEACHING

In addition to the basic information related to the subject matter, learning outcomes and previous knowledge of students, awareness regarding the criteria of good teaching is essential to carry out teaching in an effective way. The below mentioned qualities of teaching will guide you in carrying out teaching in an impressive manner.

- ❖ **Good teaching recognizes individual differences:** Good teaching always respect the individuality of students. Considering each student as unique individual, good teaching pay attention to the individual differences and develops strategies to cater the educational needs of the individual student.
- ❖ **Good teaching is a cause to learn:** Good teaching promotes proactive learning, i.e., the child is learning for himself as a result of intrinsic motivation instead of extrinsic motivation.

- **Good teaching provides opportunities for activity:** Good teaching keeps the student active and this will promote his physical and mental health.
- **Good teaching involves in guiding learning:** In learning, direction is important than speed. Good teaching helps the student to develop desirable learning habits to achieve the desired aims.
- **Good teaching is kindly and sympathetic:** Good teaching creates an atmosphere of acceptance, sympathy and understanding. Nowadays, threat is not considered as an ingredient of teaching activity. Students should feel comfortable in the presence of teacher.
- **Good teaching reduces the distance between teacher and student:** Barriers should be kept minimum between teachers and students. Teachers have to come out of the glass tower and remain approachable by conveying a sense of trust.
- **Good teaching is flexible and not tied to any method:** There is no shortage of teaching methods and teacher is free to device new methods of teaching without violating the basic principles of teaching. A good teacher not only selects teaching method according to the context but also individualize his method of teaching with a distinctive idea. Good teaching is always flexible. Instead of adhering to a single well-known method, teacher has to try other methods also as needed or indicated.
- **Good teaching incorporates cooperativeness and suggestiveness:** Teaching is a teamwork and as team-mates, teacher and students achieve more through combined efforts. Good teacher always request cooperation and encourage the students to come up with suggestions.
- **Good teaching is democratic:** Teaching is meant for all students in the class. Irrespective of the intelligence, socioeconomic status and gender, teacher has to motivate all students to think and express their ideas. Freely expressed ideas will make the class atmosphere more active and interesting. Student can be compared to a kite in the hands of the teacher. Just like the kite in the sky, student is free to think and act but teacher should keep the controlling thread intact and use it appropriately to control the student.
- **Good teaching provides desirable and selective information:** Good teaching always identify desirable and needed information from the jungle of information. While sharing information, teacher should also consider the need and level of students. Even though philosophy of education is included both in the BSc (Nursing) and MSc (Nursing) syllabus, an intelligent teacher never teaches the same content for both categories and limit the explanation according to the level of students when teaching BSc (Nursing) students.
- **Good teaching helps the child to adjust himself to his environment:** This is the very aim of teaching and good teaching helps the child to overcome the adverse situations by concentrating on his strengths.
- **Good teaching is progressive:** Good teaching will unleash the talents of students and enable them to reach good positions in life. Good teaching is progressive in the sense that it will contribute to the further development of the student.
- **Good teaching always consider the level of students:** In order to make the teaching more student-friendly and interesting, teacher has to consider previous knowledge of students, level of intelligence, receptivity and mental maturity.
- **Good teaching lead to emotional stability:** Good teaching not only trains the student to behave rationally than emotionally but also teaches to ventilate emotions in a healthy way.
- **Good teaching is diagnostic and remedial:** A talented teacher always diagnoses the problems of students, especially those related to the learning through proper assessment and evaluation. This is usually done in the beginning stage itself and helps the student overcome the problem by suggesting or implementing appropriate remedial measures.

- **Good teaching is stimulating:** Good teaching prepares the students for receiving the knowledge. Entry of a talented teacher into the class itself will send a wave of enthusiasm and makes the students active and receptive.
- **Good teaching should be on the basis of previous knowledge of the student:** Good teaching always correlates previous knowledge of the students with the present teaching. This will help the students to get a unified view regarding what is being taught.
- **Good teaching will develop initiative, independence in thinking and doing, self-reliance and confidence among students:** Good teaching never spoon-feed students with prefabricated knowledge, on the contrary it fosters initiative, critical thinking, hardwork and self-confidence. In short, good teaching equips the student to lead a socially and economically productive life.
- **Good teaching is carefully planned in advance:** Planning is essential for any activity and particularly for effective teaching. When a teacher fails to take one hour class effectively for 50 students due to inadequate preparation, total time wasted is 51 hours. Then you can imagine the enormous amount of time wasted in an academic year due to inadequate preparation from the side of a teacher. The proverb "if you fail to plan, you are planning to fail" is applicable to teaching also.

## MAXIMS OF TEACHING

Maxims of teaching are accepted truth or general rule of conduct or the laws which are essentially to be followed by the teacher while teaching. Maxims include:

- **Proceed from known to unknown:** The teacher has to correlate the learning of the students with their experiences and previous knowledge. Teacher has to start with something which is known to the student and then proceed to unknown. A class on geriatric nursing could be more convincing, if the teacher starts the class by inviting students opinion regarding the peculiarities or needs of the old age people from their own experiences and then proceeding to further details which are unknown to them.
- **Proceed from concrete to abstract:** This is simply the application of commonsense in teaching. It is quite natural that students learn first the things which are seen and handled by them. Students can comprehend new ideas only when they are taught with sufficient illustration. So, every teaching activity should be enriched with sufficient illustration. For instance, while teaching central nervous system, teacher should first teach the anatomy of brain with the help of a specimen or model (concrete aspect) then teach about the afferent impulses and efferent impulses by using diagrams (abstract aspect).
- **Proceed from simple to complex:** It is always better to teach the most simple lessons first and then the complex one. While conducting classes on pediatric nursing, the teacher has to teach simple topics like differences between pediatric nursing and adult nursing before proceeding to complex procedures and disease conditions.
- **Proceed from easy to more difficult:** This is self-explanatory. When planning to teach the nursing management of cirrhosis of liver, the teacher has to arrange the different aspects of the disease condition in an increasing order of difficulty like definition, classification, etiology, pathology, pathogenesis, etc.
- **Proceed inductively:** In inductive teaching, teaching is made effective with the help of a suitable example. Usually the topic is introduced to the students by way of stating a befitting example and through analyzing the example they would be able to understand the general rules, definitions, formulas, etc. A teacher can start the class on amputation by asking a simple question like "what do you do to save your rose plant if one of its branches is severely infected with pests or fungus and not responding to pesticides". Naturally,

students suggest the cutting down of the infected branch in order to save the entire rose plant. When the students give their answer, teacher can correlate the rose plant with the human body and can introduce the topic as follows "just like the infected branch of the rose plant sometimes the limbs of the human body can also get infected or damaged beyond repair. In such a situation in order to save the life of the patient we have to cut down the infected limb and this cutting down of the irreparably damaged limb is simply called amputation. Let us see the details of amputation". Through this example students can be easily introduced to the topic of amputation.

- **Proceed from general to specific:** While proceeding from general to specific, general rules are explained first and from that specificity is arisen. While teaching growth and development, the teacher explains the universal phenomenon of growth in general by citing animals and plants as examples and then proceeds to the specific features of growth and development exhibited by human beings.
- **Proceed from specific to general:** In certain situations, it is imperative to proceed from specific to general. When proceeding from specific to general, first the teacher has to present the specific facts to the students before the facts are taught to them in general. For instance, the role of protein in body building and repair has to be specified before generalizing the consequences of under nutrition by showing the picture of emaciated children as an example.
- **Proceed from indefinite to definite:** The ideas of students in the initial stages are indefinite and vague. These ideas are to be made definite, clear, precise and systematic by adopting effective teaching methods. In this refining process of making definite ideas from the indefinite ideas, teacher has to employ appropriate use of AV aids and other strategies as needed. A first year nursing student possess only some indefinite and vague ideas about nursing and a talented teacher transforms these ideas to a definite one by providing details of nursing such as definition of nursing, history of nursing, qualities of a good nurse, etc.
- **Proceed from empirical to rational:** Empirical knowledge is gained through observation and experience. One peculiarity of empirical knowledge is that it lacks scientific background. Rational knowledge is built upon a scientific basis and is more dignified than the empirical knowledge. As a result of their day-to-day life experiences students gain empirical knowledge. Teacher has to proceed from this empirical knowledge to rational knowledge by explaining the scientific aspects to the students. First year nursing students possess the empirical knowledge of placing a wet cloth on the forehead for reducing the temperature. While teaching the nursing management of hyperpyrexia, the teacher has to convert the above said empirical knowledge to a rational one by explaining the scientific principle of placing the wet cloth on the forehead for reducing the temperature.
- **Proceed from whole to parts:** Whole is more meaningful to students than the separate parts of the whole. The whole approach helps the students understand the relationship between different parts and the resulting correlation makes learning easier and meaningful. While teaching osteology, anatomy teacher has to give a brief description of the whole skeletal system by mentioning its functions, total number of bones, etc., before dealing with different individual bones or parts of the skeletal system like clavicle, humerous, etc. This will help the students to learn individual bones in relation to the whole skeletal system in a more meaningful way.
- **Proceed from part to whole:** In some situations, teacher has to proceed from part to whole for providing information in a meaningful way. For example, while teaching the qualities of an ideal chemical disinfectant, teacher proceeds from part to whole by explaining the qualities one by one and finally explains the whole qualities by the end of the class.

- **Proceed from analysis to synthesis:** Analysis means breaking a problem into component parts and synthesis is the reverse, i.e., putting together this separate part into a complete whole. This approach is widely used in teaching nursing. Nursing management of a disease condition is taught to the students analytically by splitting the content into component parts like definition, etiology, pathology, clinical features, medical or surgical management, nursing management, rehabilitation, etc., then they are trained to synthesis all these different components into one whole as needed in order to provide meticulous nursing care to the patient in the clinical area. A nursing student who is taught about the different aspects of cardiac arrest can easily synthesis these aspects into a usable form while caring a patient with cardiac arrest and can possibly revive the patient quickly.
- **Proceed from overview to details:** Students can easily comprehend, if the teacher proceeds from overview to details. For example, while explaining the surgical instruments needed for performing cesarean, teacher has to introduce all the instruments by listing down their names before explaining their uses and ways of handling each instrument in detail.
- **From observation to reasoning:** The teacher has to provide an opportunity for the students to see and notice the factors involved in a particular topic or context before explaining the reasons associated with it or eliciting reasons from the students. For example, in the pediatric ward, teacher has to provide a chance to the students to observe a 10-month-old child who has been admitted with complaints of developmental delay before explaining the reason by herself or asking questions to the students regarding the hospitalization of the child.
- **Proceed from psychological to logical:** This is the fundamental approach in teaching. Some of the maxims like concrete to abstract and simple to complex are based on this approach. Psychological aspect is student-centered and concerned with the receptiveness of students, reaction of students, recalling ability of students, listening to student's needs, etc. Logical aspect is teacher-centered and deals with the systematic arrangement of the content, decision regarding when to teach, etc. During teaching, teacher has to consider the psychological aspect before proceeding to logical aspects. For example, while teaching first year students, even though the teacher possesses in-depth knowledge regarding the nursing care of dying patients, in order to teach this sensitive topic without embarrassing them, the teacher has to consider the psychological status or maturity of students before proceeding logically by explaining the needed contents only in a nonthreatening manner.

Please note that the maxim of teaching is not the final word in teaching. A hard-working teacher need not be worried or preoccupied with the maxims of teaching because maxims of teaching will naturally become the part and parcel of the teaching activity in the due course of time. Moreover, most of the maxims communicate same meaning or sense even though they are spelled differently.

## TEACHING STYLES

Paul B Thronton classify teaching styles into three types namely: directing, discussing and delegating. The most effective teachers vary their styles depending on the nature of the subject matter, the phases of the course among other factors.

### Direction Style

The directing style promotes learning through listening and following direction with this style, the teacher tells the students what to do, how to do it and when it needs to be done. The teacher imparts knowledge to the students through lectures, assigned readings, audiovisual presentations, demonstrations, role playing and other means. Students gain information primarily by listening, taking notes, doing role plays and practicing what they are told to do. The only way to seek feedback is by asking "Do you understand the instructions".

## Discussion Style

The discussion style promotes learning through interaction. In this style, the teacher encourages students actively in discussion by asking students to respond to challenging questions. The teacher acts as a facilitator by guiding the discussion to a logical conclusion. Students learn by logical thinking based on facts and data.

## Delegating Style

The delegating style promotes learning through empowerment. With this style, the teacher assign tasks students work on indecently, either individually or in groups.

Instead of adopting a single style, it is advisable to use an appropriate mix of teaching styles. Structure the classes to include some good aspects of each teaching style. Using an appropriate mix of teaching styles helps students learn, grow and become more independent. Giving importance to only one style causes students to lose interest and become more dependent on the teacher.

It is advisable to use more of the directing style in first part of the academic year. In the middle part teacher can use more of discussion style and in the latter part teacher can adopt more of delegating style.

## CHARACTERISTICS OF EFFECTIVE TEACHING

The fact that educational institutions are spending a high proportion of the budget for maintaining the teaching staff and an increased focus on the performance indicators of teaching quality have motivated the teachers to practice the teaching activity in an effective way. Judy, Brophy and Good suggested the below mentioned characteristics of effective teaching:

- ❖ **Giving structured information:** Teaching is mainly concerned with transferring information. Students may not have the full idea regarding what they are learning or why they are learning, so teachers have to structure their instruction in order to help students in learning. Giving information in a structured way also help students to utilize the academic learning time effectively. Academic learning time is the time a student spends appropriately engaged with content.
- ❖ **Quantity and pacing of instruction:** The amount learned is related to the opportunity to learn. A successful teacher always organize the content effectively and pace the instruction in a comprehensible manner, according to the receptivity level of students. The teacher has to develop a routine pace of instruction by going fast while teaching simple topics and she should slow down when dealing with difficult areas so that students can get acquainted with the pace, follow easily and take notes if needed. By adopting a student-friendly routine pace of instruction, students will get time to interpret what the teacher has told and thereby she can ensure successful learning.
- ❖ **Teacher expectations:** Efficient teachers expect their students to learn well. They do not just accept student participation in teaching-learning process or any behavioral change but demand for participation and behavioral change. Lack of teacher expectation for learning can degrade the morale of students.
- ❖ **Teacher enthusiasm:** Nothing is infectious as enthusiasm. An efficient teacher is always enthusiastic and actively involved in the teaching activity. An enthusiastic teacher can

motivate the students to learn, encourage participation of students in the teaching activity and create a student-centered classroom in an easy manner.
- **Teacher clarity:** Teacher clarity is defined as the ability to explain and demonstrate correctly. Nature of subject matter and limited audiovisual resources makes teaching clarity essential for successful teaching. In order to attain this quality, teacher has to spend considerable time to prepare lessons and to practice demonstrations.
- **Teacher feedback:** Learning is a progressive activity and in between learner has to know about his or her level of performance or achievements. Teacher has to provide timely feedback, preferably through formal ways of asking questions or conducting evaluation tests. Teacher can also set target expectation for the students so that they can know easily whether the appropriate progress is being made or not. Positive feedback always motivate the students. Efficient teachers possess good questioning skills and most of the time questions elicit correct answers. If the student's response is incorrect, they have to help the student to find the right answer.
- **Emotional climate:** Neutral or warm classroom environment is essential for effective teaching. Try to avoid negative climate. A teacher need not be worried too much or about being liked or being popular with students.
- **Teacher observational skill:** Observation is an excellent method of assessing students. Efficient teachers possess both the general and specific observational skills. Being able to observe correctly is an important skill, especially in the case of nursing teachers.
- **Handling assignments:** Assignments play a major role in today's teaching-learning process. While dealing with assignments, teacher has to state clear expectations of what is expected, how to get help and what to do when finished.
- **Management skills:** Efficient teachers are first of all effective managers. They know how to manage the classroom for achieving desirable ends.
- **Ability to develop appropriate progressions:** Efficient teachers not only help students to attain progress but also consider this progress while teaching them. In order to ensure appropriate progression, teacher has to teach the content in relation to the learners background knowledge rather than blindly following the content. For instance, while teaching the impact of consumer protection act on nursing, teacher need not explain full details because students might have gained knowledge regarding the impact of consumer protection act on healthcare professions though different media like newspaper, television, etc. So considering the progress achieved by the students in the matter of consumer protection act, teacher has to teach the topic in a discussion form by eliciting students opinion instead of simply reading out the content from a prepared note.
- **Context specific:** This is the essence of teaching. An intelligent teacher always take into account the situations and teach only the relevant subject matter. Revising and highlighting the importance of universal precautions just before posting the students in the operation theater exemplifies context specific nature of teaching.

## TEACHING SKILLS

Teaching is a complex process. For conducting teaching in a successful manner, teacher has to possess a variety of teaching skills. *A teaching skill can be defined as a set of teacher behaviors which are specially effective in bringing about desired behavioral changes in students.* The Australian Advisory Committee on research and development in education has analyzed teaching into 140 skills. Allen and Ryan of the Stanford University have suggested fourteen skills. It is better to relate teaching skills with different stages of a lesson as shown in **Table 6.1**.

Even though all the skills discussed in **Table 6.1** are important, some of them deserve more attention as they are used more frequently in teaching. They are: (a) Skill of stimulus variation; (b) Skill of explanation; (c) Skill of reinforcement; (d) Skill of promoting student participation; (e) Skill of using examples; (f) Questioning skills. As we have already discussed reinforcement and promoting pupil participation elsewhere, let us discuss the remaining ones.

**TABLE 6.1:** Component of teaching skills associated with different stages of a lesson.

| Stages of a lesson | Component teaching skills |
|---|---|
| Planning stage | • Writing instructional objectives<br>• Selecting the content<br>• Organizing the content<br>• Selection of the audiovisual aids material |
| Introductory stage | • Creating set for introducing the lesson<br>• Introducing the lesson |
| Presentation stage | **Questioning skills**<br>• Structuring classroom questions<br>• Fluency in questioning<br>• Probing questions<br>• Questions—delivery and distribution<br>• The use of higher order questions<br>• Divergent questions<br>• Response management.<br>**Presentation skills**<br>• Pacing of the lesson<br>• Lecturing<br>• Explaining<br>• Discussing<br>• Demonstrating<br>• Illustration with examples<br>• Using teaching aids<br>• Stimulus variation<br>• Silence and non-verbal cues<br>• Reinforcement<br>**Managerial skills**<br>• Promoting pupil participation<br>• Recognizing attending behavior |
| Closing stage | • Management of the class<br>• Planned repetition<br>• Giving assignments<br>• Evaluating pupils progress<br>• Diagnosing pupil learning difficulties and taking remedial measures |

## Stimulus Variation

The need for this skill-varying the stimulus-arises because sustained uniformity of presentation can lead to boredom and mental inactivity. Again, it is based on research evidence, which indicates that changes in perceived environment attract attention and stimulate thought. Perrot describes the behaviors associated with this skill as follows:

- **Teacher movements:** Deliberate and timed shifts around in the class room can help revive and/or sustain interest. However, avoid nervous, fussy and irritating movements like obsessively pacing up and down the same part of the room.
- **Focusing behavior:** Communication can be aided by the use of *verbal focusing* (giving emphasis to particular words, statements or directions) and *gestural focusing* (using eye movements, facial expressions and movement of head, arms and body). *Verbal-gestural focusing,* which is a combination of the two, can also be useful.
- **Changes in speech patterns:** This involves changing the quality, expressiveness, tone and rate of speech, all of which can increase attention. Planned silences and pauses can also be effective.
- **Changing interaction:** Teacher and entire class, teacher and student and student and student—instead of teacher monologue.
- **Shifting sensory channels:** Information is processed by means of the five senses and research suggests that pupils ability to take information can be increased by appealing to sight and sound alternatively. Thus, the teacher has to judiciously use audiovisual aids while teaching.

## Explanation

Research findings indicate that clarity of presentation is something that can exert considerable influence on effective teaching. The following factors contribute to the effectiveness in explanation:

- **Continuity:** Maintaining a strong connecting thread through a lesson is a matter of greater importance. This should be perfectly clear and diversions from it should be kept to a minimum.
- **Simplicity:** Try to use simple, intelligible and grammatical sentences. A common cause of failure is the inclusion of too much information in one sentence. Keep sentences short and if relationships are complex, consider communicating them by visual means. As regards vocabulary, use simple words well within the class's own vocabulary. If specialist, subject-specific language is used, make sure the terms employed are carefully defined and understood.
- **Explicitness:** One reason for ineffectiveness in presenting new material to a class is the assumption that the students understand more than is in fact the case. Where explanations are concerned one must be as explicit as possible.

## USE OF EXAMPLES

The use of examples is a fundamental aspect of teaching and there is no need to stress its importance, particularly in the presentation of new material. Perrott offers the following guidelines for the effective use of examples: (a) Start with simple examples and work towards more complex ones; (b) Start with examples relevant to pupils' experience and level of knowledge; (c) Relate examples to the principles, idea or generalization being taught; (d) Check to see whether you have accomplished your objectives by asking the pupils to give you examples which illustrate the point you were trying to make. Teaching with the help of examples is known as **inductive teaching.**

# QUESTIONS AND QUESTIONING

Asking questions constitutes a major part of teacher's activities. Teachers use questions not only for cognitive/intellectual reasons (concerning the subject matter of the lesson) but for emotional/social reasons (to cater for different personalities) and for managerial reasons (to minimize bad behaviors and to keep students on task).

## Purposes in Asking Questions

Purposes in asking questions are: (a) To arouse interest and curiosity concerning a topic; (b) To focus attention on a particular issue or concept; (c) To develop an active approach to learning; (d) To stimulate pupils to ask questions to themselves and others; (e) To structure a task in such a way that learning will be maximized; (f) To diagnose specific difficulties inhibiting pupil learning; (g) To communicate to the group that involvement in the lesson is expected and that overt participation by all members of the group is valued; (h) To provide an opportunity for pupils to assimilate and reflect upon information; (i) To involve pupils in using an inferred cognitive operation on the assumption that this will assist in developing thinking skills; (j) To develop reflection and comment by pupils on the responses of other members of the group, both pupils and teachers; (k) To provide an opportunity for pupils to learn vicariously through discussion; (l) To express a genuine interest in the ideas and feelings of the pupil.

## Functions of Questioning

The skillful questioning of a class performs a number of important functions. *Socially,* it helps to establish relationships and integrate groups through face to face interaction. *Psychologically,* it assists in increasing, developing and maintaining a healthy emotional and intellectual climate as well as establishing appropriate levels of motivation. *Educationally,* one function of questioning is to elicit information. Thus, it may probe the extent of student's prior learning before a new subject or area of learning is introduced; or it may help to revise earlier learning; or consolidate recent teaching and learning. More than this, however, questions should have *teaching value,* that is, in asking the question a teacher is helping the pupil 'to focus and clarify and thus have thoughts and perceptions that he would not have had otherwise'.

## Framing the Question

Teacher has to prepare questions beforehand as part of or to accompany a lesson plan. There are at least three reasons for this need. First, questions should be precisely and unambiguously worded so that they elicit the answer the teacher intends. The livelihood of misunderstandings and wrong answers is greater with unprepared, impromptu questions. Second, where a connected series of questions is required, it is difficult to organize them sequentially and logically on the spur of the movement. And third, a teacher is better prepared to deal with the unexpected if he/she possesses a body of well-thought-out questions.

It is particularly useful when framing questions to distinguish two broad kinds—*questions which test knowledge and questions which create knowledge.* The former are referred to as *lower-order cognitive questions* and the latter as *high-order cognitive questions.*

Lower-order cognitive questions embrace chiefly *recall, comprehension and application;* higher-order questions by contrast, involve *analysis, synthesis and evaluation.* Low-order questions tend to be closed questions (when a known response is sought); higher-order questions tend to be open questions (when the type of response is known but the actual response is not, students being free to respond in their own way).

Some questions need to be handled carefully or in certain circumstances, avoid altogether. These include: (a) Questions inviting a *yes or no* answer not to be used excessively, for a student has as much chance of being right as of being wrong if he guesses. Where such answers are unavoidable, another question, such as *how or why* should follow in order to provide explanatory or supportive evidence for the yes or no. Occasionally, a yes or no answer can be of disciplinary assistance when attentions are wandering: For example, 'do you understand, Allen?; (b) Questions having several equally good answers should be avoided if the teacher has only one answer in mind. Questions having several equally good answers are permissible, however, when a teacher is building up a composite answer, for example, when introducing a topic or project; (c) Composite questions-those involving a number of interrogatives—present difficulties even with brighter students and should be avoided; (d) Do not use questions beginning 'who can tell me. ....? or 'does anyone know. ..? as these may lead to various members of the class shouting out answers; (e) Questions testing powers of expression should be treated with care. Similarly, those seeking definitions of words or concepts, especially abstract ones, should be handled carefully; (f) General questions that are vague and aimless should not be used (for example, what do you know about typhoid fever?) Precision and clarity should be sought from the outset; (g) Guessing questions are sometimes useful for stimulating a student's imagination and actively involving him in discussion. If used too often, however, they encourage thoughtless responses; (h) Leading questions (those framed in such a way as to suggest or imply the desired answer—Alexander Fleming discovered pencillin, wasn't he?) and rhetorical questions (those to which student is not expected to reply—do you want me to send you outside?) should be avoided because the former tend to reinforce a student's dependence on the teacher and undermine independent thought, whereas the latter may provoke unwanted or facetious replies. Questions should be asked only if the teacher wants a real answer; (i) Elliptical questions—those worded so that a student supplies a missing word or missing words are of value when used to encourage students with learning or behavioral difficulties. Provided they are not used too often, they can give variety to questioning session.

### Asking Questions and Receiving the Answer

Questions should be asked in simple, conversational language and in a friendly and challenging manner, ensuring that the student knows what kind of answer is expected. A useful procedure is as follows: put the question to the class, pause briefly, then name the student you wish to answer. A sequence of this kind encourages everyone to listen and prepare an answer in anticipation of being asked. Respondents should be name at random rather than in predetermined and systematic way, thus avoiding selective listening. As suggested earlier, it is to the teachers advantage at this point to have prepared questions with particular students in mind. The more difficult questions for brighter students and easier ones to students experiencing learning difficulties will help sustain different motivational levels and maintain the flow of the lesson. It is especially important in this respect to try to draw out the more shy members of the class. The teacher should also check the tendency to neglect students sitting at the back or sides of the classroom when distributing questions.

Once a question has been put to a student, it should be left with him/her long enough for an answer to emerge. Lack of preparation on the part of the teacher or impatience, may lead him/her to follow one question immediately with others, or to modify the original, re-word it or explain it. Such activities merely confuse students.

The techniques of *prompting and probing* are often useful in class questioning sessions. Prompting involves giving hints to help a student. In addition to eliciting appropriate answers, prompts backed up with teacher encouragement help hesitant children answer more confidently. On receiving an answer, it is sometimes necessary to probe a student for additional information and this may be especially the case after a factual question. Probing in this context may take the form of further information, directing the student to think more deeply about his or her answer, inviting a critical interpretation, focusing the response on a related issue or encouraging the student to express himself/herself more clearly. Sometimes a correct answer needs to be repeated to make sure all have heard it. Wrong answers can be of value in clearing up misunderstandings, obscurities and difficulties, provided they are treated tactfully and without disrupting the lesson to any great extent. It is very important for students to receive information on the correctness or otherwise of their answers. This is especially the case for low achievers. Feedback from the teacher is the easiest way to maintain interest and is most effective when given after an individual response. Praise and censure should be used with discrimination. Praise is quickly devalued if used too readily; and undue censure can be discouraging. Excessive criticism directed at weaker students can do nothing but harm.

Teacher should also consider the students' questions to her. Nothing shows more clearly that a teacher and class are on friendly terms than evidence of students sensibly questioning the teacher about difficult points.

## Key Factors for Effective Questioning

Some key factors for effective questioning are:

- **Structuring:** Providing sign posts for the sequence of questions and the topic, indicating the types of answers expected.
- **Pitching and putting clearly:** Considering how broad/narrow to make the question, the order of the question, low to high, the vocabulary to be used, the degree of openness or closure of the question.
- **Directing and distributing:** Going around the whole class.
- **Prompting and probing:** Considering what to say in a prompt or a probe, rephrasing, reviewing.
- **Pausing and pacing:** Allowing thinking time, particularly for more complex questions.
- **Listening and responding:** Deciding the most appropriate form of response.
- **Sequencing:** Introducing, opening out, converging, extending and lifting.

## Common Errors in Questioning

Common errors in questioning are: (a) Asking too many questions at once; (b) Asking a question and answering yourself; (c) Asking questions only to the brightest or most likeable students; (d) Asking a difficult question too early; (e) Asking irrelevant questions; (f) Always asking the same type of questions; (g) Asking questions in a threatening way; (h) Not indicating a change in the type of question; (i) Not using probing questions; (j) Not giving students time to think; (k) Not correcting wrong answers; (l) Ignoring answers; (m) Failing to see the implications of answers; (n) Failing to build on answers.

## QUALITIES OF A GOOD TEACHER

Developments in technologies for communicating and disseminating information have a large potential impact on the practice of teaching because teaching is an activity in which communicating and disseminating information are significant aspects. But Niasbitt suggested that increase in technology create a compensating need for more human touch. He also pointed out that without the appropriate human touch, the adoption of new technology on a widespread basis is rejected. This high touch-high tech vision clearly states that nothing can substitute or replace the human component or human interaction in teaching and to become a good teacher demands constant and conscious effort from the side of teacher. The traditional or recent concepts of teaching never disagree with the below mentioned desirable qualities of a teacher **(Fig. 6.1)**.

- **Desirable personal traits:** Teacher should be a person who is just, likeable, approachable, enthusiastic, caring, active, have neat appearance, dress modestly and simply, have a sense of humour and always be a helping hand to the students.
- **User of effective teaching–learning methods:** A good teacher always follow the guidelines intended for selecting the appropriate method (*see* guidelines for selecting the teaching–learning methods) and use different methods or effective and efficient combination of methods for achieving learning aims.
- **Creator of a good classroom environment:** A good teacher always makes the classroom a student-centered environment rather than a teacher-centered one by encouraging student participation in the teaching–learning process, paying special attention to weak students, controlling the students and designing teaching according to the capacities, abilities and level of students.
- **Mastery of competencies:** This include the ability to inspire students, providing counseling and guidance as needed, possess some special skills and abilities in teaching, have knowledge and effective management skills, ability to judge students fairly, possess leadership qualities, evaluate the performance of students continuously, able to perform self-analysis and ability to accept criticisms positively.
- **Professional decision maker:** By utilizing the competencies, teacher has to decide whom to teach, why to teach, where to teach, what to teach, how to teach and when to teach.
- **In-depth knowledge of subject matter:** Different from the past students have access to latest information on subject matter. Hence, teacher should possess in-depth knowledge of subject matter.

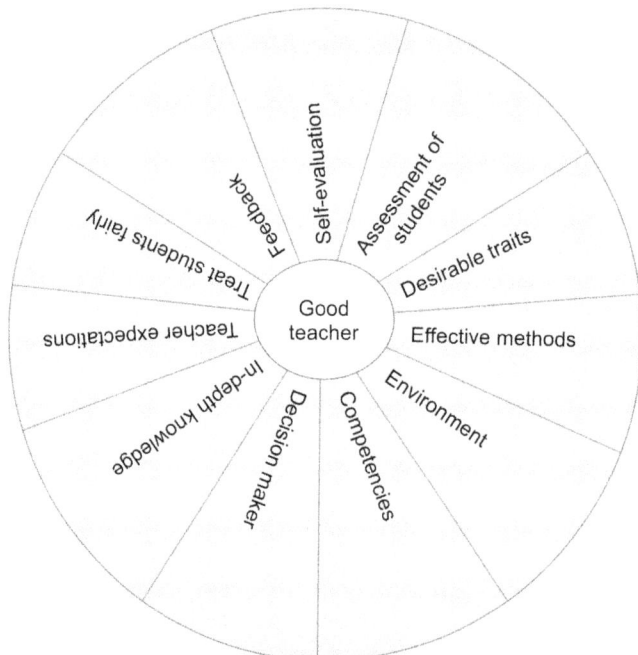

**Fig. 6.1:** Qualities of a good teacher.

- **Teacher expectations:** Teacher expectation on students is important for motivating students. Teacher need to expect more from students than giving assignments.
- **Treat students fairly:** Express a strong trust in students. Believe that students want to learn and can learn. Encourage students to explore and hunt for more knowledge. Share sources of learning material. Treat students with simple decency.
- **Provide timely feedback:** Proper feedback is essential to keep learners practice moving forward and toward improvement. Feedback should be targeted to learning goals, timely and frequent.
- **Assessment of students:** Have a systematic program to evaluate efforts of students. Avoid judging students on arbitrary standards. Assessment of students should be based on learning objectives.
- **Assist to become self-directed learners:** Students find it difficult to manage their own learning: Teachers should help students to become self-directed learners.
- **Self-evaluation:** Excellent teachers develop and improve their abilities through self-evaluation, reflection and willingness to change.
- **Teacher awareness:** According to Vaneesa R, excellent teachers have five awarenesses namely: awareness of learner, awareness of teacher-learner interaction, awareness of self as a teacher, awareness of teaching practice and awareness of context of teaching.
- **Role model:** Even though, this is last mentioned, author believes this is the first and foremost quality required by a teacher. Through role modeling she can become a great example for students regarding merits of good living.

# THE HAY MCBER MODEL OF TEACHER EFFECTIVENESS

The Hay McBer model of teacher effectiveness envisages three compulsory factors contributing to learner's progress-teaching skills, professional characteristics and classroom climate **(Fig. 6.2)**.

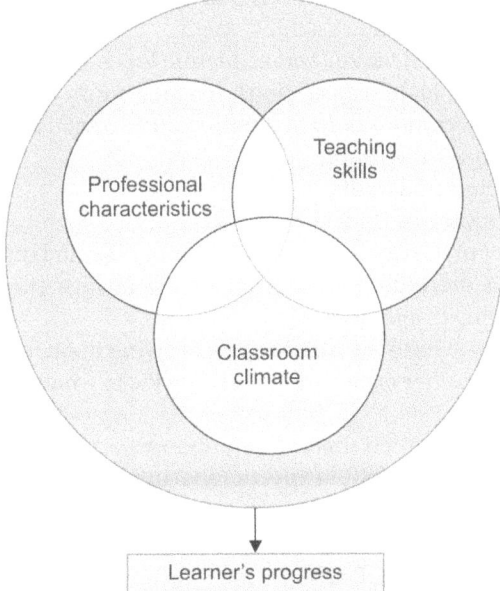

**Fig. 6.2:** Hay McBer model of teacher effectiveness.

Source: Hay McBer: Research into effectiveness: DfEE; 2000.

# REFLECTIVE TEACHER

"A reflective teacher is one who continuously evaluates performance in terms of learning outcomes of learners and enhance teaching ability through collaboration and deliberate practice". In simple words, deliberate practice is repeating a procedure with focused attention for improving performance. Deliberate practice helps to improve performance through acquiring more complex and refined cognitive mechanisms.

In Krampe's words, "deliberate practice in teaching involves more than just repetition: it requires activities that are designed to improve performance challenge the learner and provide feedback".

## Characteristics of a Reflective Teacher

- A reflective teacher continuously evaluates her performance
- A reflective teacher always strives to improve performance and give preference to learner-centered teaching strategies.
- A reflective teacher challenge the ability of learner through deliberate practice
- A deliberate teacher believes that teaching is a set of skills and mastery can be achieved through deliberate practice.
- A reflective teacher is always aware about importance of "contingent teaching". In contingent teaching, teacher conducts teaching in accordance with the progress or achievement of learners. If the learner acquire a particular level of knowledge, then teacher offer less support. If the learner has not yet acquired or mastered that knowledge the teacher provides more support.

# TEACHER EXPECTATIONS

In simple terms, teacher expectations are beliefs of a teacher about the achievement of students or learning outcomes. Teacher expectations are important because they influence the selection of teaching strategies by the teacher and can have an impact on student learning. Teacher expectation influence student's achievement.

Student behavior such as motivation and academic focus help in the formation of teacher expectations. Teacher with high expectations teaches more effectively, leading to high achievements. Teacher expectations help in building positive and respectful relationship with students which in turn promote learning.

**Teacher with high expectation usually:**
- Listen to and affirm responses from all students.
- Lead incorrect answer to the right conclusions through guided questioning.
- Give positive feedback on student's response and use positive non-verbal communication such as smiling, nodding in agreement, etc.
- Allow time for students to problem-solving before giving them feedback.
- Clearly communicate teacher expectations. Be specific in what teacher expects students to know and be able to do.
- Create an environment in which there is genuine respect for students and belief in their ability. Encourage students to fulfill expectations and offer praise when expectations are fulfilled.

# TEACHER-STUDENT INTERACTION

The interaction between teacher and learner is an integral part of teaching–learning process. According to Halstead and Billings, "teacher-student interaction is a two-way communication process intended to bring out behavior modification of the learner in accordance with the predetermined behavioral objectives by effectively processing the feedback received from students". Krause believe that positive teacher-student interaction can be achieved by shared-acceptance, affection, trust, respect, care and cooperation between teacher and student.

Teacher-student interaction is important for the following reasons:
- Create a classroom environment essential to attain learning outcomes.
- Helpful in meeting developmental, emotional and educational needs of students.
- Promote student's self-esteem, motivation and help in adopting effective learning styles.
- Essential for proper development of the student's academic self-confidence and enhancing their enthusiasm and endurance.
- Greater satisfaction for students with academic life and less chance to dropping out from institution.
- Help students to develop a sense of purpose and competencies required for a successful life.
- Positive impact on students vocational preparation and intellectual development.

Student-teacher interaction can be formal or informal, occurring either inside or outside the instructional settings. Although most interactions with teacher occurs within the formal classroom settings, informal interactions tend to be more helpful for students.

In Gebberd's opinion, at least following five factors should take into account for promoting positive teacher-student interaction in the classroom.
- Reduce the central position of the teacher.
- Appreciate the uniqueness of learners.
- Allow students to express themselves in meaningful ways.
- Give opportunities for students to explain their ideas with the teacher.
- Give students opportunities to explain their opinions.

Jia recommends following five strategies to promote teacher-student interaction.
1. Appreciate self-esteem of individual learner.
2. Understanding learner's linguistic levels.
3. Following appropriate questioning style and improving questioning strategies.
4. Building positive teacher-student relationship.
5. Reducing classroom anxiety.

## TEACHER AWARENESSES

Vanessa R explains about five awarenesses a teacher must possess in her book "The Teaching Brain". They are the following:
1. **Awareness of learner:** Teacher need to know about the cognitive development of learner. Understanding the emotional status is also very important. Emotion influence motivation and ability to process information. Awareness about learner helps teacher to follow learner-centered teaching strategies. It is also essential to assist learner to adopt effective learning styles.
2. **Awareness of teacher-student interactions:** Teacher-student interaction is an integral part of teaching–learning process. Positive teacher-student interaction can be achieved by shared–acceptance affection, trust, respect, care and cooperation between teacher and student. Good teacher-student interaction creates a classroom environment essential to attain learning outcomes.
3. **Awareness of self as a teacher:** Knowledge of self as a teacher is essential to fulfill role as a teacher in the teaching–learning process. An effective teacher is self-aware as well as aware

about the learner. Awareness of self is essential to develop an insight regarding the strengths and weakness in the performance as a teacher.
4. **Awareness of teaching practice:** Awareness of teaching practice is needed to create a good classroom environment and ensure learning. Teaching is a goal oriented task. Teachers teach others to learn. Awareness of teaching practice helps teacher to set goals of teaching and attain them in a time bound manner.
5. **Awareness of context of teaching:** Teacher should be aware about the large context of teaching activity. External context include principal, other teachers and rules of institution. All these external factors impact the teaching directly or indirectly.

## FEEDBACK IN TEACHING–LEARNING PROCESS

### Definition

In the context of education, "Feedback is the information provided to learner in order to improve his performance for attaining learning goals". As per this definition, the purpose of feedback is to help learners to move forward and toward learning goals. So feedback focuses on what students need to learn rather than what they have already learned.

### Importance of Feedback

In Bellon's opinion, feedback in education is important due to the following reasons:
* Feedback is an integral part of teaching–learning process. When given correctly, it guides the student in achieving the goals of learning process.
* Feedback is strongly and consistently related to student achievement than any other teaching behavior.
* Feedback can improve a student's confidence, self-awareness and enthusiasm for learning.
* Feedback help learner to maximize their abilities at various stages of learning. This will in turn help in achieving more knowledge and skills.
* Feedback is needed to reinforce positive aspects of student's performance and identify areas require improvement. Thus, timely guidance and reinforcement through feedback promote learning.
* Effective feedback enhances learning and improves performance of students. This will in turn reduce dropping out of students from institution.
* Feedback motivates students to perform better. This intrinsic motivation leads to proactive learning-learning initiated by the student himself.
* Feedback promotes good teacher-student relationship. This will further create a good classroom environment that facilitates learning.
* Feedback solve issues and clear misconceptions related to learning process.
* Above all timely feedback helps a student to pace learning in accordance with his abilities. Thus, helps in implementing the concept of "individual learner as the unit of teaching process".

### Characteristics of Effective Feedback

Urant Qiggin suggest following ways to provide feedback in an effective manner:
* **Effective feedback is educative in nature, specific, timely, meaningful and honest:** Feedback should focus on a skill or specific knowledge. Formative assessment provides information to give feedback on specific aspects. It should be given at the time when correction is needed then only learning goals can be achieved. Good feedback gives

meaningful and actionable suggestions to improve learning. Teacher need to be honest while giving feedback.
- **Effective feedback is goal oriented:** Feedback should always focus on the goals of learning process. Giving information becomes feedback only when it positively influences the learning process. Suggestions giving through feedback need to be relevant and achievable.
- **Effective feedback focuses on future:** Feedback focus on what students need to be learned rather than what they already learned. This is true, especially when a student commits a mistake. Instead of blaming too much for the mistake, feedback should focuses on how to avoid repetition of the mistake in the future.
- **Effective feedback is about the process, not the learner:** Feedback focus on the goals of learning process. Never criticize the learner. Always criticize the actions. When give suggestions, give suggestions about actions, not about the learner. For example, while giving feedback to a student after presentation, instead of saying "The presentation was too long and boring", good feedback would say" instead of two or three examples, limit examples to one good example to save time".
- **Effective feedback can be positive:** Effective feedback reinforce and promote good behaviors. Teachers should try to provide consistent and constructive feedback to students. Positive feedback stimulates the reward centers of the brain and help students to choose better options.
- **Adopt different ways to provide feedback:** Feedback can be given in several ways. It can be oral written, visual or done through demonstration. Use written mode when the student needs to report later. Use oral mode when there is too much information to convey. Interactive feedback in person is best as it allows student to clarify doubts. Demonstration helps to correct mistakes in the performance of a procedure.
- **Provide feedback in an appropriate manner:** Sometimes teacher need to give negative feedback. While giving negative feedback it will not discourage a student's learning effort and achievement.
- **Be sensitive to individual needs of the students:** It is important to consider the dignity of students while providing feedback. Feedback should be given in privacy, away from classmates and staff, thus maintaining confidentiality. Feedback should never discourage learning and damage self-esteem.
- **Encourage students to give feedback about the performance of teacher in classroom:** Encourage student to give feedback on how teacher is performing her role as a teacher. Let student's give feedback anonymously about: (a) What is they like about teacher's class? (b) What didn't they like? (c)If students were taking class what would they do differently? (d) What did they learn most from you as a teacher as well as a person? Students' feedback help teacher to improve their teaching skills.

## TEACHABLE MOMENTS

Teachable moments are times when learning is most achievable, when the time is right for knowledge to be shared and built. These are the movements where learner provide intentional feedback on her learning.

Time of intentional feedback by learner is the best time or opportunity for intentional teaching. Teachable movements can be nurtured by:
- Respecting existing knowledge of student.
- Responding the need for new knowledge.
- Offering assistance as needed for acquiring knowledge instead of simply transferring knowledge.

## QUALITIES OF A GOOD NURSE EDUCATOR

According to Sandra De Young, qualities of a good nursing teacher can be categorized under four headings, namely: (1) Interpersonal relationships with students. (2) Professional competence. (3) Personal qualities. (4) Student-friendly behavior in the clinical area.

1. **Interpersonal relationships with students:** A good teacher is skillful in maintaining interpersonal relationships. Interpersonal relationship is demonstrated by taking a personal interest in students, being sensitive to students' feelings and problems, conveying respect for students, alleviating students' anxieties, being accessible for conferences, being fair in all dealings with others, permitting students to express differing points of view, creating an atmosphere in which students feel free to ask questions and conveying a sense of warmth. Sandra De Young believes that nursing faculty can help students to maintain self-esteem and minimize anxieties by using three basic therapeutic approaches namely: *empathic listening, acceptance and honest communication.* Through empathic listening teacher can view the world through students' eyes. Second approach is to accept students as they are, whether or not one like them. By adhering to honest communication, the teacher can easily discuss the students' abilities and performance with them and create a relaxed atmosphere in which students are able to see the teacher as a role model. Most important aspect of honest communication is clearly identifying the students' responsibilities in the learning process by letting the students to know exactly what is expected of them and what they have to do to succeed.

2. **Professional competence:** Sandra De Yong views professional competence as the second essential quality of a good nurse educator. Professional competence is evidenced by knowledge regarding educational theory and research, thorough knowledge of the subject matter, ability to present material in an interesting, clear and organized manner, displays confidence in professional activities, ability to inspire students', creativity, ability to elicit students' interest in the subject and demonstration of skills with expertise is rated high. In addition to the lessons from life experiences and suggestions from students, Sandra De Young recommends reading, research, clinical practice and continuing education for maintaining and expanding knowledge of teacher. Professional competency can also be enhanced by a willingness to learn new roles, new styles of interacting and new teaching methods besides the ability to critique one's own performance.

3. **Personal qualities:** Teacher qualities valued by students include enthusiasm, willingness to admit errors, cheerfulness, consideration, honesty, calmness and poise, a sense of humor, lack of annoying mannerisms, patience and a neat appearance.

4. **Student-friendly behavior in the clinical area:** In Sandra De Young's opinion, a good nurse educator has to exhibit certain student friendly behaviors in the clinical area in order to promote self-confidence and security feeling among students. These behaviors include being available in the clinical area, providing conference time, being willing to help, answering questions freely, allowing students to recognize and correct errors, giving verbal encouragement, showing interest in patients and their care, conveying confidence in the learner and supervising without taking over.

## TEACHING–LEARNING METHODS

Teaching methods refer to the orderly, logical course of action taken to accomplish a particular educational goal. The actual selection and use of a particular method or strategy should be based on expected outcomes, principles of learning and learner needs (see guidelines for the selection and practice of teaching learning methods).

A teaching–learning method will help the teacher to conduct teaching in an agreeable, student-friendly and successful manner by initiating and maintaining link between the subject matter and the student. A method is essential for the construction and organization of knowledge. Critical thinking is essential to device a teaching method (The terms teaching–learning method and teaching method are used synonymously throughout this book).

## Classification of Teaching Methods

Based on the degree of dominance enjoyed by the teacher or learner in the teaching–learning process, teaching methods can be classified into *teacher-centered and learner-centered methods*. In teacher-centered method, teacher plays an active role and student's role is minimized to a passive listener, on the contrary, in the learner-centered methods; learners actively participate in the teaching–learning process. Teacher-centered methods include lecture, demonstration, bedside clinic, etc. Learner-centered methods include free group discussions, care plan, care study, return demonstration, role play, project work, self-learning methods, etc., with some conscious efforts and by the effective use of teaching aids, a talented teacher can easily transform a teacher-centered method into a more admirable learner-centered method.

Depending on the utility of teaching methods in meeting the learning needs of a particular number of students, teaching methods can be classified as *large group methods, small group methods and individual methods*. Large group methods include lecture, panel discussion, etc. Small group method is meant for a group comprising less than 20 students and includes group discussions, demonstrations, seminars, bedside clinics, etc. Individual learning method is meant for individual learning purpose and include assignments, computer assisted learning, project works, self-instruction modules, etc.

Understanding both classifications is essential for good teaching, as it helps the teacher to select the method according to group-wise and motivates her to adopt measures for bringing down the demerits of a teacher-centered method by eliciting student participation in the teaching–learning process. Irrespective of the type of teaching method, teacher should try to create a student-centered classroom by reaching to all students in the classroom.

## Teaching Strategies and Teaching–Learning Methods

Even though strategies and teaching methods help the teacher to carry out teaching and facilitate learning, one has to differentiate between teaching strategies and teaching methods. Learner-centered teaching strategies include feedback, reinforcement, review and practice. Teaching strategies can be implemented through various actions. For example, review of a topic can be conducted by asking questions or giving assignments. Compared to strategies, methods are more complex and each method use several strategies to attain the objectives. While teaching a procedure through demonstration method, teacher uses different teaching strategies like feedback, reinforcement and practice in order to ascertain the acquisition of skills by the students.

## Guidelines for the Selection and Practice of Teaching–learning Methods

Selection of appropriate teaching–learning methods requires critical thinking and decision making. Even though some guidelines are synonymous with the principles or maxims of teaching, the below mentioned guidelines will assist the teacher in the selection of fruitful teaching–learning methods.

❖ **Method should be suited to objectives and content of the subject matter:** Objectives and content play a major role in the selection of teaching method. An intelligent teacher can very easily identify the suitable method by verifying the objectives and content. As different teaching methods achieve objectives in different ways, teacher has to follow different methods in order to attain predetermined objectives. A competent teacher, who is well versed in various teaching methods, can follow this guideline in a meticulous manner.

- **Methods should suit to the level of students:** Teacher has to consider the psychological status, receptiveness, intellectual maturity and previous knowledge of students while selecting the method of teaching. Teacher can assess the level of students through analyzing their previous achievements, asking questions and giving assignments. Employing methods suitable to the level of students help the teacher to become an efficient teacher, by reaching to all students in the class. This will in turn convert the usually teacher-centered classroom atmosphere into a more desirable student-centered one.
- **Method should be based on sound psychological principles:** Methods with a psychological basis will make the teaching more rewarding and student-centered. Principles and marks of good teaching discussed elsewhere in this chapter highlights the importance of psychological principles in the teaching–learning process.
- **Method should be used creatively:** It is not a must that the teacher should follow only the conventional methods of teaching. Without violating the fundamental aspects of teaching, a talented teacher can create new teaching methods by utilizing the technological developments in the field of communication and information technology. Teacher can also arouse interest among students through most effective and efficient combination of existing teaching methods.
- **Method should suit to the teacher's style:** Able believes that style in teaching is an outgrowth of teacher's personality and character. Style is much more than exhibiting certain skills and behavior pertaining to good teaching. It is the style that transforms good teachers into inspiring teachers. Method should suit to the teacher's style in order to make the teaching more memorable, interesting and worth listening.
- **Teacher has to rely on his or her strength or assets while selecting methods:** As innovations are occurring on a regular basis, there is no difficulty in modifying the existing teaching methods or devising a new one. A teacher who is excellent in a handful of teaching methods, need not be worried about his or her weakness in dealing with a particular method. There is no single best method of teaching but only methods. Moreover, it is very difficult to attain proficiency in all teaching methods. In the journey towards a successful career, teacher has to rely more on strengths rather than worrying about the weaknesses. But it is well and good, if the teacher puts conscious effort to overcome the weakness without undermining his/her strengths.
- **Method should address the challenges:** Major challenges usually faced by the teacher in the selection of teaching methods include: (a) Maintain the quality of teaching and learning; (b) Reduce the cost of instruction; (c) Responding to technological developments in communicating and information technology. By addressing these challenges teacher can carry out quality teaching in a cost-effective way by utilizing the technological advances without neglecting the human component of teaching.
- **Selection should consider the available resources:** Teacher has to consider the available resources while selecting the teaching–learning methods and should use the available resources to the maximum extent possible. If there is a model of heart is available, teacher has to use it along with the chart while teaching anatomy of the cardiovascular system. This guideline is particularly important for nurse educators as they have to utilize the rich and varied facilities available in the clinical area for teaching students.

# LECTURE METHOD

Lecture method is the oldest method of teaching. The term lecture was derived from the Latin word *'lectare'* which means to *'read aloud'*. Despite severe criticisms leveled against it, lecture still continues as the most preferred teaching method. Regarding the criticisms, it is now understood that the fault mainly lies with the users and not with the method. With the emergence of this viewpoint, the validity of lecture as a teaching method has been increased considerably.

## Definition

According to authors, "lecture is a teaching activity whereby the teacher presents the content in a comprehensible manner by explaining the facts, principles and relationships, during which the teacher is expected to elicit student participation by employing appropriate techniques".

Even though teacher talks more or less continuously to the class, lecturing is not simply a one way transmission of information. In addition to listening and writing notes, effective lecturing allows the students to interact with the teacher.

## Purposes of Lectures

Authors firmly believe that a thoughtfully delivered lecture can serve the following purposes:

- **To provide structured knowledge:** Providing structured knowledge by integrating and synthesizing knowledge from different fields or sources is the prime function of lecture. As knowledge is flooding day by day in this era of knowledge explosion, it is difficult for the students to locate all sources of knowledge and synthesize it. Through lecture it is easy for the teacher to provide relevant knowledge by selecting and organizing the content in a learner-centered way. For instance, it is difficult for the first year students to collect all information regarding the history of nursing, whereas a knowledgeable teacher can very well teach it by adopting the lecture method.
- **To motivate and guide in hunting knowledge:** As teacher alone cannot satisfy the knowledge requirement of students, he/she has to explain the various sources of knowledge. An efficient teacher by means of clarifying lecture motivates the students to collect more information and guide them properly through the jungle of information. This purpose underlines the importance of giving references to the students after completing a particular topic. Teacher has to give *main references* as well as *general references*. Main references will provide a list of books which are commonly followed for learning a particular topic. Books come under the heading of general references provides additional information, if needed. For a lecture on nursing management of myocardial infarction, one or two textbooks on medical-surgical nursing can be included in main references, whereas general references constitutes some books on pathology, medicine and pharmacology.
- **To arouse students interest in a subject:** By following lecture method, teacher can orient the students to a subject by explaining the need for studying it, ways of learning and revision, mode of writing university examination, etc. Once the students understand the need for and ways of learning a particular subject, they will be motivated naturally.
- **Introduce students to new areas of learning:** Innovations are occurring on a regular basis in the diagnosis, treatment and nursing management of disease conditions. These innovations have created new learning areas and lecture method will help the teacher introduce these areas to students before resorting to the most suitable method. For example, teacher has to give a brief lecture about the evolution of MRI scan, merits of it and patient care implications before taking the students to the radio diagnosis department for teaching the functioning of MRI machine and the responsibilities of the nurse posted in the MRI room.

- **To clarify difficult concepts:** Lecture method is highly suitable for clarifying concepts. Teacher should use enough examples and illustrations to clarify the concepts. For instance, by adopting lecture method teacher can very well clarify the concept of interpersonal relationship by citing examples from the day-to-day life of nurses or other healthcare professionals.
- **To assist in preparing students for a discussion:** Before discussion teacher has to provide a concrete idea to the students regarding the topic of discussion, aims of discussion, etc. As a means of providing this information, lecture method helps the teacher in creating a conducive atmosphere for discussion.
- **To promote critical thinking:** Of course, compared to other methods formal lectures usually give less emphasis to critical thinking, but a thoughtfully designed and delivered lecture can challenge students to think critically and analytically by modeling the thinking process according to the characteristics of the discipline. Critical thinking can also be encouraged through incorporating challenging questions throughout the lecture. Nursing is a discipline dealing with the health problems of patients and critical thinking is essential for finding solutions to these problems. Hence nursing teachers have to promote critical thinking by way of effective lectures. For example, based on student's experience in the clinical area like practice of aseptic techniques, proper waste disposal, etc., teacher can easily teach the factors involved in the hospital infection, then by asking thought provoking questions in relation to these factors teacher can easily initiate critical thinking. Through critical thinking students will find out the relationship between factors involved in hospital infection and ways to eliminate or control these factors in order to avoid hospital infection.

## Lecturing Techniques

A thoughtfully prepared content along with appropriate techniques helps the teacher deliver lecture in a more interesting and comprehensible manner. Even the most impressive way of applying techniques is not sufficient to replace a thoughtfully prepared content. Good content is essential for the dissemination of balanced information. If the teacher prepares the content in a haphazards way, no technique can help her in attaining the purposes of lecture. In authors, point of view, the below mentioned techniques will help the teacher to practice lecture in a student-centered manner. Value of lecture as a teaching method largely depends on how well these techniques are followed by the teacher.

- **Voluntary dissemination of information or spontaneity:** This is the essence of lecturing. Instead of reading continuously from a prepared note teacher has to converse freely with the students. Of course, looking in between at the prepared note is needed, as it helps the teacher maintain the sequence, but reading continuously from the note will hamper spontaneity and reduce the interest of students. Student-friendly vocabulary and language, effective preparation of lecture note, widespread reading, objective evaluation of life experiences and thorough practice are essential to develop spontaneity. Practising one or two times before entering the class is regarded as the best way to nurture spontaneity, especially in the case of beginners. Spontaneity is not merely a recollection of learned lessons but it is a sudden outflow of information, which is enriched with the life experiences of the teacher as well as the students.
- **Voice gradation and voice quality:** Voice gradation is the periodical alteration of both pitch and volume while lecturing and with some conscious efforts voice gradation will become the part and parcel of the teaching activity. Among information disseminated through lecturing some require more highlighting in order to attain the objectives and voice gradation serves this purpose meticulously. Moreover, lecturing in a monotone make students more passive.

Teacher can depend on recent developments in educational technology to maintain the voice quality. If there is any deficiency in the voice quality, teacher is free enough to use a microphone attached to a sophisticated sound system in order to rectify the deficiency.

- **Adequate pacing:** Too slow a pace and too fast a pace are not advisable as the former creates boredom and the latter leads to confusion. A successful teacher always organizes the content effectively and pace the lecture in a comprehensible manner in accordance with the receptivity level of students. The teacher has to develop a routine pace of going fast while teaching simple topics and has to slow down when dealing with difficult areas so that students can get acquainted with the pace, follow easily and take notes if needed. By adopting a student-friendly routine pace, students get time to interpret what the teacher has told and thereby teacher can ensure successful learning.
- **Proper body language:** Action often speaks louder than words, the teacher has to keep this in mind and be aware about the body language while lecturing. One can maintain proper body language by practising principles of effective communication. Maintaining eye contact with students is very essential and avoids looking out of the window, at the wall and over the students' head as these are considered as impersonal behaviors. Occasionally, move towards the students rather than continuously standing behind the podium. Modest use of hands is recommended but avoids keeping the arms crossed or hands clasped behind. Practising in front of a mirror will help a lot in the development of proper body language.
- **Control annoying mannerisms:** Annoying mannerisms are very distracting to the students. Crushing or tossing chalk, breaking the knuckles, waving hands unnecessarily, pinching the nose and repeatedly saying 'so', 'right', 'okay' and 'uh' are the common annoying mannerisms. Usually, teachers are unaware about these mannerisms and realize the extent of damage caused by them only through the feedback provided by the superiors or colleagues during an evaluation session. Very easily mannerisms will become the part of the lecturing activity and once acquired it is very difficult to get rid of them so prevention is better than cure. Practising in front of a mirror, recording the lecture and then listening to it objectively are some of the measures to prevent the occurrence of annoying mannerisms.
- **Judicious use of audiovisual aids:** In addition to blackboard, charts and graphs, advancements in educational technology offers help through a handful of sophisticated audiovisual aids to the teacher in facilitating learning by way of the lecture method. Judicious selection of visual aids is important, as they are very useful in delivering lectures effectively. For example, a chart showing the picture of gas exchange between alveoli and capillaries is the vital one among visual aids used for teaching respiration and without this particular chart the purposes of using visual aids cannot be achieved fully while teaching respiration.
- **Simple plans and key points:** When planning for a lecture always go for a simple plan instead of complicated ones. Select some of the key points from the content and build the whole lecture around them. This will help students recollect the taught lessons in an easy manner. For instance, while delivering a lecture on the nursing management of myocardial infarction, arranging the content under key points like definition, etiology, predisposing factors, warning signs, symptoms, investigations, medical management and nursing management will help the students follow the lecture and recollect the learned lessons as and when needed.
- **Elicit feedback from students:** Even though feedback is a vital technique, due to the hurry in finishing the content, many teachers neglect it while lecturing. To a certain extend feedback assists the teacher to assess the amount of knowledge received by the students and the progress they have achieved. An intelligent teacher always critically analyzes the feedback from the students as a means for evaluating the effectiveness of her lecture and

the subsequent diagnosis of any defects. After assessing the defects properly she can take appropriate remedial measures. In this sense, feedback is diagnostic as well as remedial not only for the students but also for the teachers. Feedback can be obtained by asking thought provoking questions, inviting suggestions regarding both the content and technique and even by simply instructing a student to repeat the sentence which you have just completed.

❖ **Providing further clarifications:** One of the purposes of lecture is to clarify difficult concepts by citing examples or through illustrations. Even then, after initial clarification teacher has to assess the need for further clarification inbetween the lecture and if needed provide it. You can assess the need for further clarifications by asking "any more explanation needed", "so far is clear to you", "anything to be further clarified", "any doubts to be rectified", etc. It is better to provide further clarifications before proceeding to the next topic or session. For instance, while teaching pragmatism as an educational philosophy, teacher should provide further clarifications, if needed regarding pragmatism and curriculum before proceeding to pragmatism and discipline.

❖ **Time management:** Time factor is very important in lecturing. Certain teachers cover the content within the stipulated time while some others find it very difficult to do so. When time exceeds than expected, tension slowly invades the teacher and damage the entire lecture. Hence, skill in managing time is essential for conducting lecture in a smooth way. Through time bound practice by using a clock, teacher can easily develop a proportion between time and content. Keeping this proportion in mind she can determine the amount of content she can cover within the allotted time. Restricting the tendency to deviate from the main objectives of lecturing is also helpful in saving time.

## Advantages of Lecture Method

Lecture method is the most economical method of teaching. Provided with all facilities lecture can be conducted even with a teacher to student ratio of 1:200. For students, lecture method is economical in terms of time, as they get more information by attending lecture than reading books. Moreover, reading from a book is impersonal compared to lecture method. Contrary to the popular misconcept that lecture makes student passive, a well-designed and thoughtfully delivered lecture stimulate the students and promote thinking process. Lecture method enhances the listening capacity of students. It can be employed to meet the learning needs of any group of students. Above all, students usually prefer lecture method.

## Disadvantages of Lecture Method

It is a fact that teachers can practice lecture method without adequate preparation. With mere confidence in hand and neglecting the importance of adequate preparation, many teachers enter the class and deliver lectures. Invariably, these lectures will fail to attain the objectives. To conduct a demonstration or bedside clinic, teacher prepare well, but when it comes to lecturing, they simply go to the class, even without a prepared note. *As a method of teaching nursing*, this high possibility or increased chance of practising lecture without adequate preparation is its major limitation or disadvantage. By and large, this limitation is the root cause of many other disadvantages also. Unfortunately, many educators misinterpret this disadvantage as simplicity of the lecture method and consider this disadvantage as an advantage. From the above discussion, it is clear that the teacher who performs the lecture is responsible for many of the below mentioned disadvantages.

As lecture method is more concerned with the teaching of facts and information, compared to other methods, less attention is given to problem-solving, critical thinking and decision making in formal lectures. This does not mean that lecture is incapable of promoting critical thinking. Through a thoughtfully designed and delivered lecture teacher can easily promote critical thinking (see Purposes of Lecture). Opponents of lecture method believes that lecture makes the students passive and decrease their participation in the teaching–learning process. This is true only when the teacher is ill-prepared and carry out the lecture in a haphazards manner. A well prepared and thoughtfully delivered lecture can easily make the students active in the class.

Lecturing is not conducive for meeting the students individual learning needs. This major disadvantage is more or less inherent in the lecture method and commonly occurs in large lecture classes. Laurillad believes that lecture does not provide opportunities for students to engage in continuing dialogue with lecturer, where their conceptions can be shaped through feedback. Nor does it allow students to actively apply and experiment with their conceptions.

## Strategies to Overcome Disadvantages

Gibbs, Habeshaw, Newble and Cannon recommend the below mentioned strategies to overcome the disadvantages.

- **Emphasize higher-level intellectual skills:** Ensure that the teaching objectives specify more than just facts and technical skills by emphasizing higher-level intellectual skills, such as problem-solving, critical thinking and the exploration and development of appropriate attitudes. Lecturers can challenge students to think critically and analytically by modeling the thinking process according to the characteristics of the discipline. Critical thinking can also be encouraged by the use of challenging questions throughout the lecture.
- **Signposting for clear direction:** As well as organizing and ordering the content, tell learners what you are doing by providing good signposts about the structure and direction of the lecture. Include such things as: (a) links between sections like what is coming next and what has just been completed, (b) summaries, (c) reviews, (d) statements, which indicate a change of topic, and (e) highlight principles or key ideas so that they stand out from the details and examples.
- **Make lectures more interactive:** Include teaching activities that promote cognitive challenge and require learners to demonstrate a deep understanding of the subject matter and relevant problems. This may mean using small group activities during the lectures so that learners have an opportunity to interact with each other and to explore issues, discuss, analyze, and report back to the class. This helps learners to internalize the material and work with it to relate to their own context. Also arrange for learners to use the lecture material immediately following the lectures so that they actively process it and do not forget it (see Interactive Lecture).
- **Less memorizing of facts and more construction of meaning:** Decrease the amount of factual material that has to be memorized. When learners are pressed for time and overloaded with content, they will usually take a surface approach. Learners need to know what to listen for, how the lecture links to and supports subsequent learning activities and what they should be doing with what they hear. You need to let them know what sort of notes are likely to be useful and what follow-up learning activities you expect them to undertake. Spend more time in helping learners to understand and use basic principles rather than memorizing facts. Ask students to explain answers to questions instead of just accepting the correct answer.

## INTERACTIVE LECTURE

Interactive lecture is a combination of lecture, discussion and questioning. It is the modified version of the traditional lecture method and developed by retaining the merits and deleting the demerits of the lecture, discussion and questioning. Sandra De Young has beautifully explained the interactive lecture in the following way, "The techniques of lecture, discussion and questioning can be effectively blended together into an interactive lecture, utilizing the advantages of all the methods and reducing their disadvantages. Class time can be logically and efficiently divided into sections for lecture, informal discussion, questioning, more lecture and so on. In this way, subject matter is presented for discussion, problem-solving can take place and questions can stimulate student thinking and clarify difficult points. Students become periodically active in the class, which eliminates some of the objections to pure lecturing. Changing tactics every 15 to 20 minutes may also help recapture students' attention at points when it naturally seems to wander. The class becomes more interesting and it is to be hoped, more memorable."

## DEMONSTRATION

Possession of psychomotor skills is very essential for good nursing practice and by virtue of its effectiveness in teaching psychomotor skills, demonstration enjoys a dominant position among teaching methods employed in teaching nursing. By definition, "demonstration is a method of teaching by exhibition and explanation combined to illustrate a procedure or experiments". According to Gullibert, purpose of teaching is to help students: (a) acquire, retain and be able to use knowledge, (b) understand, analyze, synthesize and evaluate, (c) achieve skills, (d) establish habits, and (e) develop attitudes. As far as nursing is concerned, demonstration is the apt method of teaching to achieve many of the purposes enlisted by Guilbert.

### Phases of Demonstration

Entire demonstration can be divided into three phases, namely: the planning and preparation phase, performance phase, and evaluation phase.

### *Planning and Preparation Phase*

In the planning and preparation phase, teacher prepares herself, arranges necessary articles and creates a conducive learning environment suitable to the number of students. During this phase the teacher has to: (a) Set well-defined objectives based on the theoretical knowledge and need of students; (b) Review related knowledge; (c) Based on scientific principles or rational basis split the demonstration into appropriate steps so that students can easily follow the demonstration; (d) Do rehearsals as needed for attaining the proficiency required for conducting demonstration; (e) If the demonstration involves the presence of a patient or mock patient, plan for their comfort and safety. Obtain necessary permission in the case of patients; (f) Create a conducive learning environment by providing adequate facilities, especially the facility to observe the demonstration; (g) Plan for maximum student participation; (h) Ensure adequacy and good working condition of equipment, assemble equipment in a convenient order; (i) Plan for return demonstration; (j) Give necessary guidance to the students for achieving the objectives of demonstration. This can be done by listing the objectives and explaining what is expected from the student in order to achieve them; (k) Prepare a checklist regarding the articles and steps so that teacher can avoid shortcomings in the performance phase; (l) In the planning phase itself teacher should foresee the importance of providing opportunities for students to practice the skills and make arrangements for the same; (m) Preparation of procedure manual at the institutional level by the faculty or at the regional level by collaborating with other institutions not only brings uniformity to procedures but also reduces the workload of teachers in the preparation phase.

## Performance Phase

In this phase, teacher performs the demonstration. Throughout this phase she has to maintain a positive approach by telling *"what to do"* rather than *"what not to do".* She should also exhibit a fine coordination of head, heart and hand than simply repeating as per the procedure manual. Following steps will help you perform demonstration in an impressive way: (a) Based on the principle of proceeding from whole to parts, briefly narrate the whole procedure before explaining the individual steps in detail. This can be done either by asking few questions or by briefing yourself; (b) Explain the name and use of articles kept ready for performing demonstration; (c) Start the demonstration slowly so that students can follow easily; (d) Explain the purposes and scientific principles associated with each step; (e) Pace the steps and verbal explanations in a student-friendly manner; (f) Make sure that students have understood each step, repeat if they have not understood it; (g) Wherever possible involve students in the performance phase; (h) In between ask questions and encourage to seek clarifications in order to get a feedback from students, complete the procedure with a summary; (i) Replace the articles, demonstrate the after care of them and wash hands; (j) Show the way of recording the procedure; (k) Conclude the performance phase with a discussion. Discussion will help provide any further clarifications.

## Evaluation Phase

Evaluation is done mainly through return demonstration and asking thought provoking questions.

## Advantages of Demonstration

- Through demonstration teacher illustrates the coordination of head, heart and hands, which is essential for the development and refining of psychomotor skills.
- Students are very much interested to see the application of the theory which they have learned in the previous classes. This interest along with the use of multiple senses promotes learning and brings out the correlation between theory and practice.
- Amount learned and retained is directly proportional to the students' interest and senses involved so the amount learnt and retained is high in demonstration compared to other methods.
- Accompanying explanation helps the student understand and clarify the scientific principles involved in each step of the procedure.
- Observational skill is important in assessing patients' condition and demonstration is a good means for developing the same.
- Return demonstration helps the teacher to evaluate the knowledge and skills acquired by the student. If she is not satisfied with the return demonstration, she can redemonstrate the procedure for making it more clearly to students. This provision for immediate evaluation and rectification of noted shortcomings by employing appropriate remedial measures is considered as the greatest advantage of demonstration. In fact, through return demonstration teacher can correct students then and there as needed. Thus, return demonstration ensures competency of student in carrying out nursing procedures and thereby protect the patient from ill-prepared students.
- Gratification gained through the application of theory motivates the students to attend demonstration classes.
- Demonstration demands adequate preparation from the side of nurse educator and immediate feedback from the students through return demonstration will serve as a means to critically evaluate her competency in handling this teaching method.

❖ Exploring the scientific principles underlying the steps in demonstration foster critical thinking.

## Disadvantages of Demonstration

Demonstration is a teacher-centered, small group teaching method but return demonstration is student-centered. As a method of teaching nursing skills, obviously there is no clear-cut disadvantage for demonstration. Theoretical background and a good explanation from the side of teacher reduce the possibility of blindly following the procedure book. As already stated, demonstration is the apt method for developing psychomotor skills and by realizing the importance of psychomotor skills in clinical practice, students are less likely to remain inattentive while attending demonstration.

## DISCUSSION

Discussion is a student-centered teaching method, and it is very useful in teaching nursing.

### Meaning

According to Aggarwal, discussion is a thoughtful consideration of relationships involved in the topic or problem under study. These relationships are analyzed, compared and evaluated for drawing conclusions.

Sandra De Young believes that discussion involves an interchange of informed opinions and reactions, group consideration of a problem or issue, sharing of ideas and information and exchange of questions and answers.

Discussions may be *formal or informal*. Formal discussion is pre-planned and guided by preset rules in order to achieve predetermined goals. Informal discussion is characterized by free verbal exchanges between the participants in the absence of preset rules or predetermined goals.

### Purposes of Discussion

Discussion method is commonly used for teaching selected topics and to enrich lectures, observation visits and case presentations. Discussion will serve the following purposes:

❖ **To teach context specific interpretation and application of principles, theories and concepts:** Usually principles, theories and concepts are explained in general and at times it will be very difficult to interpret these principles, theories and concepts in a way suitable to particular situation or context. Discussion will help interpret the principles and theories as suitable to a context. To achieve this purpose, students should possess prior knowledge regarding the topic selected for discussion. They can attain prior knowledge either through self-reading or attending lectures. For example, the concept and principles of interpersonal relationship is known to third year BSc (Nursing) students but it is impossible to apply these principles in same manner during pediatric nursing and medical surgical nursing postings. A discussion under the leadership of teacher will help students realize the peculiarities of adult and pediatric care so that they can interpret and apply the principles of interpersonal relationships in a way suitable to their respective areas of posting.

❖ **Assist students to develop, express and validate their opinions or beliefs regarding legal, ethical and controversial issues in nursing:** In the light of social changes and technological advancements in patient care, legal and ethical issues are gaining much attention than ever before. Adequate help have to be rendered to students in order to address and tackle these issues in a professional manner. First step towards equipping student in this regard is helping them to develop an opinion related to these issues. Discussion serves this purpose in a meticulous way. In discussion, pros and cons of an opinion is critically analyzed by the group members in order to decide its validity. Naturally, group will agree to a valid opinion and an invalid opinion is rejected by pointing out the existing lacunae. Thus, discussion assist students to develop, express and validate an opinion.

- **To clarify information and concepts:** Discussion following lectures usually aims this purpose. Discussion helps the teacher not only assess the knowledge gained by students but also provide an opportunity for further clarifications. For example, a discussion on the feasibility of aims of education postulated by idealism after a lecture on educational implications of idealism will help the students clear any remaining doubts and provide more information regarding the merits and demerits of idealism.
- **To share information:** This universally accepted purpose of discussion is naturally accomplished along with other purposes. Exchanging of ideas or viewpoints and the conclusions drawn at the end of discussion ultimately results in sharing of information.
- **To foster democratic values:** Discussion help the students develop an ability to tolerate the most contradicting opinions or viewpoints and to defend their own viewpoints assertively. In this way, students become familiar with the democratic ways of getting things done.
- **To develop team building and social skills:** Teamwork always divide the task and double the success. As potential members of health team, student nurses have to develop team building and social skills. Through discussions under the leadership of teachers students learn the essentials of team building and social skills like how to elicit cooperation from others, value the contribution of others and the group process.
- **Development of right attitudes:** In nursing, nothing can be accomplished properly in the absence of right attitude. Optimum utilization of skill and knowledge is possible only in the presence of right attitude. As attitudes are mainly caught by the students rather than taught by the teachers, inculcating proper attitude among students is really a challenging task. Through listening a discussion or participating in it, students get a chance to compare their own attitude regarding an issue or situation with others. This will motivate them to do a self-analysis and ultimately results in the inculcation of right attitude appropriate to the issue or situation under consideration. In broad sense, discussion change the attitude of students as desired and teach them how to change the attitude of others also.
- **To develop problem-solving skills as a group:** Discussion is the best method to draw group involvement in solving a problem. A detailed discussion under the leadership of teacher after dividing the whole group into subgroups and assigning a particular aspect of problem to each subgroup will help find a solution through pooling the expertise of group members and consolidating their thinking process. For example, a discussion aimed to solve the problem of hospital waste disposal can be conducted as follows: First teacher has to divide the whole class into five subgroups then divide the problem also into five interrelated components like safe handling of waste, segregation and collection, safe transport, safe disposal and overall responsibilities of nurses in the safe disposal of hospital waste and assign single component to each subgroup. Each subgroup have to discuss their respective component and find a solution pertaining to it. In the final round discussion all the five subgroups presents their ideas, critically analyze them and draws the solution under the guidance of the teacher.
- **To arouse students' interest:** Discussion facilitates expression of ideas and interaction with the teacher. This opportunity for expressing themselves motivates students to prepare well through self-learning. Facility to interact with the teacher and peers helps them clarify the doubts in a more democratic and authentic way. Above all, discussion allows the students

to find a solution for their learning problems or difficulties through collective effort. All these will arouse students interest and motivate them to participate actively in the teaching-learning process.

### Classroom Discussion Techniques

Teacher can make the discussion a successful one by employing proper techniques. Techniques can be categorized under three headings, namely: proper planning, preparing students for discussion, and discussion guiding techniques.

#### *Proper Planning*

As all the topics cannot be dealt through discussion, planning is mainly concerned with selection of apt topics, formulation of objectives and setting guidelines. Controversial issues, ethical issues and legal issues like professional status of nursing, impact of Consumer Protection Act on nursing, etc. are preferred by the teachers for conducting discussion. Another set of topics include recent challenges to nursing, recent trends and developments in nursing, commonly occurring problems in the clinical area, curriculum-related issues and malpractice from the side of students like plagiarism. In order to arouse students' interest, preference should be given to topics related to their experiences. Planning is also concerned with arranging the discussion in a conductive environment at a convenient time. While planning discussion pertaining to clinical problems, it is well and good to invite the concerned nursing staff to guide the discussion in addition to the nurse educator. A well ventilated spacious room with chairs arranged in a way to limit the barriers not only promotes communication but also allows the teacher to oversee the course of discussion, especially when the whole class is divided into subgroups. By all means, environment should be nonthreatening to students.

#### *Preparing Students for Discussion*

Unlike other methods, discussion demands certain amount of preparation from the side of students and preparation starts one or two weeks before the date of discussion. Students cannot blindly attend a discussion. Teacher can prepare the students through: (a) Providing some basic information related to the topic to be discussed by means of an introductory lecture and helping students acquire knowledge through their own effort by giving references or introducing to experts; (b) Clearly stating the objectives and guidelines; (c) Clarifying the role of the teacher, students and student leaders. Teachers role is limited and main role is played by the students. After two or three discussions, under close supervision teacher can allow students to act as leaders or chairpersons. If class is divided into subgroups, the role of group leaders have to be emphasized. Clarifying the roles will help the students realize their responsibilities and act accordingly.

The task of preparing students is comparatively less, if the topic is related to their day-to-day experiences. The topic, objectives, venue and time of discussion should be displayed in the classroom notice board much ahead of time so that students can prepare for the discussion.

#### *Discussion Guiding Techniques*

Teacher can open the discussion session with a keynote address. In the keynote address, she has to give a brief introduction regarding the topic of discussion and dictate the objectives and guidelines. Keynote address ends with an invitation for the students to express their ideas or viewpoints. Once the students actively involved in the discussion, teacher has to assume the role of a leader or facilitator. One student with good writing skills should be entrusted to record the proceedings.

Ensuring participation of all students is very important. This can be achieved by controlling and discouraging over talkative students and motivating passive students to express their opinions. Allotting specific time to each student, allowing to talk on a rotational basis, at times ignoring an over talkative student and inviting opinion from a passive student by calling him by name are some of the other measures to bring out fair participation. While leading or guiding the discussion, teacher has to clarify any difficult or controversial statements put forward by students in order to avoid misinterpretation and confusion. Appropriate use of positive reinforcements is essential to motivate the students. After two or three discussions, teacher can handover the leadership or chairmanship to the students with an intention to instill leadership qualities among them. When a student is leading the discussion teacher has to closely supervise and provide adequate guidance so that the discussion will proceed in the desired manner.

Teacher has to make sure that the opinions or viewpoints are exchanged between the group members instead of exchanging opinions directly to the teacher or the student leader. Throughout the discussion she has to emphasize the importance of the assertive style of communication and restrict any aggressive style of communication. When a student requests some time for thinking, it has to be granted and silence prevailing this time can be utilized by other members also to enrich their thinking process. In between the discussion, if the teacher notices any deviation from the pre-determined objectives or wasting time by unnecessary exploration of facts, she has to redirect the course of discussion as intended.

If subgroups are involved in the discussion, group leaders have to summarize the viewpoints of their respective groups to the teacher or student leader. Under the guidance of teacher the pros and cons of these viewpoints are analyzed and a consensus is reached by consolidating their merits.

Discussion ends with a concluding note delivered by the teacher. Concluding note invariably contains a summary of the discussion, statement regarding the fulfillment of objectives, evaluation regarding the performance of students and the student leader if present, a few words of appreciation to encourage students and suggestions for improving the forthcoming discussions. In addition to give suggestions for improvement, a democratic teacher also invites suggestions from the students. A thoughtfully prepared concluding note not only provides feedback to students but also motivates them to prepare well for the forthcoming discussions.

## Discussion Skills

A reflective teacher may find it useful to consider the following points **(Box 6.1)**.

### *Advantages of Discussion Method*

- ❖ When properly conducted, discussion is an excellent student-centered method. Active participation not only results in better learning but also promotes retention and recalling ability of students.
- ❖ Acceptance of students' opinion and suggestions during the discussion enhances their self-esteem.
- ❖ If the purposes are accomplished properly, discussion help the students to develop problem-solving skills, critical thinking ability, self-confidence, ability to compare and contrast, democratic values, team building and social skills, proper attitude, awareness regarding group process, self-expression skills and comprehensive knowledge on a particular topic or issue.

**Box 6.1:** Discussion skills of a nurse educator.

1. **Do the participants take turns or do they frequently talk over or interrupt?**
   - Do they invite contributions, redirect contributions for further comments, give encouragement?
   - Do they listen to each other? Are they willing to learn from each other (i.e. respond and react to each other's contributions)?
   - Or do they indulge in 'parallel' talk (i.e., continue their own line of thinking)? Does conflict emerge or is harmony maintained (at all costs)?
   - Are the ideas disputed?
   - Is the speaker attacked?
   - Is conflict positively handled?
   - by modifying statements, rather than just reasserting them?
   - by examining the assumptions, rather than leaving them implicit?
   - by explaining/accounting for the claim, rather than ignoring the challenge?
2. **Do they elaborate, rather than answer in monosyllables?**
   - by giving details of events, people, feelings?
   - by providing reasons, explanations, examples?
   - Do they extend ideas, rather than let ambiguity go unchallenged?
   - by asking for specific information?
   - by asking for clarification?
   - Do they explore suggestions?
   - by asking for alternatives?
   - by speculating, imagining and hypothesizing?
   - Do they evaluate?
   - by pooling ideas and suspending judgement before making choices?

*Source*: Pollard and Tann

### Disadvantages of Discussion Method

- First and foremost disadvantage is its time-consuming nature. Routine time allotment for a period is 45 minutes or one hour, and it is very difficult to complete the discussion in a desirable manner within this short time.
- Success of discussion depends mainly on the preparation of students. Sometimes, teacher may feel helpless when the students make it a habit to attend discussions without adequate preparation in spite of her repeated requests. This helplessness in turn reduces her interest in discussion. Teacher has his or her own limitations in preparing students for discussion, students have to realize these limitations and cooperate with the teacher through attending the discussion only after considerable preparation.
- When both the teacher and students come ill-prepared for a discussion nothing good can be achieved except some meaningless verbal exchanges between the students.
- If the teacher or student leader is incapable of controlling the group, few talkative students can hijack the discussion by making others passive or inattentive.
- Discussion is less efficient, if the number of students exceeds 20. When the number of subgroups increases, it will be difficult for the teacher to ensure fair participation of all students and guide the course of discussion in the right direction.

## SEMINAR AND SYMPOSIUM

Seminar and symposium are the two common forms of discussion employed in teaching nursing. Lot of confusion exists regarding the way of conducting seminar and symposium. Some educators even use these terms interchangeably. Even though seminar and symposium share some common features of discussion, each has its own entity as a teaching method. Seminar and symposium are usually used for teaching higher level students like postgraduates, research scholars, etc. Let us see in detail regarding seminar and symposium.

## SEMINAR

Based on the level of organization, seminar can be classified into four types, namely: mini seminar, main seminar, national seminar and international seminar. Seminar conducted in the classroom is called mini seminar, main seminar is organized at the departmental or institutional level. As names indicate, national seminar and international seminar are conducted at the national and international level respectively. In classroom seminar, one student presents a particular topic or problem and the group will conduct a detailed discussion based on the presentation under the guidance of the teacher. Below mentioned characteristics of seminar are more applicable to other types of seminar.

### Meaning

A seminar as an instructional technique involves generating a situation for a group to have guided interaction among themselves on different aspects or components of a topic, which is generally presented by one or more members.

From the meaning, it is clear that seminar is a discussion based on information presented by experts under the guidance of an eminent resource person for the benefit of group members. The person who guides the seminar is the chairperson, experts who present the information are speakers and the group members who are benefited from the seminar are the participants. For example, cardiology nursing department in association with medical surgical department of the college of nursing can conduct a seminar on 'innovations in cardiovascular nursing' for MSc (Nursing) students and staff nurses. Here, cardiology nursing department and medical surgical department are the organizers, MSc (Nursing) students and nursing staff are the participants, an eminent nursing person from a cardiology institute will guide the seminar as the chairperson and speakers panel will include one cardiac surgeon, cardiac physician and two nursing personnel specialized in cardiovascular nursing. The topic innovations in cardiovascular nursing' is divided into four interrelated components, namely: (a) innovations in the management of cardiac diseases, (b) innovations in cardiac surgery, (c) innovations in the nursing management of patients with cardiac diseases, and (d) role of nurse in the rehabilitation of cardiac patients. The first two components will be dealt by the physician and surgeon while the rest will be dealt by the nursing personnel.

### Role of Different Personnel

As said earlier, personnel involved in the seminar can be categorized into organizers, chairperson, speakers and participants.

### *Role of Organizers*

It is the organizers who decides the topic of seminar. Usually topics are related to the current trends or recent developments in the clinical practice or nursing education. Once the topic is decided and objectives are formulated, organizers start searching for a suitable chairperson and select an eminent person who is well versed in the concerned topic as the chairperson. In consultation with the chairperson, organizers modifies the objectives if needed, finalize the various aspects of the topic and select speakers. Date and time is fixed according to the convenience of the chairperson and speakers.

In case of national or international seminars, large scale preparation is needed and organizers have to form various committees like invitation committee, finance committee, academic committee, etc., and coordinate effectively for the successful conduction of the seminar.

### Role of the Chairperson

Chairperson should possess in depth knowledge regarding the topic, and it is his duty to guide the seminar in a fruitful manner. Seminar begins with an introductory speech by the chairperson. In the introductory talk, he justifies the topic selection by stating its relevance and importance in the current context and introduces the speakers by highlighting their achievements. After the introductory speech chairperson invites speakers according to the order. When one speaker completes his speech, he gives a brief summary of it and invites next speaker to to present his viewpoints. Once all the speakers complete their presentations, chairperson opens the discussion session by inviting participants to come out with their doubts, clarifications and contributions. Some chairpersons prefer discussion after each speaker completes the presentation. Even though this is good, it is not advisable always due to its time-consuming nature.

### Role of Speakers

Success of a seminar depends on how well the discussion session is utilized by the participants. The quality and quantity of the information presented by the speakers have a direct role in preparing the participants for the discussion session. In this sense, success of the seminar is largely determined by the performance of the speakers. Speakers have to prepare and handover the study materials to the organizers in advance so that organizers can compile all study materials in a user-friendly way. Normally, study material is given to the participants one or two hours before the seminar. Speakers are expected to present the relevant information in an interesting and comprehensible manner with the help of suitable audiovisual aids.

### Role of Participants

Objectives of seminars are framed in accordance with the learning needs of the participants. Always participants make the seminar very live and interesting. They have to prepare themselves well in advance and the study material issued by the organizers before the seminar will also provide the required information in a condensed form. They have to utilize the discussion session by asking questions, seeking clarifications and expressing their viewpoints. Participants should use discussion to enrich their knowledge rather than testing the knowledge of the speakers or the chairperson.

### Seminar Technique

Organizers make necessary arrangements for the seminar and distribute study material to the participants one or two hours before the seminar. Seminar begins with an introductory speech by the chairperson. Chairperson then invites the speakers to present the latest information about different aspects of the seminar topic. After each speech chairperson has to summarize it before inviting the next speaker. After all speakers presented the information on various aspects of the topic, chairperson opens the discussion session by inviting questions, clarifications and contributions. Questions and clarifications should be addressed to the chairperson instead of addressing directly to the speakers. Chairperson then invite the concerned speaker to give the reply. If the doubt persists even after the clarification by the speaker, chairperson himself can clear the doubt. Seminar will come to an end after the discussion session with a concluding note by the chairperson. In the concluding note, chairperson summarizes the whole information exchanged in the seminar and congratulates organizers, speakers, and participants.

# SYMPOSIUM

Symposium is a form of discussion in which different viewpoints or opinions regarding the single aspect or component of a topic is discussed under the guidance of a chairperson. Symposium is the most preferred method to discuss controversial issues, such as professional status of nursing, impact of Consumer Protection Act on nursing and the like.

Even though the topic Consumer Protection Act has various aspects like importance of consumer protection in a consumer-driven society, Consumer Protection Act and healthcare system, etc., in a symposium on Consumer Protection Act and nursing practice. We discuss mainly the viewpoints or opinions prevailing among the nursing community regarding the impact of Consumer Protection Act on nursing practice. Thus, in symposium our discussion is centered around only one aspect or component of a topic by giving minimum attention to remaining aspects.

Just like seminar, personnel involved in the symposium can also be categorized into organizers, chairperson, speakers and participants **(Table 6.2)**.

## Role of Different Personnel

With few exceptions, role of different personnel in the symposium are similar to that of the seminar. In symposium, chairperson has to exert more control over the speakers in order to restrain them from crossing the limit while expressing or challenging contradictory opinions. In order to make the symposium a success, chairperson has to maintain a nonjudgmental attitude and provide equal opportunities to all speakers to express their feelings. Study material may not be issued to participants, as they have to participate in the discussion held at the end with their own viewpoints and opinions. Thus, symposium demands more preparation from the side of participants.

## Symposium Technique

Symposium begins with the introductory speech of the chairperson. After the introductory speech he invites speakers to present their viewpoints. Once the speakers complete their presentations, the chairperson opens the discussion session by inviting the participants to express their opinions regarding the various viewpoints put forward by speakers. In addition to exchanging their opinions with the chairperson, to a certain extent participants can also converse directly with the speakers. In symposium, more time is allotted for the discussion

**TABLE 6.2:** Difference between seminar and symposium.

| Seminar | Symposium |
|---|---|
| • Topics are related to recent trends and developments in nursing | • Topics are related to controversial. issues in nursing |
| • Multiple aspects of the topic under consideration is discussed | • Single aspect of the topic is discussed |
| • Chairperson has to exert less control | • Chairperson has to exert more control |
| • Less time for discussion involving participants | • More time for discussion involving participants |
| • Comparatively less preparation from the side of participants | • Demands more preparation from the side of participants |

involving participants compared to the time allotted for speakers. Finally, under the leadership of chairperson a consensus is reached after verifying the pros and cons of different viewpoints expressed by the speakers as well as the participants.

The chairperson, speakers and participants have to take utmost care to maintain a cordial atmosphere by adopting an assertive style of communication.

### Disadvantages of Seminar and Symposium

Disadvantages levelled against symposium and seminar includes: (a) Shortage of resource personnel; (b) Autocratic attitude of chairperson did not allow fair presentation of information by speakers or participants; (c) Inadequate preparation from the side of resource personnel. In authors' point of view, these disadvantages are not withstanding due to the following reasons: (i) Since there is a tremendous increase in the number of nursing institutions and nursing programs in the recent years, getting a suitable resource person is not a matter of concern, (ii) Chairpersons are usually well-known popular figures with pleasing manners. A chairperson with an autocratic attitude will not be entertained in further seminars or symposiums, (iii) As symposium and seminar are restricted mainly to postgraduate students and research scholars, resource persons will not take a chance and prepare well to safeguard their reputation.

## SIMULATIONS

### Meaning

According to International Dictionary of Education, simulation is a teaching technique used particularly in management education and training in which a 'real life situation' and values are simulated by 'substitute' displaying similar characteristics.

Some educators consider simulation as a technique in teacher education in which student act out or role play teaching situations in an attempt to make 'theory' more practically oriented and realistic.

From the above said meanings, it is very clear that simulation creates an environment resembling real-life situation which helps the students practice and gain experience as in a real-life situation so that they can practice confidently when exposed to real-life situation.

### Types of Simulation

There are three types of simulation, namely: simulation exercise, simulation game and role playing.

1. **Simulation exercise:** A controlled representation of a piece of reality that learners can manipulate to better understand the corresponding real situation.
2. **Simulation game:** A game that represents real-life situations in which learners compete according to a set of rules in order to win or achieve an objective.
3. **Role playing:** A form of drama in which learners spontaneously act out roles in an interaction involving problems or challenges in human relations.

A variety of simulation is available for nursing and health care education. Ziv classified the simulations available for nursing in the following manner:

- Simple models or mannequins
- Simulated/standardized patients
- Computer screen-based clinical case simulators
- Realistic high-tech procedural simulators (task trainers)
- Virtual reality
- Realistic, high-tech interactive patient simulators.

## Purposes of Simulation

Simulation can serve the following purposes:
- Simulation is intended to help students' practice decision making and problem-solving skills and develop human interaction abilities in a controlled and safe setting.
- Through an active involvement in a simulation exercise, a game or a role playing situation, the student achieves cognitive, affective and psychomotor outcomes.
- Simulation provides a chance to apply principles and theories students have learned and to see how and when these principles work.
- Through simulation students can learn how to learn and test various approaches in a setting where patients cannot be hurt and where wrong decisions can always be reminded. It is hoped that the knowledge gained through simulation can be easily transferred to the real patient care settings.

## Value of Simulation

- **Simulation ensures safe nursing practice by nursing students through bridging the gap between theory and practice:** In the simulated environment of the fundamentals laboratory, students learn safe practice of nursing through the perfect application of learned theory under the guidance of the teacher. Thus, simulation bridges the gap between theory and practice.
- **Simulation is an effective technique to learn psychomotor skills:** In the simulated environment of the fundamentals laboratory, by the use of mannequins and other equipment students learn psychomotor skills essential for giving nursing care in the clinical situation.
- **Simulation helps the students develop critical thinking abilities and problem-solving skills:** Simulation is the most effective way for developing problem-solving skills. The acquisition of problem-solving skills will in turn help students apply the nursing process by gathering and analyzing data, identifying the problems, setting priorities, selecting and modifying interventions and evaluating outcomes.
- **Simulation not only helps the students learn the decision making process but also provide feedback regarding the consequences of the decisions made:** In the simulated environment, students learn decision making process by making decisions rather than simply grasping the related theory. They also get the feedback regarding the consequences of the decision from the teacher and classmates. In this way, students become aware of their ability to make effective decisions.
- **Simulations, especially the role play enables students to empathize with the real-life situations:** Empathy is the most desirable quality as far as a nurse is concerned and through participating in a role play or viewing it students develop this most desirable quality. By means of empathy, students place themselves in others' position, this will help understand others' feelings and to interact effectively by employing appropriate communication styles suitable to the situation. As interaction is taking place in a simulated environment, students get an immediate feedback regarding their way of interaction and communication style. In short, simulation is a good means for developing communication skills and understanding the complexity of human relationships.
- **By way of simulation teacher can easily inculcate proper attitude among nursing students:** As said elsewhere, inculcating proper attitude is a difficult task but a nurse educator cannot ignore this aspect because proper attitude is essential for good nursing practice. Simulation helps students recognize the need of proper attitude in giving

comprehensive nursing care and helps them to cultivate a positive attitude essential for a successful nursing career.

- **Simulation can also be used to evaluate students:** Questions in the simulated form are very useful in assessing the knowledge related to the practical aspects of a subject. For example, the teacher can evaluate the student's knowledge regarding the various aspects of the lecture through a simulated form of question like you are appointed as a nursing tutor in a school of nursing and instructed to take a two-hour class on 'history of nursing in a class of 50 students under the supervision of the principal then:
    i. Which teaching method would you select?
    ii. Justify your selection?
    iii. List down the techniques you would adopt in order to make the teaching more interesting and comprehensible.
    In the evaluation session principal commented that you are looking frequently to a black spot on the wall and pinching the nose occasionally. From the principal's opinion:
    iv. Identify the techniques in which you are lacking proficiency.
    v. Explain the measures that will assist you in attaining proficiency in the identified techniques.

As a whole, we can say simulation motivates students by making real-life situations less threatening, exciting and interesting.

### Role of the Teacher

Teachers' role in simulation has three facets namely: planning, facilitating and debriefing.

While planning, teacher has to purchase a simulation package or develop an appropriate simulation capable of achieving course objectives. Before using teacher should ensure the usefulness of the simulation. Teacher can cooperate with other faculty members in the development and use of simulations. She can help students prepare themselves for simulation by providing references and directing to other sources of information. Irrespective of the type of simulation, teacher should try to involve all the students in one way or the other as actors, discussion members and observers. She has to encourage shy or reluctant students to participate in the simulation.

Once the simulation progresses as desired, teacher adopts her role as a facilitator. She has to observe carefully the behavior of students and take down the important pieces of conservation among them so that she can substantiate or modify the viewpoints of students in a better manner during the debriefing session. When the simulation is based upon a problem, as a facilitator, teacher has to maintain a nonjudgmental attitude by not giving quick suggestions or advice.

As purposes of the simulation are mainly achieved in the debriefing session, teacher has to play an important role in this session. Debriefing session should be conducted immediately after the simulation. Initially, teacher summarises the whole event and then encourages the participants to do a self-analysis and give their opinion regarding the roles played by them and the value of experience they gained through enacting the roles. Self-analysis helps students not only rationalize their actions or behavior but also realize their drawbacks, thereby making them sensitive to the suggestions made by others. In the case of emotion laden simulations, debriefing should allow ventilation of feelings. Next, observers are allowed to express their opinions regarding the performance of participants, experience gained and how they would perform, if they were the participants. Finally, teacher explains the concepts and principles applied in simulation and how the students are benefited from the experience gained through simulation.

## Advantages of Simulations

According to Ried, simulation simplifies the complexity of real life to a level that can be handled by the beginners. In the simulated environment of fundamentals laboratory, first year students learn how to deal with patients. Even though the environment in the fundamentals laboratory is controlled, it is somewhat similar to a hospital ward. Experience gained from fundamentals laboratory helps the students get acquainted easily with the real-life situation during their clinical postings. Simulation is highly student-centered because of its very interesting and motivating nature, effectiveness in teaching slow learners as well as fast learners and all type of students.

Even though there is a teacher to guide, simulation always facilitates peer learning, which is considered as an excellent way of learning. Various roles played by the students in simulation, such as participants, discussion members and observers provide them an opportunity to learn.

Simulation offers an excellent opportunity to learn from mistakes, especially from those which are detrimental to the nursing students, if committed in the real-life situation. For those who believe in the proverb "to err is human but repeating is foolish," simulation is an excellent method of learning. Through simulation students also become aware of possible ways and chances of committing mistakes so that they can avoid mistakes by taking precautions.

According to Dekker and Donatti, simulation help students acquire concrete meanings for abstract terms. By conducting a simulation, teacher can easily make the students understand the concepts like interpersonal relationship, assertive communication style, etc. As simulation provides a realistic experience, students can easily apply these concepts in the clinics.

Simulation fosters critical thinking and problem-solving skills. Through simulation teacher can provide a controlled environment in which students can test different solutions arising out of critical thinking until a suitable solution is reached. This will enable them to solve the problems, especially in the clinical situation. When different students suggest different solutions to solve a problem or to overcome a difficult situation, students get an idea regarding the usefulness of a multipronged approach in solving problems or overcoming crisis situations.

## Disadvantages of Simulation

Students may generalize the result of a single simulation; however, teacher can prevent this by providing proper explanation. While explaining the purpose of simulation, teacher should make it clear that the lessons or solutions learned from a particular simulation cannot be blindly applied to another situation or problem. This is essential because the fruitful implementation of solutions require careful analysis of the factors involved in the problem or situation. When the teacher teaches the application of principles or concepts through a simulation, she should highlight the need of context-specific application of general principles or concepts so that students will not apply principles or concepts learned from a particular simulation to other situations in the same manner. For example, a student posted in the pediatric ward cannot apply the concepts or principles of interpersonal relationship in the same manner as learned from a role play intended to teach interpersonal relationship in an adult ward.

Simulation is expensive in terms of time, money and energy. Even though the induction of computers in education reduced the cost of preparing simulations, still simulations, especially the commercially prepared ones are very expensive. Teachers have to spend a lot of time to prepare a simulation. As a teaching method also it is very time consuming. Since a lot of time is required to prepare and practice simulations, many teachers prefer other methods.

Emotion laden simulations may cause mental trauma to the participating students. Simulations, especially role plays can cause mental trauma to students who are handling negative roles like drug addicts or alcoholics. To avoid this, teacher should make sure that the feelings are ventilated properly during the debriefing session.

Since simulation trains students in the real life like situations, students may undervalue the complexities waiting for them in the real world. This is a major drawback of simulation and do more harm than good. In order to avoid this drawback, teacher should not be too flexible while conducting simulation and should immediately notice and correct mistakes. Moreover, teacher should have a sense of authority while giving corrections or guidance.

If the group dynamics is not good as expected, simulation may fail to attain objectives. Inadequate preparation and the tendency of some students to excel at the cost of others can trouble group dynamics. Adequate preparation from the side of the teacher and students, giving proper direction to students and controlling an over enthusiastic student are some of the ways to maintain proper group dynamics.

## ROLE PLAYING

By definition, "role playing is a form of drama in which learners spontaneously act out roles in an interaction involving problems or challenges in human relations for subsequent discussion by the whole class".

From the definition, it is clear that role playing is a spontaneous acting out of roles. Based on the written or verbal explanation of the simulated situation, participants spontaneously act out the roles without a script or rehearsal, but at times if needed, teacher can plan for role playing and guide the participants by giving necessary instructions. Role playing is advised only when the learners have a background knowledge regarding the simulated context or situation and the roles assigned to the participants. Role playing is very useful to nursing students as it helps them acquire skills in matters related to human behavior and human relations like conflict resolution, interpersonal relationship and therapeutic relationship. Through role playing teacher can prepare final year students for the forthcoming job interviews and evaluation interviews. Since role playing is very helpful in analyzing social problems, it can be effectively used to teach community health nursing. Another purpose of role playing is to assist student in giving health education in an attractive manner. Since educative approach is regarded as the best approach to promote public health, this purpose is very much admired by the health workers all over the world. Through role play students also develop empathy (see value of simulation).

When the teacher feels that role playing is very effective in attaining teaching objectives or in dealing with topics involving human interactions, she can employ role playing by giving verbal or written explanation of the context and assigning roles to a few students as participants. It is well and good, if the students voluntarily take up the roles, otherwise she will have to select students in her own way. Then the participants will act out the roles according to the situation and the remaining students have to observe and critically analyze the characters acted out by the participants. Once the participants finish the acting, teacher opens the discussion session by inviting observers to express their opinions. In role playing, only five to ten minutes is allotted for acting out the roles and most of the time is utilized for discussion. The discussion should focus on the role of characters in the particular context instead of criticizing the participants. Discussion helps the students understand the principles and concepts underlying human interactions and enables them to apply these principles as and when needed.

## MICROTEACHING

Teaching is a very complex activity involving simultaneous application of multiple skills. It is very difficult for a student teacher to attain these skills and refine them at a stretch. In the same way, it is difficult for the teacher also to properly assess all the teaching skills of a student teacher at a time and give necessary corrections. By way of scaled down teaching in a controlled environment, teacher can easily identify the deficiencies of the student teacher in performing a particular teaching skill and help him attain proficiency in that skill by providing assistance to rectify the identified deficiencies. In simple sense, this scaled down teaching by a student teacher in a controlled environment under the supervision of a teacher in order to attain proficiency in a particular teaching skill is called microteaching.

## Definition

- According to Bush, "microteaching is a teacher education technique which allows teachers to apply clearly defined teaching skills to carefully prepared lessons in a planned series of five to ten minutes encounter with a small group of real students, often with an opportunity to observe the result on video tape".
- Singh believes that microteaching is a scaled down teaching encounter in which a teacher teaches a small unit to a group of five pupils for a small period of five to twenty minutes. Such a situation offers a helpful setting for an experienced or inexperienced teacher to acquire new teaching skills and to refine old ones.

## Simple Outline of Microteaching

Microteaching helps student teacher or trainee acquires hard-to-attain teaching skills in a simplified manner through a scaled down teaching situation. Scaled down teaching situation is created by reducing class size to a small group of four to six pupils, reducing the length of teaching time to five to ten minutes and by focusing on the refining of a particular teaching skill rather than trying to attain proficiency in various skills. The skill under consideration may be questioning, leading a discussion, eliciting student participation, effective use of teaching strategies, appropriate use of audiovisual aids, classroom management, etc. Based on the objectives, the student teacher prepares the lesson and takes class under the supervision of the teacher. It is well and good, if there is a provision to record the class on a video camera and to show it to the student teacher immediately after the class. This will provide an authentic feedback and helps the student teacher do a self-analysis objectively. The pupils are instructed to fill in rating questionnaires pertaining to the specific aspects of the teaching activity. Based on supervisor's suggestions, pupils' remarks and self-analysis, student teacher restructures the lesson by rectifying the noted defects and reteaches immediately to a new group of pupils under the supervision of the same supervisor. Student teacher receives the reefed back and usually feels confident in handling a particular skill within two microteaching cycles. Subsequent microteaching cycles will help the student teacher attain proficiency in some other teaching skills. Forthcoming discussion on phases of microteaching will give you an idea regarding the way of conducting microteaching in an organized manner.

## Phases, Activities and Components of Microteaching

According to JC Clift, microteaching has three phases, namely: (a) Knowledge acquisition phase, (b) skill acquisition phase, and (c) transfer phase. JC Aggarwal explains the three phases as follows:

### *Knowledge Acquisition Phase*

In this phase, the student teacher attempts to acquire knowledge about the skill—its rationale, its role in classroom and its component behaviors. For this, he reads relevant literature. He also observes demonstration lesson—mode of presentation of skill. Thus, the student teacher gets theoretical as well as practical knowledge of the skill.

### Skill Acquisition Phase

On the basis of the model presented to the student teacher, he prepares a micro lesson and practices the skill and carries out the microteaching cycle. There are two components in this phase, namely: microteaching setting and feedback. Microteaching setting includes conditions like size of the micro class, duration of the micro lesson, supervisor, types of students, etc.

### Transfer Phase

Here the student teacher integrates different skills. In place of scaled down situation, he teaches in the real classroom and tries to integrate all the skills.

The three phases involve certain steps as detailed below:

1. **Orientation of student teachers:** This involves providing necessary information and theoretical background about microteaching on the following aspects like: (a) Concept of microteaching; (b) Rationale or significance of using microteaching; (c) Procedures of microteaching; (d) Requirements and setting for the adoption of microteaching technique.
2. **Discussion of teaching skills:** Under this step the knowledge and understanding of the following steps is to be developed: (a) Analysis of teaching into component teaching skills; (b) Discussion of the rationale and role of these teaching skills in teaching; (c) Discussion regarding the component teaching behaviors comprising various teaching skills.
3. **Selection of particular teaching skill:** Each skill needs to be practised at a time. Student teachers should be given necessary background for the observation of a model of demonstration lesson on the selected particular skill.
4. **Presentation of a model demonstration lesson on a particular skill:** Demonstration lesson is given by the teacher for the student teachers on the practice of a particular skill. This is also known as *'modelling'.* Demonstration can be given in a number of ways like: (a) By exhibiting a film on a video tape; (b) By providing written materials such as hand books, guides, illustrations, etc. (c) By making the trainees listen an audiotape; (d) By arranging a live demonstration by the teacher or some experts.
5. **Observation of the model lesson:** An observation schedule designed for the observation of the specific skill is distributed for the guidance of the student teachers for observing the lesson.
6. **Criticism of the model lesson:** A critical appraisal of the model lesson is made by the student teachers.
7. **Preparation of the micro lesson plan:** For the preparation of the micro lesson plan on the skill to be demonstrated, help may be taken from the sample lesson plans and from the teacher.
8. **Creation of microteaching setting:** The Indian model of microteaching developed by NCERT gives the following setting:
   a. Number of Pupils: 5-10
   b. Types of Pupils: Real pupils or preferably peers
   c. Type of Supervisor: Teacher and peers
   d. Time duration of a microteaching cycle: 36 minutes.
   This duration is divided as detailed below:
   - Teach 6 minutes
   - Feedback 6 minutes
   - Replan 12 minutes
   - Reteach 6 minutes
   - Refeedback 6 minutes

9. **Practice of the skill (teaching session):** During this step, the student teacher teaches the prepared lesson for six minutes to a micro class of five to ten real pupils or peers (student teachers). The teaching activity is supervised by the teacher and other student teachers (peers). Where possible, the student teacher may also have the lesson taped on a video or audio tape.
10. **Providing feedback:** The peers and teacher observing the micro lesson may provide immediate feedback. Where possible, mechanical gadgets like the video tape, audio tape, closed circuit television, etc., may be used for providing feedback.
11. **Replanning (replanning session):** In the light of the feedback received, the student teacher replans his micro lesson. He is given 12 minutes for this purpose.
12. **Reteaching (reteaching session):** This session lasts for six minutes and the student teacher reteaches his micro lesson on the basis of his replanned lesson.
13. **Providing refeedback (refeedback session):** The student teacher is provided refeedback on the re-taught micro lesson.
14. **Integration of teaching skills:** This is the last step and is concerned with the task of integrating several skills individually mastered by the student teacher. It is helpful in bridging the gap between training in isolated teaching skills and the real teaching situation faced by a teacher.

## Merits of Microteaching

- Microteaching help student teachers to acquire hard-to-attain teaching skills by providing a real situation for practising skills.
- Since microteaching focuses on a particular skill at a time, student teachers can attain proficiency in teaching skills in a phased manner.
- Provision of immediate feedback makes microteaching more interesting and reliable.
- Since main role is played by the student teacher, it is regarded as a student-centered method.
- As gadgets like video camera and tape recorders are used extensively in microteaching, it exemplifies the effective use of technology in the field of education.

## Demerits of Microteaching

- Microteaching is time consuming, especially in the case of an ill-prepared student teacher.
- Because of modeling (see Step 4) there is a risk of simply imitating a teaching skill by the student teachers. Since a teaching skill can be attained and nurtured in different ways other than imitating, to a certain extent microteaching is hampering the creativity of the student teacher.
- Even though microteaching can be successfully employed in classroom teaching situations, more research is needed to ascertain its usefulness in other teaching situations.

# TEACHING NURSING

## Definition

In author's opinion, "Teaching nursing is a dynamic process of transforming nursing students to good human beings with qualities of a competent professional nurse through behavior modification by way of appropriate teaching–learning process."

This definition comprises three vital components:
1. **Dynamic process:** Teaching nursing is a dynamic process. Aims of nursing education change in accordance with development in cognitive neuroscience, trends in general education and trends in health care.

2. **Competent professional nurse:** Competent professional nurse is capable of promoting health, preventing illness, restoring health and alleviate sufferings depending on the context of care.
3. **Appropriate teaching–learning process:** Appropriate teaching–learning process enables nursing students to acquire relevant attitude, knowledge and skills essential to become a professional nurse.

## Principles off Teaching Nursing

Even though every nurse educator follows his or her own principles while teaching, following principles can serve as a general guidelines for teaching nursing.

- **Strategies of teaching nursing are influenced by the latest developments in cognitive neurosciences, trends in general education and trends in health care industry:** This principle underlines the dynamic nature of teaching nursing. Nurse educator need to be aware about latest trends in related areas and try to integrate these while preparing teaching material.
- **Teaching nursing enables students to acquire relevant skills, attitudes, knowledge and values through ongoing behavior modification:** Teaching nursing enables students to proactively acquire new or modify existing skills for maintaining competency in nursing care. This can be achieved through ongoing behavior modification of nursing students.
- **Teaching nursing promotes collaboration than competition:** This principle is based on the latest trend in education. Through collaboration much more can be achieved than engaging in competition.
- **Clinical area is a goldmine of learning experience:** This principle underlines the importance of providing adequate clinical experience as well as clinical teaching in teaching nursing. Clinical area offers a variety of learning opportunities for becoming a competent professional nurse.
- **Providing adequate provision for translating theory into practice is the key of teaching nursing:** This principle highlights the need of providing enough opportunities to develop competencies required for nursing practice. Simultaneous provision of adequate clinical exposure and effective clinical supervision, etc., will help to follow this principle.
- **Technology only makes teaching easier not better hence, student-teacher interaction is most important in teaching nursing:** This principle highlights the importance of effective student-teacher interaction in teaching nursing for achieving objectives.
- **Nurse educators need to assist students in developing mastery orientation among students in order to achieve learning outcomes:** As learning takes place in a variety of situations mastery orientation is a must for attaining learning outcomes in nursing education. Students with mastery orientation believes in hard work, have a goal of learning, focus on developing new skills and acquiring knowledge. In short, students with mastery orientation become self-directed learners. Self-directed learners believes in effort and practice rather than "intelligence" or "talents".
- **Successful implementation of students support and guidance programme (SSGP) is an integral part of teaching nursing:** By providing adequate support for learning through guidance and support services teachers can enhance learning ability of students.
- **Teaching nursing prepares students for expanded or evolving professional roles in health care and education:** In accordance with the trends in health care, the traditional roles of nurses will change. Teaching nursing need to empower students to attain these roles in their upcoming professional life.

* An eclectic approach to discipline with emphasis to preventive discipline and discipline with dignity is desirable in teaching nursing.
* Students perform better when they understand what they are expected to do; hence nurse educators need to explain teacher expectations well in advance.
* Nursing students need constructive and timely feedback for attaining Learning goals.
* Becoming a reflective teacher helps nurse educator to become an expert teacher through collaboration and effort.
* Teachings nursing always try to inculcate values among students that uphold professional status of nursing.

## Teaching Psychomotor Skills

In simple terms, skill is the practical expertise to do something. In nursing, psychomotor skill can be defined as a system of goal directed or well organized behavior that is essential to provide meticulous nursing care in a wide range of situations. The goal may be promoting health, preventing illness, recovering health or alleviate suffering.

National guidelines for educating EMS instructors recommend four steps for teaching a psychomotor skill they are:
a. Overview by briefly explaining about what to do before performing a skill, how to perform a skill and what to do after performing a skill.
b. Demonstration by following whole to parts and then parts to whole approach is useful to students.
c. Assisting students to perform the skill by effectively supervising return demonstration.
d. Providing timely and constructive feedback for improving proficiency in performing a skill.

## CLINICAL TEACHING

Clinical area really poses a great challenge to nursing teachers. In nursing, psychomotor skills enjoy a dominant position and professional competency of a nurse is recognized mainly by the demonstration of clinical skills. Developing clinical skills demands more effort from the side of teachers and students compared to teaching and learning theoretical knowledge. Irrespective of the theoretical knowledge, students usually feel insecure and incompetent if they lack adequate clinical skills. Introduction of sophisticated equipment on a regular basis to assist patient care again adds to the complex nature of clinical teaching. Considering the increased mechanization of the patient care, while teaching clinical skills teacher has to motivate the students to follow the *"high tech-high touch"* approach in order to preserve the human component of nursing care. Through appropriate clinical teaching methods an intelligent teacher always helps the student to develop an appreciable level of nursing skills. In the case of a studious student, clinical area is a gold mine of learning opportunities and experiences.

### Definition

In authors' opinion "clinical teaching is the process of assisting nursing students to develop attributes essential for professional nursing practice in a real life situation by adopting appropriate methods of teaching and supervision".

This definition highlights the following:
* **It is a process:** Clinical teaching is a process involves lot of preparation from students and teachers. As a process clinical teaching has three important phases namely: planning or preparation phase, during which objectives of clinical postings are laid down and communicated to all concerned. Second is the implementation phase or actual clinical

posting is carried out with adequate supervision and ongoing evaluation. Third phase is the evaluation phase for assessing the achievement of objectives of clinical posting.
- **Attributes for professional practice:** Attributes for professional nursing practice can be divided into core professional skills and soft skills. Relevant attitude, knowledge and skills are essential for competent nursing practice.
- **Methods of teaching and supervision:** Adopting appropriate methods of teaching and supervision is essential for achieving objectives of clinical teaching.

## Objectives of Clinical Teaching

A well structured clinical teaching will help students achieve the following objectives: (a) Understanding of health, illness and healthcare system; (b) Developing an awareness of own attitudes, values and responses to health and illness; (c) Understanding of the interrelated roles of healthcare team; (d) Developing clinical competencies like reasoning, psychomotor and interpersonal and communication skills; (e) Creating an ability to provide a scientific rationale for interventions; (f) Developing self-management skills, especially related to time and work load; (g) Developing ability to process, record and use data effectively; (h) Developing ability to evaluate critically and improve own performance; (i) Developing ability to review and investigate the quality of clinical practice; (j) Develop professional accountability; (k) Acquire commitment to develop and maintain professional competence.

## Principles of Clinical Teaching

- **Clinical teaching is a vital and irreplaceable component in preparing the nursing students for professional practice:** This principle underlines the importance of providing adequate clinical experience to students. Infrastructure of nursing institutions should be evaluated on the basis of the clinical facility available for students. If clinical facility is inadequate in the parent hospital, institution head need to arrange facilities through affiliated hospitals.
- **Clinical education should reflect the nature of professional practice:** Professional practice requires critical thinking and problem-solving abilities, specialized psychomotor and technological skills and a professional value system. Clinical education should assist students to acquire above said qualities in an admirable manner.
- **Clinical teaching is important than classroom teaching:** Unlike classroom teaching, clinical teaching provides real life experiences and opportunities for transfer of knowledge to practical situations. Faculty who teach in the clinical setting can help students achieve objectives in a successful manner. According to Halstead, effective clinical teachers are clinically competent, know how to teach, have collegial relationships with students and are friendly, supportive and patient.
- **The nursing student in the clinical setting is a learner, not a nurse:** The students learn through doing hence opportunity shall be provided for the student to practice various activities to enable effective learning.
- **Sufficient learning time must be provided before performance is evaluated:** Most of the teachers perceive their role as "to evaluate" and majority of the students also perceive the same about teachers. The teacher cannot expect the students to perform competently in their first attempt. Skill acquisition is a complex process that involves making mistakes, learning how to correct and overcoming those mistakes.
- **Clinical teaching must be supported by a climate of mutual trust and respect:** To support learning and student growth in clinical practice, the teacher must respect the students as learners and trust their motivation and commitment to the profession. The students must respect the teacher's commitment to both nursing education and society.

- **Clinical teaching and learning should focus on essential knowledge, skills and attitudes:** Clinical teaching primarily must focus on essential curriculum which includes the knowledge, skill and attitude which are essential for safe and competent practice. Enrichment curriculum which enhances further learning is of importance but is secondary. For example, before giving a test dose of an antibiotic which may trigger an anaphylactic reaction, nursing student must make sure that a syringe loaded with adrenaline is kept ready for emergency use if needed. Here knowledge about the drug reaction of a particular drug, its dose and action is regarded as essential knowledge and comes under essential curriculum. Whereas the structure of the drug and its metabolism comes under enrichment curriculum.
- **Quality is more important than quantity:** The length of time spent in clinical area is no guarantee of the amount or quality of learning that has taken place. The proposed duration may be insufficient for some students and unnecessarily long for others to acquire a particular skill.
- **Nursing students experience stress and anxiety in clinical learning situation:** The effective clinical teacher recognizes students' need for supportive and collegial relationships and develops an interpersonal style that promotes a conducive learning environment. A safe and stress free learning environment has been created when students feel comfortable in speaking openly. Negative relationships with faculty can contribute to anxiety. Positive relationships are nurturing and can enhance learning. Caring behaviors and caring environment are essential for reducing the stress of students.

## Outcomes of Clinical Teaching

According to Katheen and Marityn the outcomes of clinical teaching include knowledge, skills, professional attitudes and values essential for safe and competent nursing practice.

1. **Knowledge:** Clinical teaching activities enable students to transfer knowledge learned in classroom and in self-directed learning to real life situations. In clinical practice, theory is translated into practice. By observing and participating in clinical activities students acquire knowledge. Knowing how to practice nursing involves cognitive skills in problem-solving, critical thinking and decision making.
2. **Skills:** Skills are another important outcomes of clinical teaching. Nurses must possess adequate psychomotor, interpersonal skills, communication skills and organizational skills in order to practice effectively in a challenging clinical environment. Among these skills most important one is psychomotor skills. Psychomotor skills enable nurses to perform as desired in the clinical area. These skills are purposeful, complex, movement-oriented activities that involve an overt physical response.
3. **Professional attitudes and values:** Clinical learning also produces important outcomes in affect-beliefs, values and attitudes that are essential for professional nursing practice. Affective outcomes represent the humanistic and ethical dimensions of nursing.

## Challenges in Clinical Teaching

Each nurse educator perceives challenges in a different manner but may have to face following challenges in clinical teaching:
- Providing an ideal clinical environment with adequate resources to practice what is taught in the classroom. In other words, finding it difficult to provide an ideal environment for translating theory into practice.
- Clearly defining clinical objectives and teacher expectations.
- Patient-related challenges. Patient may be too sick or unwilling to participate in teaching.

- Giving individual attention to students.
- Strictly following objectives of clinical posting by preventing students from performing non-nursing activities in clinical area.
- Eliciting active participation from students in attaining objectives of clinical posting.
- Insufficient time for adequate clinical supervision due to excess written assignment.
- Finding time for direct observation of learners and providing individual feedback.
- Integrating clinical practice with rest of curriculum.

## Selection of Clinical Area

De Young Sandra recommends following criteria for selecting appropriate clinical area:

- **Opportunity to achieve learning objectives:** Clinical area should provide an opportunity to achieve predetermined learning objectives. Achievement of learning objectives can be ascertained by ensuring: (a) conducive clinical environment for learning, (b) communicating learning objectives to the concerned personnel like nursing staff, hospital managers, etc. (c) rectifying any problems noticed during previous postings of students, (d) providing timely appropriate feedback to students in the clinical area, (e) ensuring adequate supervision and (f) ensuring student-friendly behaviors in the clinical area. In short clinical area should provide an opportunity to students for translating theory into practice.
- **Level of learners:** Clinical posting is always carried out by considering the level of learners. A first year student is never posted in maternity wards or a second year student is never posted in psychiatry wards. Clinical postings always consider the cognitive abilities of the learners.
- **Degree of control over students by faculty:** It is advisable to post students where faculty have total control over students. This will ensure discipline among students and help in timely completion of clinical assignments.
- **Availability of role model for students:** This criterion is really a challenging one for nurse educators. First, the clinical setting should be an ideal one as taught in the classroom. Second staff nurses need to provide nursing care in an ideal manner. Setting teaching wards with enough supplies and equipment and adequate nursing staff helps to meet this criterion.
- **Geographical consideration:** It is not advisable to provide clinical postings regularly in faraway places from college. Based on this criterion apex bodies like Indian Nursing Council stipulates certain distance from nursing college to parent hospital.
- **Physical factors:** Physical factors influence the learning outcomes of clinical posting in a significant way. Physical facilities should ensure adequate learning opportunities, safety of students as well as patients and adequate supervision.
- **Staff relationship with teachers and students:** Better relationship with staff of clinical area is very important in achieving objectives of clinical postings. This is true, especially when students are posted in affiliated institutions.
- **Opportunity for interdisciplinary communication:** Presence and cooperation of other health care professionals enhance learning ability of nursing students. For example, if the physician allows nursing students to accompany him during medical rounds it will provide another learning opportunity for students.
- **Costs:** Cost involved in clinical posting also need to consider, especially when posted in tertiary care areas. For example, cost of posting students in operation theater is much more than posting in a general ward. Hence, nurse educators should always try to achieve objectives of postings in high cost incurring areas within the stipulated period.

# Clinical Teaching Methods

## Classification of Clinical Teaching Methods

Clinical teaching methods can be classified in **Table 6.3** for the convenience. This classification is not a final one as nurse educators can develop innovative clinical teaching methods by using his/her own expertise.

**TABLE 6.3:** Classification of teaching methods. (see also innovative teaching methods in chapter 7)

| Written assignments | Learner-centered methods | Teacher-centered methods | Digital teaching methods |
|---|---|---|---|
| Care plan | Return demonstration | Demonstration | Pre-existing videos of clinical area |
| Care study | Case presentation | Nursing care conference | Live streaming of procedures |
| Clinical logs | Individual conference | | Video conference |
| Concept maps | Group conference | | |
| | Clinical post conference | | |
| | Clinical questioning | | |
| | Activated demonstration | | |

Let us discuss some of the commonly used clinical teaching methods in nursing.

## Nursing Care Plan

Besides providing assistance in rendering comprehensive nursing care, nursing care plan is also used as an excellent clinical teaching method. Rendering nursing care through nursing care plan help the students develop basic nursing skills like assessing the patients' condition, formulating nursing diagnosis, prioritizing patients' needs, planning care, implementing the care with rationale and evaluating the care. Nursing care plan based care help students to recognize the importance of delivering continuous and comprehensive care in a systematic way. Moreover, effective use of nursing care plan as a clinical teaching method fosters professionalism and creativity among students. In short, as a clinical teaching method, care plan help the students become familiar with the nursing process approach of delivering nursing care.

Before teaching care plan, teachers have to conduct a discussion and reach into a consensus regarding the format and content, preferably in accordance with the guidelines formulated by internationally recognized bodies like NANDA so that a unified view regarding care plan can be developed by nullifying confusions.

Considering the transnational career opportunities of nurses, nursing teacher has to maintain an international perspective while preparing the care plan format and motivate the students to follow the same.

To enrich the value of nursing care plan as a clinical teaching method, teacher has to give sufficient help and guidance students in preparing and implementing care plans. Students can discuss the care plan with the teacher as well as with the classmates for clarifications. Students should be given sufficient time to prepare, implement, evaluate and modify the care plan according to the patient needs. Beginning students who are learning the nursing process need to write simple, short care plans on simulated or real patient situations. They can learn the process without writing comprehensive lengthy plans. After a few weeks of clinical posting, the number and complexity of care plans can be increased gradually. When used judiciously, nursing care plan is an excellent, cost-effective and learner-centered clinical teaching method.

With no compromise on reliability, nursing care plan can be implemented in all clinical settings. This advantage of universal application along with the merits of a learner-centered method has created widespread popularity to this most admired clinical teaching method.

### *Nursing Care Study*

According to authors, "nursing care study is the blueprint of nursing care rendered by a nursing student to a selected patient, for a particular period by following nursing process approach, with an intention to develop comprehensive nursing care abilities".

To make students familiar with this method, well in advance teacher has to issue guidelines necessary for conducting the care study. Guidelines pertaining to the format and content, criteria for patient selection, involvement of patient's family in the care, role of teacher, role of other health team members, duration of care, available resources, evaluation of care study and peer group involvement in the aftermath discussion are essential for the successful practice of this method.

Format and content should ultimately focus on the nursing care issues and all information related to the patient is expected to serve as a background knowledge for providing comprehensive nursing care. In consultation with teacher, student can select the patient in accordance with the guidelines. Patient's immediate environment should be conducive for providing continuous care.

After selecting the patient, student has to give continuous care for a minimum of seven to ten days and, if there is an opportunity to assess the patient's condition during the first follow up visit in the hospital, teacher has to make necessary arrangements for the same. Student has to plan and deliver care in a systematic way by following the nursing process approach. Student can involve patient's family in the care and is free enough to seek appropriate help and cooperation from other health team members during the tenure of care for a better cause.

Student has to gather information related to the patient's disease condition with special reference to nursing care. For this, student can refer textbooks, journals, research studies and related websites. Discussion with experts will also help in gathering information. In fact, student has to hunt for literature related to the patient's condition.

In between teacher has to see that care study is progressing as planned and give necessary guidance as and when needed. Teacher can enquire with the student periodically regarding the progress or outcome of the care. Continuous interaction between the teacher and student is a key factor for the fruitful practice of this clinical teaching method.

By the end of the stipulated days of care or after the discharge of the patient, one week time can be given to the student for submitting the care study. Teacher should conduct a discussion on the care study in the class and encourage other students to participate actively. If there is time, student has to present the entire care study before the classmates so that they can actively participate in the discussion. Teacher should direct the discussion in such a way that all students should be benefited from the care study. Predetermined criteria will help the teacher evaluate care study in a creative manner.

There is no prescribed format and content for the care study, but an ideal care study invariably contains description regarding patient bio data, health profile, disease condition, investigations, line of management, related literature, nursing care planned and implemented according to the nursing process approach, discharge summary if present, etc. This list is not an end in itself and teacher can include more aspects, if seems relevant.

Number of care studies per clinical block or academic year is determined by the institutional policy, but a minimum of two care studies are recommended for each clinical subject in an academic year. With some modifications in the format, nursing care study can be successfully implemented in all healthcare settings.

Nursing care study provides an opportunity to learn nursing skills through problem-solving approach. Through care study students learn to identify and define patients' problem. After analyzing the problem, student tries different ways to solve it. This process of solving the patient's problem will ultimately result in meeting the patient's needs. Since problem-solving approach is regarded as the best approach to teach nursing, nursing care study is definitely a student-centered method.

Care study trains the student to locate, gather and process the information required to solve the patient's problems. The interaction with the patient's relatives and coordination with other health team members promote team building skills, especially the skill associated with initiating and maintaining interpersonal relationships.

The sense of accomplishment resulting from providing individualized comprehensive care to a patient will promote positive attitude towards patient care. Quite naturally, this method contributes to the development and refining of nursing skills.

Validity of any teaching method in nursing is judged by its ability to assist the learners in acquiring knowledge, skills and inculcation of proper attitude. Since nursing care study meticulously meets these criteria, it is regarded as an inevitable component in the art of teaching nursing.

## Bedside Clinic

Bedside clinic is an organized clinical instruction in the presence of the patient. Based on the type of topic, bedside clinic can be medical, nursing or combined. This is a teacher-centered method meant for a small group of students and can be conducted by a nurse educator, doctor or a ward sister. The name of the patient, other details and the venue should be informed to students prior enough so that they can study the case sheet of the patient, review the related literature and actively participate in the bedside clinic. Depending on the convenience of the patient, clinic can be conducted at the bedside or in the nearby clinical teaching room. Prior permission should be taken from the patient or relatives for conducting bedside clinic. Patient selected should have typical signs and symptoms rather than unusual or confusing symptoms. The usual duration is 30 to 45 minutes and students have to gather around the patient in an informal way in order to avoid tension to him. Patient should be taken into confidence and nothing should be done or told throughout the clinic which may humiliate or embarrass him. If patient's condition permits, it is better to motivate him to give a brief description regarding his condition.

The learning experience is essentially discussion with a focus on the total care of the patient, specific nursing care, observations and recorded data and their implications, the patient reactions, response to care and progress. The medical and surgical treatment and consequences regarding how they relate to and effect the nature of nursing care are the key factors in the learning exercise and include the solving of patient care problems.

Presence of the patient during the entire period is not a must. Before going to the patient's side, teacher has to explain some of the details which does not require his presence like bio-data, family background, past medical history, etc. Condition of the patient, signs and symptoms, line of management and nursing care are discussed in the presence of the patient.

While discussing, teacher can also involve the students, especially the student who is looking after the patient. After the explanation by the teacher students are allowed to interact with the patient for further clarifications. Once this interaction is over, patient is set free and in the further discussion students' doubts and questions are clarified or answered. Bedside clinic ends with a summary, recapitulation of important aspects and feedback from students.

Even though bedside clinic is a teacher-centered method, measures, such as informing students much ahead of time, selecting patients with disease conditions of common interest, ensuring patient's or relative's cooperation, proper timing and encouraging student participation will bring out student involvement.

### Nursing Care Conference
Nursing care conference has all the characteristics of the bedside clinic except the presence of the patient. When the teacher as well as the students are well acquainted with the patient's features this is the preferred method.

### Nursing Rounds
In the hospital, nursing rounds is mainly concerned with judging the adequacy of nursing care received by the patients and it is conducted under the leadership of senior nurses or nurse administrators with the active participation of nursing teachers, staff nurses and nursing students.

As a clinical teaching method, nursing rounds is a modified compact version of the bedside clinic. In bedside clinic, a detailed discussion regarding the nursing care of a single patient is carried out by taking 30 to 40 minutes, whereas in nursing rounds only a few minutes is spend with each patient. In short, nursing rounds is intended to discuss briefly the nursing management of all patients in the ward by sparing few minutes for each patient. The ideal duration of nursing rounds in a ward is 45 minutes and this time is sufficient to know about 20 to 25 patients. For a successful nursing rounds, students have to know all patients in the ward. The patients' dignity have to be preserved throughout the rounds. The time of the rounds should be informed to the students if there is no stipulated time for daily rounds.

In nursing rounds, the nursing teacher or head nurse who knows the details of the patient briefs the nursing care. The staff nurse or the nursing student who has been taking care of the patient for a few days are allowed to contribute some genuine points and have to answer the questions of the group. The group then discuss the nursing care aspects in brief and the senior nursing personnel in the group or the nurse administrator concludes the discussion by giving some opinions, needed guidance and instructions. One staff nurse records all the instructions and suggestions given by the administrator in the nursing rounds register maintained in the ward. Then the group move towards the next patient. Group members have to encourage students for actively participating in the discussion. Nursing rounds focus mainly on the nursing care and in the nursing care only the cardinal aspects are discussed. For instance, the importance of maintaining an intake-output chart in the case of a patient receiving diuretics is highlighted. In the same manner, the necessity of accurate assessment and recording of the pulse rate is stressed in the case of a patient receiving digoxin.

Demonstration of nursing care by senior members during the nursing rounds will help students develop psychomotor skills and inculcate proper attitude among them. By attending nursing rounds, students are motivated to learn more about the nursing management of patient in the ward by referring related literature and through discussion with experts. Moreover, interaction with senior members promotes team spirit and professionalism.

Authors believe that the unique feature of nursing rounds is its ability to nurture the discriminating power of students. Through nursing rounds, students develop an ability to discriminate or classify the patients into high risk, risk and no risk categories depending on the severity of illness. When students are assigned to a number of patients at a time or when they become staff nurses, this discriminating power will help them identify patients who required constant or immediate attention.

## Group Conference

In group conference, a subject of common interest related to the clinical area is discussed by the students under the guidance of the nurse educator. This is a small group teaching method. Subjects selected for group conference should have a clinical orientation and enrich the clinical skills of students. Subjects like nursing management of patients with a particular disease, common errors likely to be committed by students in the clinical area, any deficiencies noted in the nursing care delivery by students, updating of procedures, patient care implications while administrating drugs, cost-effective use of supplies and equipment, infection control, proper waste disposal, ward routines, interpersonal relationship with patients, interpersonal relationship with other health team members, ethical and legal issues related to nursing care and other genuine topics or issues identified by students or teacher can be discussed in the group conference.

Discussion should be based on relevant information and directed towards achieving some desirable ends. Students are allowed to participate actively in the discussion, preferably by explaining their own experiences in the clinical area. Nursing teacher has to encourage the students to express their viewpoints and guide them as needed. While discussing problems pertaining to the clinical area, sometimes, it is impossible to solve them by adopting ready-made solutions prescribed by the textbooks, so the teacher has to motivate students to come forward with innovative ideas suiting to the problem or situation. During the discussion, the teacher has to assess the pros and cons of suggestions put forward by students before giving the opinion. From the suggestions derived from the various group conferences, those which are relevant to the ward situation can be put into the notice of the head nurse in a friendly manner. Group conference helps the students develop problem-solving skills, team building skills and the ability to express oneself assertively. By providing an opportunity to express the innovative ideas and to refine clinical skills, group conferences make the clinical area a more interesting place for teaching and learning.

## Individual Conference

Individual conference is a clinical teaching method which focuses on the overall development of the individual student with special emphasis to the development of clinical skills.

Depending upon the context, felt need of students and preparation from the side of the teacher and students, individual conference can be classified into *unplanned or incidental conference and planned conference*. In addition to the nursing teachers, Staff nurses with adequate teaching skills are also allowed to conduct individual conference.

When the teacher/staff nurse recognizes the need for prompt guidance incidentally by observing the student's performance or when the student realizes the necessity of immediate guidance and seeks for it, unplanned conference takes place. Unplanned conference is very short and emphasis is given to solve the problem or to deal with the situation of immediate concern. The remaining general aspects of the problem are discussed afterwards informally or in a planned conference. Planned conference is more systematic and predetermined. In each clinical area, individual student should have the prescribed number of planned conferences and more, if the student's performance is not good as expected. For conducting planned conference, prior intimation to the student is a must and the time and place should not be changed as far as possible.

Individual conference mainly deals with the student's nursing care ability, level of performance, achievements, activities and assignments related to the clinical experience.

Even though routine instruction helps the teacher find out the subject for individual conference, individual conference is much more than the routine instruction. In routine instruction, the clinical instructor may not get sufficient time to address the individual needs of the students. For example, nursing teacher teaches Ryle's tube insertion to whole students in the ward through demonstration as a part of routine instruction but only through an individual conference the teacher can help the student who is finding it difficult to acquire the skill of Ryle's tube insertion.

Individual conference provides an opportunity for the students to know about his achievements and to express the difficulties or problems he is facing, especially in relation to the acquisition of clinical skills. The teacher has to respect the individuality of the student and allow the student to express his or her concerns freely. This will help the teacher identify the students' attitude and insight regarding the problem. This informal approach also assists the teacher to decide upon the kind of help required by the student. Individual conference should be held in an atmosphere comfortable to the student. After the conference, a brief record of the conference should be maintained by recording the nature of the problem, events led to the conference, student's attitude towards the problem and the kind of help rendered by the teacher.

By way of providing an opportunity to sharpen the clinical skills and to know about the progress, individual conference boost the self-confidence of the students. An increase in the self-confidence will in turn boost the sense of security. As a perfect combination of teaching and guidance, individual conference is regarded as one of the best individual instruction methods.

## ASSIGNMENT

Assignments play a major role in the teaching–learning process. Assignment is a work allotment. It is a sort of self-study which supplements classroom teaching. The success and effectiveness of assignment depends upon the amount of independent work done by the students.

### Guidelines for Preparing Assignments

Teacher has to follow certain guidelines in order to assign good assignments. They are: (a) More dictation of questions or problems is not an assignment. The teacher has to suggest along with it the books to be consulted and the references to be studied. Elaborate hints have to be given for the successful completion of assignments; (b) the assignments should preferably raise out of the activities, needs and interests of the students; (c) it must motivate, remove doubts or misunderstandings and develop insight; (d) the task of assignments should be clear and to the point. It is not possible to achieve desired results by indefinite, vague and lengthy assignments; (e) the assignment should be a cooperative activity in which the teacher and students taken an active role; (f) weekly assignments are preferable to daily or monthly ones.

### Principles of Assignment Planning

The principles of assignment planning are: (a) It should correlate with previous knowledge and experience; (b) it should motivate the students; (c) it should be related to purpose; (d) it should challenge not threaten; (e) it should provide for individual difference; (f) it should be cooperatively made.

## Types of Assignments

The teacher can use four types of assignments, namely: *preparatory assignments, study assignments, revisional assignments and remedial assignments.*
1. **Preparatory assignments:** These are meant to prepare the students for the classes which is to follow on the coming days. This type of assignments will enable the teacher to lead the class with ease and understanding. An assignment on anatomy of heart before teaching cardiovascular diseases is an example of this type of assignment.
2. **Study assignments:** These can be varied—care plans, assignments for the preparation of a topic in the light of reference provided, assignments for listing points in favor or against a given argument, etc.
3. **Revisional assignments:** These assignments are given for checking students retention and understanding of facts. Assignment on answering previous university questions is an example of this type of assignment.
4. **Remedial assignments:** These assignments are devised in the light of students' reactions to the above mentioned assignments. The purpose of these assignments is to remove weak points and clear misunderstandings.

## Planning Assignments

If the teacher wants to see whether students can think analytically, assign a short essay in which they have to analyze a particular patient problem or an issue related to the course. This kind of assignment forces students to use their own analytical powers and not just copy someone else's ideas from the literature. If teacher wants to test students' ability to use resources to answer specific questions, ask them the questions, let them investigate the answers and have them write up the answers in a short paper.

There are other types of creative yet worthy assignments. Students could be asked to devise assessment forms or patient-teaching materials. They could be asked to solve a problem in the real world of nursing and report on the solution. They could do personal interviews, formulate ideas for research or keep logs and journals.

It is important to keep the students' workload in mind when designing assignments. Nursing care plans are an indispensable part of nurse educator's assignments. Beginning students who are learning the nursing process need to write simple, short care plans on simulated or real patient situations. They can learn the process without writing comprehensive lengthy plans.

Whatever the assignment for a course, it is the teacher's responsibility to read all student-work carefully and soon after it has been handed in. Student papers receive not only a grade but comments as well. If the teacher weighs his or her own workload when planning assignments, student work can be given due attention and returned promptly. In short, teacher has to state clear expectations of what is expected from assignments, how to get help and what to do when finished.

## SUMMARY

Transferring knowledge is equally important as generating knowledge. Teaching is not only concerned with imparting knowledge but also preparing the student to adjust with their environment. Teaching–learning process is a three way communication between the teacher and student in order to facilitate learning. Teaching is an art as well as a science. Principles of teaching, maxims of teaching and marks of good teaching will guide the teacher in carrying out the teaching activity in a fruitful way. Knowledge regarding the qualities of a good teacher and characteristics of effective teaching assists the teacher in attaining teaching objectives. A teaching skill can be defined as a set of teacher behaviors which are especially effective in bringing about desired changes in students. It is better to relate teaching skills with different stages of lesson.

Even though teaching strategies and teaching-learning methods are concerned with attaining teaching objectives, one has to differentiate between them in order to develop teaching skills. Based on the degree of dominance enjoyed by the teacher or learner in the teaching-learning process, teaching-learning methods can be classified into teacher-centered and learner-centered methods. Depending on the utility of teaching-learning methods in meeting the learning needs of a particular number of students, they can be classified into large group methods, small group methods and individual methods.

Lecture, demonstration, discussion, symposium, seminar, simulation exercises, simulation games, role playing, microteaching, nursing care plan, nursing care study, bedside clinic, nursing care conference, nursing rounds, individual conference and group conference are some of the methods used for teaching nursing. Teacher has to follow certain guidelines while selecting teaching-learning methods. Knowledge regarding the advantages and disadvantages of each method will help the teacher to carry out the teaching activity in a better way by limiting the disadvantages. Assignments play a major role in the teaching-learning process.

## MULTIPLE CHOICE QUESTIONS

1. **Teaching with example is called:**
   a. Inductive teaching
   b. Reflective teaching
   c. Lecture
   d. Discussion

2. **Contingent teaching is based on:**
   a. Previous knowledge of students
   b. Progress of learners
   c. Skill of learners
   d. Learn style of learners

3. **Which is an example of teacher-centered teaching method:**
   a. Lecture
   b. Role play
   c. Project work
   d. Return demonstration

4. **Interactive lecture is a combination of lecture and:**
   a. Discussion
   b. Demonstration
   c. Role play
   d. Project work

5. **Which is an example of learner-centered teacher method?**
   a. Return demonstration
   b. Lecture
   c. Bedside clinic
   d. None of the above

6. Which is an example of learner-centered clinical teaching method?
    a. Return demonstration
    b. Demonstration
    c. Nursing care conference
    d. Video conference
7. Which is a teacher-centered clinical teaching method?
    a. Demonstration
    b. Return demonstration
    c. Care study
    d. Group conference
8. Which is the best quality of a teacher?
    a. Role modelling
    b. Effective teaching
    c. Good teacher-student interaction
    d. Listening
9. Clinical log is an example of:
    a. Assignment
    b. Receiving feedback
    c. Remedial teaching
    d. None of the above
10. Which is the most difficult aspect in teaching?
    a. Role modeling transferring knowledge
    b. Developing attitude
    c. Developing skill
    d. Listening

## ANSWER KEY

| 1. a | 2. b | 3. a | 4. a | 5. a | 6. a |
| 7. a | 8. a | 9. a | 10. b | | |

# CHAPTER 7

# Teaching and Learning Nursing in Digital Age

## LEARNING OBJECTIVES

**After completing this chapter, reader will be able to:**

- Define digital teaching in nursing education.
- Identify components of digital teaching in nursing education.
- Follow principles of teaching nursing in digital age.
- Explain approaches to teaching in digital age.
- Design teaching methods in digital age.
- Identify role of teacher in digital age.
- Develop teaching skills in digital age.
- Practice online teaching and learning methods.
- Practice innovative teaching methods in nursing education.
- Prepare students for online learning
- Appreciate challenges in online teaching.
- Practice evidence-based teaching in nursing.

Society is changing very fast and so as the trends in education. Education is highly influenced by the changes in the society. This is because aims of education is derived from the needs of the society. All are concerned with providing quality cost effective education to masses by utilizing advancements in technology. General education as well as professional education is taking advantage of technological advancements in providing good quality education. Nursing education also utilizes advancements in technology to achieve its aims.

## ONLINE EDUCATION

According to Oliver Shikten "online education is a form of education which is delivered and administered using the internet". The purposes of online education are:

- For supplementing classroom learning
- Replace classroom learning in unusual circumstances like COVID-19
- Distance education
- Conducting examinations
- Re-learning, revision
- Recurrent programs

## DIGITAL TEACHING

### Definition

Digital teaching in nursing education can be defined as "the process of teaching nursing through an ever-growing and diversified combination of methods, internet, technology, media and devices without undermining the human component in the teaching–learning process by ensuring maximum student participation".

It includes traditional methods as well as technology enabled teaching–learning process involving online teaching, online learning and blended learning. Digital teaching does not mean ignoring traditional methods as it utilizes technology even for making traditional methods more learner-centered and interesting.

## Principles of Teaching and Learning in Digital Age

Digital technologies provide increasingly powerful tools and offer a variety of educational opportunities that can improve teaching and learning. National Association of Independent Schools suggests following principles of teaching and learning in the digital age.

- Teachers research, evaluate and use technology to provide differentiated personalized instruction and to achieve curricular goals.
- Teachers need to design environment to transform the relationship between teacher and learner in a desirable manner, engaging students in higher-order thinking skills, creation of content and critical thinking.
- Teachers embrace technologies that promote a culture of participatory and collaborative approaches to learning such as inquiry-based, student-centered, flipped classroom, project and problem-based learning.
- Teachers model and empower students to effectively practice media and information literacies inside and outside the classroom as content creators and learners.
- Teachers promote networking opportunities for their students and colleagues to collaborate locally and globally.
- Teachers evaluate opportunities to leverage online and/or hybrid learning environments and implement them when they enhance student learning.
- Teachers explore technology enriched and adaptive formative assessments for sophisticated evaluation that reveal growth over time and that inspire intrinsic motivation to improve learning.
- Providing prompt feedback is an integral part of digital teaching and learning.
- The institution recognizes that quality digital teaching can be achieved only through teachers sustained professional growth by creating a culture of continuous growth and adequate support for innovation and learning.
- Institution encourages teachers to seek out opportunities to build learning networks and to explore and evaluate digital tools.
- The institution considers technology integration as an essential component of development and need to provide the necessary time and resources for it and ensures that teachers acquire and demonstrate essential skills and proficiencies.
- Teachers' use of technology for teaching and learning is included in the institution's teacher evaluation process as appropriate for the institution's mission and philosophy.
- The institution provides adequate staffing and infrastructure for conducting digital teaching in an appropriate manner.
- The institution develops a policy regarding faculty and student interactions on social media sites.
- Teachers teach model and expect safe, healthy, ethical, legal and responsible use of digital resources and social media by students and parents.
- The institution establishes a curriculum-based digital responsibility program that includes ongoing discussions of online behavior, cyber bullying and respectful and legal use of online tools.
- The institution updates on issues, events and concerns related to online behavior and informs faculty, students and parents when appropriate.
- The institution provides up-to-date information on fair use, copyright and creative common information and requires compliance by faculty, staff and students.

## Approaches to Teaching in Digital Age

According to Tony Bates, "teaching is a highly complex occupation which needs to adapt to a great deal of variety in context, subject matter and learners. He suggested following approaches to teaching in the digital age".

- No single method is likely to meet all the teaching requirements teachers face in a digital age. It is argued that academic knowledge is different from other forms of knowledge and is even more relevant in a digital age. However, academic knowledge is not the only kind of knowledge that is important in today's society and as teachers we have to be aware of other forms of knowledge and their potential importance to our students and make sure that we are providing the full range of contents and skills needed for students in a digital age.
- Nevertheless, some forms of teaching fit better with the development of the skills needed in a digital age. In particular, methods that focus on conceptual development such as dialogue and discussion and knowledge management rather than information transmission and experiential learning in real world contexts are more likely to develop the high level conceptual skills required in a digital age.
- It is not just conceptual skills that are needed. It is the combination of conceptual, practical, personal and social skills in highly complex situations that are needed. This again recommends combining a variety of teaching methods.
- Nearly all of these teaching methods are media or technology independent. In other words, they can be used in classrooms or online. What matters from a learning perspective is the efficacy and expertise in appropriately choosing and using the teaching method than the technology.
- Even then it is a fact that new technologies offer new possibilities for teaching, including offering more practice or time on task, reaching out to new target groups and increasing the productivity of both teachers and the system as a whole.
- It is not enough to look just at teaching methods; we need to look at designing an appropriate learning environment to help foster and develop the knowledge and skills that students will need. We shall see that technology can be particularly helpful in providing such rich learning contexts.

The ultimate purpose of approaches to teaching in digital age is to enable teachers to identify the teaching methods that are most likely to support the development of the knowledge and skills that students or learners will need in a digital age. Of course teacher also need to consider other factors such as the nature of the learners and their prior knowledge and experience the demands of particular subject areas and the learning environment or institutional context where learning take place while selecting methods of teaching.

## Teaching Skills in Digital Age

Tony Bates beautifully explained about the skills needed for teaching in the digital age. Types of skills needed for teaching can be classified as follows:

- Conceptual skills such as knowledge management, critical thinking, analysis, synthesis, problem solving and creativity/innovation.
- Developmental or personal skills such as independent learning, communication skills, ethics, networking, responsibility and teamwork.
- Digital skills embedded within and related to a particular subject or professional domain.
- Manual and practical skills, such as machine or equipment operation, safety procedures observation and recognition of data patterns and spatial factors.

## Design of Teaching Methods in the Digital Age

In Tony Bate's opinion design of teaching methods means deliberately planning methods of teaching and a broad learning environment that will facilitate the development of knowledge and skills that our students need. While design teaching methods teacher need to consider following factors:

- The teacher needs to be able to identify/recognize the skills they are hoping to develop in their students within a particular course or program.
- These skills are often not easily separated but tend to be contextually based and often integrated.
- Teachers need to identify appropriate methods and contexts that will enable students to develop these skills.
- Students will need practice to develop such skills.
- Students will need feedback and intervention from the teacher and other students to ensure a high level of competence or mastery in the skill.
- An assessment strategy needs to be developed that recognizes and rewards student's competence and mastery of such skills.

When we say teaching methods in digital age it doesn't mean that we are avoiding methods we followed till date. Teaching methods in digital age include all methods that help students to acquire the knowledge and skills as per the objectives of course or program. Thus, it includes teaching methods from lecture to webinars.

One peculiarity of teaching in the digital age is that it uses a combination of methods as a single method for achieving objectives of teaching. For example, to overcome disadvantages of traditional lecture, discussion and role play is also integrated into lecture for making it into a more student-centered teaching method.

## Role of Teacher in the Digital Age

In this digital age, the role of teacher has become more crucial than ever before and irreplaceable. Teachers are no longer primary source of information for students but only a teacher can help students in contextualizing the information and guiding students in the practical application and use of the information. For example, a student get information about mannitol as an osmotic diuretic from the internet but only a teacher can contextualize the information by teaching students that mannitol is used mainly to reduce cerebral edema based on the site of action of a mannitol. Contextualization of information is very important, especially in professional education. Moreover, education is not only gaining knowledge and skill but also involves developing other attributes essential for a good living. A teacher can help students to attain qualities essential for a good living in many ways. This is the reason why the role of teacher is irreplaceable even in the advancement of technology.

The role of teacher in the digital age can be referred as "evolving role" as factors influencing educative process, especially technology is evolving everyday demanding more professional development as a teacher. It is a fact that use of technology changed the role of teacher from traditional knowledge provider into a facilitator and mentor. Teacher guide the student's learning process and engage in joint problem solving with students. Technology provides opportunities for more interaction between teacher and students.

Teacher need to be skilled enough to perform her role meticulously in this digital age. It is extremely important for the present day teacher to be more skilled, knowledgeable and efficient for performing her role. Technology is evolving every day; therefore, teachers must develop the ability to learn new things more quickly as compared to students. Technical skills and critical thinking enable teacher to develop following qualities essential for fulfilling **"evolving role"** in this digital age of teaching.

- Facilitating better learning in the classrooms and online environment. This can be done by: (a) contextualizing information with suitable examples and considering learning as a shared experience between the teacher and students, (b) guiding students properly. As learning experiences are usually designed and planned before the commencement of classes teachers can devote more time to guide students, (c) motivating students by providing constructive feedback. Teachers need to find appropriate ways to convey positive messages along with necessary criticism, (d) promoting interaction between teacher and students through effective communication and (e) communicate teacher expectations properly before the commencement of classes.
- Creating a learner-centered classroom by effectively utilizing digital media tools to enhance students learning ability. This makes students more responsible and self-directed learning thereby promoting proactive learning. Self-directed learning help students to develop a passion for learning which in turn result in better learning outcomes.
- Mentoring students to build a career and good life. Teachers need to help learners develop high level of confidence. Teachers have to provide massive support to students and help them to deal with stress in a positive manner. Teacher also assist students to develop "life skills" along with teaching subject matter.
- Collaborating with students and help them to utilize new learning opportunities. Present day teachers need to be good collaborators. In the digital age teachers are learning with students through co-learning and collaboration. Students should be given enough opportunities to collaborate on assignments and project.
- Continuous professional development as a teacher for enhancing competency in teaching and guiding students. Teachers can utilize new technologies and various educational platforms for updating skills in addition to collaborating with other teachers.
- Be a role model to students. This is an essential role of teachers in the digital age. Be a role model, especially by becoming a lifelong learner. Present day teachers need to be good learners themselves. This is because teaching techniques change often due to technological advancements.
- Teachers need to be creative and innovative. They also needs to promote creativity among students. Becoming a lifelong learner is the best way to remain creative and innovative.
- Appreciating change in the teacher-student relationship. In the past, the relationship between teacher and learner was hierarchical in nature. The teacher was the dispenser of knowledge and communication between student and teacher was one-way. That model no longer provides the best learning experiences for students. In the digital age, teachers are learning with their students through co-learning and collaboration. This provides a basis for personalized learning.
- Appreciating recent developments in cognitive neurosciences and incorporate it into teaching practice, especially to assist students in developing self-regulated learning skills. Teachers need to promote collaboration than competition. New digital technologies allow teachers to engage in professional development, strengthen teaching skills and create learning communities that cultivate professional relationships outside of school. Collaboration in the digital age enables teachers to reach out and connect with like-minded educators.

# ONLINE TEACHING IN NURSING EDUCATION

## Definition

Online teaching in nursing education can be defined as "the teaching intended to attain predetermined objectives through internet by using the most appropriate as well as convenient device, online platforms or Apps and social media". The device may be a smart phone or laptop or computer. Online platforms or Apps that enable two way communication if not, simultaneous communication is required to conduct online teaching. Social media like WhatsApp and YouTube can also be used in combination with online platforms or individually to conduct online teaching.

## Classification of Online Teaching

Online teaching in nursing education can be classified according to: (a) on the basis of content of online teaching and characteristics of learners and (b) on the basis of kind of interaction between teacher and student possible through the online platform chosen for conducting online teaching.

## Classification Based on Online Content and Characteristics of Learner

1. **Fully online program with the nurses as learners:** The number of participants is less than thousand. For example, an online program conducted by a nursing college on nursing leadership attended by less than thousand nurses.
2. **Fully online course with huge number of nurses as learners (MOOCS):** For example, huge number of nurses worldwide attended massive open online course (MOOC) conducted by John Hopkins University on COVID-19 management.
3. **Non-formal (distant) nursing education with 30% traditional classroom teaching and 70% online teaching:** In this program also learners are nurses. This program is mainly conducted in India by Indira Gandhi Open University for nurses with diploma program in order to achieve BSc nursing degree.
4. **Formal nursing education with 30% online and 70% traditional teaching:** In this program nursing students are the learners. This program is conducted by institutions recognized by a university and other apex bodies related to nursing education. The percentage of online content may vary according to the guidelines of apex bodies.

In this chapter we are discussing only about online teaching in the formal nursing education.

## Classification Based on Interaction

1. **Synchronous online teaching:** It enables teachers and students to participate in a teaching–learning activity together at the same time from different places. Real-time synchronous online teaching involves online chats and videoconferencing. Teachers and students can interact simultaneously. Teachers allow students to ask questions and clarify doubts. Online platforms like Zoom and Google classroom are widely used for synchronous online teaching as they facilitate real time interaction between teacher and students. In synchronous online teaching, teaching takes place as per fixed time table or schedule.
2. **Asynchronous online teaching:** It is opposite of synchronous teaching. In asynchronous online teaching, teacher and students are not engaged in teaching–learning activity at the same time. There is no real time interaction with teacher and students. The content is sent to students via email, web or WhatsApp. Students can learn in their own time and schedule.
3. **Interactive online teaching:** It adopts a midway between synchronous and asynchronous online teaching. Interactive online teaching allows senders to become receivers and vice versa, effectively enabling a two-way communication between the teacher and students.

Online teaching through WhatsApp is an example if both teacher and students engage in two-way communication through posts and voice messages. From the messages sent and received, the teacher and students can make changes in the teaching–learning methods.

4. **Linear online teaching:** It is carried out by sending recorded lectures and other training materials to students through television and radio programs. Many state governments adopted this method for training school children during COVID-19 pandemic. The limiting factor is that it does not allow two way communications between teachers and students. This type of online teaching does have its place in education, although it is becoming less relevant with time.
5. **Blended teaching:** It combines face-to-face and online teaching into one cohesive experience. Particular amount is taught online and remaining through face-to-face interaction in classroom settings. The online teaching may be synchronous or interactive in nature. Online teaching in formal nursing education is best example of blended teaching.

## Principles of Online Teaching in Formal Nursing Education

- Meticulous integration of online teaching and face-to-face classroom teaching is essential for achieving the aims of formal nursing education.
- As it is difficult to attain objectives of formal nursing education through online teaching, teachers should try to provide authentic learning experiences in the maximum possible manner through online teaching.
- A blended curriculum with learning objectives better achieved through online teaching and face-to-face interaction forms the basis of online teaching in formal nursing education.
- Online teaching in formal nursing education is not just transferring a portion of content through online. Instead, it involves developing challenging and engaging online teaching-learning activities that complement face-to-face teaching in the classroom.
- Online teaching requires meticulous planning which is a time consuming process. All on a sudden commencement of online teaching when institutions are closed due to unforeseen reasons like COVID-19 pandemic may be better termed as **"emergency remote teaching"** than online teaching.
- Commencement of online teaching in formal nursing education cannot be described as "transition from traditional teaching" because traditional teaching remains as the main component of teaching in formal nursing education. Online teaching only complement tradition face-to-face teaching in formal nursing education.
- Online teaching should be based on clearly stated objectives.
- Online platforms chosen for conducting online teaching should allow at least two way communication if not synchronized communication.
- Practicing proactive teaching strategies by teacher is important for achieving the aims of online teaching.
- As in the classroom teaching, during online teaching also teacher need to clearly express teacher expectations to students and encourage their participation.
- Teacher should always try to provide a learning experience rich in interaction, addressing needs of student and essential for achieving learning outcomes.
- Online teaching should be based on clear guidelines with specific description regarding the roles and responsibilities of apex bodies, management, principal, teachers, supporting staff and students.
- Timely feedback from the teacher regarding to a student inquiry is very important in ensuring active participation of students and achievement of learning outcomes.
- Equal importance to be given for formative and summative assessment strategies.

## Steps in Conducting Online Teaching in Formal Nursing Education

Steps in conducting online teaching can be divided into: (a) planning, (b) implementation and (c) evaluation.

### Planning the Online Teaching

- Formation of a committee with principal as chairman and vice-principal as chief learning officer for online teaching. All faculty members and supporting staff are members of the committee. Sub-committees are formed under department heads to coordinate content preparation and other activities.
- Preparation of a blended curriculum for blended teaching which involves face-to-face classroom teaching and online teaching. Clearly divide content into two portions: (a) that can be taught by face-to-face interaction and (b) that can be taught by online teaching. Blended curriculum also lists down the teaching methods and assessment strategies for both classroom and online teaching. Another important aspect of blended curriculum is the formulation of educational objectives for both types of teaching.
- Plan for meticulous integration of online teaching and face-to-face classroom teaching.
- Formulating guidelines for conducting online teaching based on the educational objectives. Educational objectives clearly address the needs of students and faculty members in relation to online teaching.
- Provide training for the teachers and supporting staff in the conduct of online teaching. Training can be arranged through a workshop conducted at the college or through webinars by experts.
- Provide orientation to students regarding online learning and how to engage in the teaching-learning process.
- Selection of online platform by considering safety, convenience and appropriateness. Online platform should allow at least two way communication if not synchronized or real time communication.
- Arrange resources at the institution level and for teachers and students.
- Prepare a schedule with detailed timetable.
- Communicate clear expectations of teachers to students in a very comprehensible manner.
- Principal communicate to faculty members regarding the expectations of institution.
- Establish a contingency plan whenever we are working with technology. We can never guarantee that it will always work well as we desired. Prepare an alternative way for students to contact teachers such as a different email address and phone number.
- Prepare a quality checklist for ensuring smooth conduct of online teaching.

### Implementation of Online Teaching

- Conducting online teaching on a trial basis for two days to check the effectiveness of conducting online teaching.
- Collect feedback from teachers and students regarding their experience on online teaching.
- Taking measures to improve efficiency of online teaching based on feedback.
- Conducting online teaching in full-fledged manner with active participation of students as per schedule.
- Class coordinators submit weekly report to principal and principal submit report to university is needed.
- In between principal and teachers evaluate quality of online teaching through quality checklist.

- Focus on the integration of the online and face-to-face teaching. Connecting what studied in classroom and in online is important in achieving aims of nursing education.
- Every Monday and Saturday principal need to conduct a webinar regarding the progress of online classes.

### Evaluation of Online Teaching

- Principal collect feedback from students and teachers on regular basis.
- Principal also collect self-assessment from teachers regarding their performance.
- Principal evaluate the conduct of online teaching and motivate faculties by conveying appreciation and suggesting ways to improve online teaching further.
- By evaluation principal ensures the conduct of online teaching as per the schedule and objectives are achieved as planned.

### Practical Guidelines for Conducting Online Teaching in Formal Nursing Education

- Classify and specify learning objectives which would be better achieved by online teaching and which would be better achieved by face-to-face classroom teaching.
- Meticulously integrate face-to-face and online components of teaching into a unified purposeful teaching activity.
- Always commence online teaching after giving adequate training to faculty members and orientation to students regarding the successful conduct of online teaching.
- Select safe and appropriate online platform which allows at least two way communication if not real time communication. Teachers can use a mix of online platforms according to the nature of content. For example, even if using WhatsApp for teaching, teachers can use other online video conferencing platform for teaching topics require active discussion and live demonstration. In such circumstances teachers need to inform students earlier. Irrespective of the online platform using once in a week teacher need to conduct discussion with students using appropriate video conferencing App to assess effectiveness of teaching.
- Principal need to actively monitor online teaching by becoming a member in all groups constituted for online teaching.
- Principal and faculty members need to conduct video conference on every Monday and Saturday to ensure effective implementation of online teaching.
- Conduct online teaching for a maximum four to five hours per day with adequate cooling off time. Remaining time can be utilized for preparing assignments and assessment.
- While preparing timetable, mentioning topics along with subject matter help students to prepare for classes in advance.
- All class coordinators should send weekly report to principal on Saturdays and the principal need to compare it with schedule to ensure progress.
- Online teaching is not a lecture conducted in online platform. It is an active learning session. Online teaching should be a mix of discussions, collaboration, video and audio clips and hands on exercises with text and possibly brief video lectures. In short, teachers need to **chunk lessons** while taking online classes.
- If possible, use photographs in the prescribed textbook while teaching online. Never send pages of textbook or lengthy videos as it fails to engage students.
- Provide timely feedback or "rapid feedback" to students. This doesn't mean teacher need to be available 24 × 7 while conducting online teaching.
- Be present during the time of online teaching. Teacher should have a "social presence" in their online classrooms and encourage students to do the same.

- Consider online teaching as a group activity with active participation of all concerned individuals. The role of principal, faculty members, supporting staff and students need to be explained well in advance and should cooperate each other for the successful conduct of online teaching.
- Encourage students to participate in online class discussion. To ensure participation from students, teachers need to insist on a minimum number of "posting" from each student every week.
- Establish a contingency plan whenever we are working with technology. We can never guarantee that it will always work well as we desired. Have an alternate way for students to contact teacher such as a different email address or phone number.
- Manage students' expectations properly. Make all assignments and other expectations as clear as possible.
- Focus on content and teaching not technology. Develop new learning activities that capitalize on the strengths of technology.

## Advantages of Online Teaching in Formal Nursing Education

- It ensures teaching–learning activity to a certain extent when it is difficult to conduct face-to-face classroom teaching due to unforeseen reasons like COVID-19 pandemic.
- It reduces the gap between the planned curriculum and received curriculum. This advantage is a continuation of the above said advantage.
- Provide opportunity for personalized learning. This is the most important advantage of online teaching.
- Students have access to relevant and most updated content. In online teaching it is easy to make available updated content than in the traditional teaching.
- Help teachers in up skilling and thereby become more efficient teachers.
- Increased flexibility of time and location so that students from diverse geographical regions can learn.
- More convenient as online teaching does not require any travelling by teacher and students.
- Easier access and sharing of information. It is easy to access and share resources in the digital format.
- Online teaching is comparatively easy to organize and manage when compared to classroom teaching if provided with enough resources.

## Disadvantages of online Teaching in Formal Nursing Education

- Major disadvantage of online teaching is the difficulty in providing all authentic learning experiences related to teaching nursing. To a certain extent this problem can be solved by judicious selection of online content by preparing a robust blended curriculum.
- More focus on theory than practical aspects and information overload as it is easy to access and share information. This can be solved by preparing quality content and follow principles of selection of learning experience.
- Need strong motivation from the part of students for actively participating in the online teaching program. A good orientation program before the commencement of online teaching motivates students to actively participate in the online teaching program.
- Difficulty in providing resources to students like safe and appropriate online platforms and devices is another disadvantage. This limitation leads to selection of available resource than appropriate one. This disadvantage can be overcome to a great extent by choosing cost effective Apps like WhatsApp which allows two way communications.

- High possibility for misinterpreting online teaching inferior to traditional classroom teaching. Due to this students may not give adequate importance to online teaching. Again, proper orientation to students will help to solve this problem.

## Challenges of Online Teaching

Online teaching, especially very unexpected with no adequate time to getting prepared or planning and arranging enough resources give rise to lot of challenges to teachers, students parents and other stakeholders of education. Even, well planned and implemented online teaching possesses lot of challenges. Let us discuss some of the challenges and possible solutions. These challenges are not all inclusive as each teacher and student faces unique challenges in online teaching.

- **Developing appropriate teaching strategies and approaches to teaching for attaining objectives of educational program:** Following principles of teaching and approaches to teaching in the digital age helps teachers to overcome this challenge. By ensuring collaboration, effective communication and active learning teacher can make sure that students are receiving valuable and engaging learning experience through online teaching. This will help in achieving objectives of the educational program.
- **Preparing teachers and students to perform their new roles effectively in the online teaching and learning environment:** The shift to online teaching and learning can be difficult. It require restructuring course components using new pedagogical approaches, learning activities and teaching tools that may be new to teachers and students. Training teachers for developing skills essential for online teaching and assisting students as needed for attending online classes helps to overcome this challenge.
- **Ensuring active participation of students in the teaching–learning process:** Engaging students in online teaching is one of the most challenging aspects in online teaching. This challenge can be managed by motivating students in a proper manner. Teacher need to maintain personal contact through email or chat. Try to engage students through group work, class discussion and collaborative activity. Another way to engage students is making the course content or subject matter more relevant and comprehensible to students. Interactive questions during classes also help to teach content in a comprehensible manner. Selection of appropriate technology tools, methods and media like multiple videos, discussions and various forms of sources of knowledge such as journal articles, blogs, etc., also help to engage students properly. Conducting ongoing assessment in different ways, providing prompt and meaningful feedback and encouraging collaboration with other students are also essential for ensuring active participation of students in online teaching.
- **Conduct of assessment in online teaching:** Assessment of learning outcomes in online teaching includes evaluating, measuring and documenting of learning progress of students based on the educational objectives. Authentic assessment of learning is an integral part of online teaching. Authentic assessment not only helps to know learning progress of students but also about relevant problems they are facing in online teaching. Thus, end goal of better assessment is better learning. Using assessment tool as a learning tool rather than measuring tool enhance learning experiences. Teachers need to follow good assessment practices for the successful conduct of online teaching. According to DUUS, in online teaching assessment plays a key role in moving from a low end learning to high end learning. Low end learning is just transferring of content like serving food. High end learning ensures more participation and critical thinking from the side of learners. Teachers can use a variety of assessment techniques suitable for online teaching like written assignments, short essays, multiple choice questions, student presentations, quiz, etc. Providing specific, effective and immediate feedback is an important aspect of assessing students' performance.

- **Ensuring quality of teaching resources:** Preparing authentic and relevant course material or content is a very challenging task. Teachers cannot simply use the content prepared for classroom teaching in online teaching. Teachers need to modify instruction suitable for the online format by choosing content carefully and activities that enhance student engagement in online teaching. Good content boost students' critical thinking and engagement in learning. Including lot of examples and encouraging students to come up with suitable examples make learning more interesting and comprehensible. Teacher can use a variety of multimedia resources. Providing video, audio, reading and interactive content can make learning more engaging. Seeking opinion of students about the benefits and drawbacks of content also helps in preparing authentic and relevant course material.
- **Ensuring teacher-student interaction in a desirable manner:** Deeper and meaningful teacher-student interaction is the basis of online teaching. In an online classroom, much of the learning is completed asynchronously and students often feel disconnected from their teacher as well as classmates. Effective communication and maintaining personal contact through email or chat helps in enhancing teacher-student interaction. Providing effective feedback is the best way to ensure student-teacher interaction in the online classroom environment. When students complete a task, they get feedback and make progress accordingly. Feedback should be encouraging and based on learning objectives. Providing specific and immediate feedback also help teacher to evaluate students' performance.
- **Encouraging collaboration:** Interaction among students is one of the most important elements of successful online teaching or education. Collaborative engagement motivates learning and promotes a deeper and productive approach to online teaching. Unfortunately, collaboration is one of the most difficult things to achieve when students are not physically present together. Problem-based learning is a collaborative learning strategy that gives students the opportunity to apply subject matter to real-world case studies in small groups. This method whether used in group or individual learning, helps students build upon their creativity and critical thinking skills.
- **Solving technical difficulties with online teaching:** Not every home will always have a reliable internet connection or readily available device for students to use. An initial email or message to parents will give students the opportunity to solve these issues. Students should be allowed to contact teacher through phone to solve technical issues related to online teaching.
- **Making students responsible for learning:** Students may not be responsible for learning or proactive in learning in online teaching compared to classroom teaching. Teachers need to put more effort to encourage students for proactive learning. This can be done by clearly communicating teacher expectations to students and teaching based on clear and measurable goals. In short, in online teaching, learning outcomes should be made clear to students before teaching subject matter.
- **Learners may have inappropriate expectations:** Learners may have expectations as in a classroom teaching. This problem can be solved by clearly communicating expectations, policies and routines like reasonable waiting time for feedback, estimated teaching hours per week and role of teachers and students in online teaching.
- **Providing meaningful assignments:** Giving assignments in online teaching is entirely different from classroom teaching. One assignment description is not enough; more clarification regarding assignment is necessary. Assignments should be in line with the predetermined objectives. Teachers should explain clearly expectations regarding assignments like date of submission, possible reference materials, etc. Teacher need to find innovative ways of giving assignments so that students are motivated to utilize vast resources available for preparing assignments.

## ONLINE LEARNING

Online learning is the learning taking place primarily through internet by using the most appropriate as well as convenient device, online platforms or Apps and social media. It helps learners to learn at their own pace according to their own convenience. It is also referred as "e-learning" in certain contexts. Students engage in online learning for completing a MOOC, a non-formal (distance) education programs or a hybrid program in which classroom teaching is more than online teaching. In addition to internet, online learning can also be accomplished with CD-ROMS and DVDS, streaming audio or video and other media.

### Increasing Student Engagement in Online Learning

According to edglossary.org, "In education, student engagement refers to the degree of attention, curiosity, interest, optimism, and passion that students show when they are learning or being taught, which extends to the level of motivation they have to learn and progress in their education". When students are engaged with the lesson being taught, they learn more and retain more. Katrina a Meyer suggest following ways to enhance student engagement in online learning.

- Teaching students how to learn online by helping them developing self-discipline and other self-regulatory behaviors, motivation to succeed, the ability to defer gratification and skills for active online learning.
- Teachers need to be very clear about learning outcomes and what students are expected to achieve. Teachers need to be competent in online teaching and should understand how students learn through online.
- Teachers have to prepare content by focusing on active learning, collaborative learning, authentic and experiential learning for engaging students in learning.
- While online teaching, teacher need to give importance to student effort in order to engage them effectively. This include using assignments that require students to do something—such as work in a group, solve a problem, prepare a project and experience a situation—will more likely enhance student engagement. For example, giving assignment to students to teach family members about hand washing technique to prevent COVID-19 is an example of active assignment.
- Make interactions with educational purpose in mind. Be it for online discussions, group work or simple email exchanges, students need to know the goal and reason for the learning activity.
- Promote critical thinking among learners by asking questions, critique student responses and providing additional context.
- Teachers have to evaluate online classes over and over again to ensure effectiveness of online teaching. This will help to identify elements that promote student engagement and what does not. Then, teachers can modify teaching accordingly.
- Assess student engagement by using appropriate strategies and motivate students who are not actively engaging in online classes to actively participate.
- Providing short lecture segments than lengthy lectures. In between lectures, teachers need to pause for breaks, summarize key points and soliciting questions to keep student engaged.
- Use maximum number of suitable examples (inductive teaching) while teaching online. This will improve comprehension.
- Encourage students to support each other by creating groups. Learners can create groups on WhatsApp and face book to provide support and share recourses with one another. Students may feel more comfortable to ask help to peers than to their teachers.

## Online Learning and Teaching Methods

### Classes Using Lecture Capture

In this method, teacher records the lecture and made available to students before or after conducting the lecture. **Flipped** classrooms, which pre-record a lecture for students to watch on their own, followed by discussion in class is the most effective form of classes using lecture capture.

### Learning Using Learning Management Systems

Learning management systems (LMS) are software that enable instructors and students to log in and work within a password protected online learning environment. Learning management systems used by universities and institutions replicate a classroom design model. They have weekly units or modules, the instructor selects and presents the material to all students in the class at the same time, a large classroom enrollment can be organized into smaller sections with their own instructors. There are opportunities for online discussion, students participate and learn almost at the same pace and assessment is by tests or essays. In short learning management systems are digital platforms where:

- Content (subject matter) are created
- Contents are stored
- Contents are systematically shared
- Student interactions are done
- Online classes conducted
- Assessments performed
- Certification completed

## The ADDIE Model

According to Morrison, ADDIE stands for:

### Analyze

Identify all the variables that need to be considered when designing the course such as learner characteristics, learners' prior knowledge, resources available, etc.

### Design

This stage focuses on identifying the learning objectives for the course and how materials will be created and designed. The content is decided in the form of text, audio and video and arranged in a prescribed order suitable for learning.

### Develop

This stage includes the creation of content, whether to develop by the institution or outsource, copyright clearance for the third party materials, loading of content into a website or LMS and so on.

### Implement

This is the actual delivery of the course, including any prior training or briefing of learners, support staff and student assessment.

### Evaluate

Feedback and data is collected in order to identify areas that require improvement and this data is used into the design, development and implementation of the course in the next time.

## Online Collaborative Learning

Collaborative learning is an e-learning approach where students are able to socially interact with other students and teachers. Collaborative learning is based on the principle that students can enrich their learning experiences by interacting with others and benefiting from one another's strengths. Learners work together in order to expand their knowledge of a particular subject or skill. In e-learning environment this is typically done through live chats or instant messaging.

This method can be done asynchronously or synchronously. It allows students to learn from the ideas, skill sets and experience of others enrolled in the course. By engaging in a shared task like project students learn a variety of skills such as group analysis and collaborative teamwork building skills. In collaborative group discussions, learners learn to listen attentively to each other and value the efforts of shared knowledge and input. Online discussion also helps learners respond to questions, participate and offer peer feedback to support the sharing of new information.

## Competency-based Learning

Competency-based learning begins by identifying specific competencies or skills and enables learners to develop mastery of each competency or skill at their own pace, usually working with a mentor. Learners can develop just the competencies or skills they need or can combine a whole set of competencies into a full qualification such as a certificate, diploma or a full degree.

Learners work individually, usually online rather than in cohorts. If learners can demonstrate that they already have mastery of a particular competency or skill through a test or some form of prior learning assessment, they may be allowed to move to the next level of competency without having to repeat a prescribed course of study for the competency. Competency-based learning attempts to break away from the regularly scheduled classroom model, where students study the same subject matter at the same pace in a cohort of fellow students. Mainly competency-based learning is being used for education requiring more abstract or academic skills development, sometimes combined with other cohort-based courses or programs.

## Communities of Practice

According to Tony Bates, communities of practice are groups of people who share a concern or a passion for something they do and learn how to do it better as they interact regularly. Communities of practice are everywhere. Nearly everyone belongs to some community of practice. For example, WhatsApp group of teachers working in a college or principals group of all nursing colleges are examples of communities of practice. In Wenger's opinion although individuals learn through participation in a community of practice, more important is the generation of newer or deeper levels of knowledge through group activity.

One of the significant developments in recent years has been the use of massive open online courses (MOOCs) for developing online communities of practice.

## Educational Webinars

Educational webinar is a presentation, lecture, workshop or a seminar conducted over the internet using videoconferencing software or Apps. During which the host uses conferencing equipment and multimedia to connect to viewers or listeners interactively, including voice communications, live or pre-recorded videos, online presentations, product demonstrations, text chats and more. Basically, webinars for online education have following six significant benefits.

1. **Flexibility:** Webinar enable students to access learning material anywhere at any time, which is good for those who do not have time or are far away from accessing learning materials.
2. **More opportunities for students:** Students learning through webinars are able to choose even those degree programs that they couldn't otherwise take due to distance limitations. It is now possible for students to complete degree programs offered in a different country.
3. **Learning timetable availability:** The learning timetables of classes offered on campus are usually rigid and do not offer much flexibility to students. Webinars have made it possible for students to attend classes in a flexible manner through webinars.
4. **Cost effective:** Students who use webinars for education find it cheaper since travelling costs and other expenses needed for on campus learning are excluded. Books that traditional classes require might not be necessary when students use webinars.
5. **More interaction:** Teachers are more approachable online and students are more comfortable communicating with teachers through chats and discussions than face-to-face interactions. This is because in webinars all attendees have equal opportunity to contribute in the virtual class.
6. **Better understanding of content:** According to a study by the US Department of Education "on average, students in online learning conditions performed modestly better than those receiving face-to-face instruction".

Then it is no surprise that webinars are getting more and more adopted worldwide as a new form of online education. Based on the features, institution can decide upon best webinar software or App suitable for conducting webinars.

## EVIDENCE-BASED TEACHING IN NURSING

The concept of evidence-based practice has its origins in medicine. Socket describes evidence-based practice as "integrating individual clinical expertise with the best available external evidence from systematic research". Thus, in evidence-based teaching in nursing, the nurse educator need to integrate her reliable and valuable evidence from personal experience with evidence from systematic, external research. According to Geoffmaster, evidence-based teaching involves the use of evidence to:

❖ Establish where students are in the learning or their previous knowledge.
❖ Decide on appropriate teaching strategies and interventions.
❖ Monitor student progress and evaluate teaching effectiveness.

### Evidence to Identify Starting Points for Teaching and Learning

At first, essential form of evidence for teaching is information about level of attainment by learners or their previous knowledge. Their previous knowledge is the starting point for teaching and to ensure that learners are provided with well targeted learning opportunities and appropriately challenging learning goals. Understanding where learners are in their learning is important to clinical teaching as understanding a patient's symptoms and health is important for providing effective nursing care.

In evidence–based teaching, assessments are undertaken to gather evidence and draw conclusions about where students are in their learning. The objective is to use observations of students' performance and work to draw inferences about their current level of attainment. A thorough understanding of where a student is in their learning may require a detailed analysis of errors they are making or the misunderstandings they have develop. This understanding serve as essential evidence for removing obstacles for further progress and a key element in providing effective clinical teaching. Instead of grading, this evidence is used to identify what students know, understand and can do.

### Evidence to Decide on Appropriate Teaching Strategies and Interventions

From the teaching experience of the teacher and systematic research teacher can collect evidence to find answers to the following questions for deciding on appropriate teaching strategies and intervention.
- Which interventions are likely to improve students' level of understanding and skills?
- What teaching strategies help in attain clinical teaching objectives?
- For which learners?
- Under what conditions?

In general, evidence provides best ways to implement effective teaching strategies and interventions in subject-specific contexts.

### Evidence to Evaluate Student Progress and Teaching Effectiveness

A third form of evidence for teaching is information about the progress students make in their learning over time. This is important information for evaluating learning success and for making judgements about the effectiveness of teaching strategies and interventions.

Evidence about the progress students make is crucial information for teaching. It provides a basis for establishing whether and how effectively students are learning. Low levels of progress may indicate lack of student effort and /or ineffective teaching and demands remedial action. Information about progress provides the most direct indicator of teaching effectiveness as well as necessary for the evaluation of educational policies, progress and teaching methods.

## INNOVATIVE TEACHING METHODS IN NURSING

### Definition

In author's opinion, "An innovative teaching method in nursing can be defined as a modified traditional method or a wholly newly developed method based on pedagogical theories by way of optimum utilization of resources capable of attaining learning outcomes by ensuring maximum student engagement". This definition depicts the following:
- A traditional method can become innovative method by adding some learner centered teaching strategies.
- A wholly newly developed method may not be considered as an innovative one if it fails to engage students in learning.
- Resources include research findings, man power, technology, devices, internet textbooks, search engines like Google, etc.
- Method should engage students in learning and capable of attaining learning outcomes.
- As it is based on pedagogical theories it should address the learning needs of students.

## TYPES OF INNOVATIVE TEACHING METHODS IN NURSING

### Integrated Lecture

Integrated lecture involves teaching students through a combination of lecture, videos if needed 3D animated videos, role play, discussion, soliciting questions from students and PowerPoint presentations. Teacher avoids board work to ensure full time face-to-face interaction with students during class. PowerPoint presentations are used instead of board work. 3D animated videos are used to teach procedures in the classroom. A talented teacher can integrate even role play in integrated lecture. The time for lecturing is less and lecturing time is mainly used to guide students and facilitate learning. Role play can be wisely used to develop attributes like proper attitude or teach how to behave in complex situations.

## Concept Mapping-based Lecture

Concept mapping is a great way to build upon previous knowledge by connecting new information to it. When new knowledge is integrated with and connected to existing knowledge that new knowledge is easier to understand and to remember.

A concept map is a visual organization and representation of knowledge. It shows concepts and ideas and the relationships among them. You can create a concept map by writing keywords and then drawing arrows between the ideas that are related. Then you add a short explanation by the arrow to explain how the concepts are related.

For example, while teaching qualities of a professional nurse, teacher tells students to prepare a concept map based on their knowledge regarding a nurse. After conducting a discussion on the concept map of students, teacher prepares the concept map showing all qualities of a professional nurse by adding new branches in the concept map prepared by students.

## The Flipped Classroom

In flipped classroom the content is sent previous day to students online as videos. Next day students come prepared and more time can be used for discussion and collaborative work. Knewton points out following benefits for flipped classroom.

- Students receive instant feedback as teachers have more time to help students and explain difficult concepts.
- Teachers can understand which concepts are more difficult to students. After each lesson, students write the questions they have and the teacher analyzes the students' feedback individually to explain concepts that students do not understand.

## Webinars by Experts

As online teaching is common now, it is easy to conduct webinars by experts for students. Webinar is a seminar or other presentation that takes place on the internet, allowing participants in different locations to see and hear the presenters, ask questions and sometimes give answers. Teachers can arrange webinar even after the class time so that normal classroom teaching will not get affected.

## Activated Demonstration

Activated demonstration is a clinical teaching method. It is given to a student when she is confused in between providing nursing care to the patient. When the patient's presenting problem is unfamiliar to the student, learning may become passive by simply observing the patient. Teacher then help the student by understanding the student's needs and make the passive situation into active learning experience. Activated demonstration provide learner with a supervised active experience.

## Clinical Questioning

According to Susan Bannister, when used strategically, questioning can engage learners by stimulating active participation in the learning process, guide them towards the understanding of deeper concepts, promote peer collaboration and build their confidence. Moreover, through questioning in the clinical area teachers can promote critical thinking and life-long learning.

Questioning is a challenging teaching method and even experienced teachers occasionally make mistakes. Different learners and teaching situations require different types of questions. The best approach is to constructing questions based on learner's ability. Clinical teachers can follow **Dreyfus** model of skills acquisition to assess level of learners. The four Dreyfus stages most relevant to clinical teachers are: **novice** (learners function by using a limited rule-based knowledge system without a clinical context), **advanced beginner** (learners have some knowledge of clinical rules and may just be getting exposed to a clinical environment), **competent** (learners greatly involved in actual care of patients), and **proficient** (learners show increasing initiative in patient care and use intuitive clinical reasoning based on their previously gained clinical experience). Generally, **most students will be in the novice to advanced beginner stage.**

Due to limited clinical experience, novice learners benefit mostly from simple questions focused on factual knowledge. These questions are often phrased in a direct manner and have a single best answer. Advanced beginner learners are working on linking facts they may have learned in isolation, so questions should prompt them to connect information and demonstrate understanding of concepts and comprehension. Competent and proficient learners are applying information to common clinical situations, so questions can be more complex that prompt them to apply theoretical knowledge to a specific clinical situation in the decision making process.

While questioning in the clinical area teacher should minimize discomfort by creating a positive learning environment. Avoid asking questions in a rapid-fire sequence and instead ask questions one at a time. To further promote a positive environment, teachers can ask open ended questions that increase the chance of finding an acceptable answer. If the learner's response to a question is incorrect, guide her while maintain confidence in her abilities, especially in front of patients. When used appropriately, clinical questioning facilitates the development of critical thinking, decision making and problem solving among students.

### The Few Minutes Preceptor Model

The few minutes preceptor method of clinical teaching can be done by staff nurses in the parental hospital. As many hospitals are now employing graduates and postgraduates as staff nurses, it is easy to implement this method of clinical teaching. This method involves identifying the needs of each individual learner, teaching and providing feedback by following a five step approach.

1. Allow learner to explain about the condition of patient and possible nursing diagnosis.
2. Probe for underlying reasoning or alternative explanation.
3. Teach a general principle.
4. Provide positive feedback about what the learner did right.
5. Correct any errors by making suggestions for improvement.

### SNAPPS in Teaching Community Settings

SNAPPS is a learner-centered teaching approach which can be used successfully in community settings, especially during home visits. SNAPPS consists of six steps.

1. Summarize briefly the medical history of patient and findings of physical examination to the teacher.
2. Narrow the nursing diagnosis to two or three important problems and possible nursing interventions.

3. Analyze the problems and discuss how patients condition support or refutes the nursing diagnosis.
4. Probe the teacher by asking questions about patients' condition to clear doubts or confusion.
5. Plan management for the patients' health problems.
6. Select a learning issue related to patient condition. Discuss the findings from the learning issue with the teacher.

This method is recommended for community postings of final year students. The teacher takes the role of a facilitator by promoting critical thinking, empowering the learner to have an active role in their education and serving as a knowledge "presenter" rather than a knowledge "source".

## SUMMARY

Digital teaching in nursing education can be defined as the process of teaching nursing through an ever growing and diversified combination of methods, internet, technology, media and devices without undermining the human component in the teaching-learning process. Online nursing education is the teaching intended to attain predetermined objectives through internet by using the most appropriate as well as convenient device, online platforms or Apps and social media. Online teaching can be classified as synchronous online teaching, asynchronous online teaching, interactive online teaching, linear online teaching and blended teaching.

Understanding principles of online teaching helps to conduct online teaching in an effective manner. Innovative teaching methods in nursing include integrated lecture, concept mapping-based lecture, the flipped classroom, webinars by experts, activated demonstration and clinical questioning, the few minutes preceptor model and SNAPPS.

## MULTIPLE CHOICE QUESTIONS

1. **Knowledge management is an example of:**
   a. Conceptual skill
   b. Developmental skills
   c. Manual skill
   d. None of the above
2. **Teamwork is an example of:**
   a. Personal skill
   b. Developmental skills
   c. Manual skill
   d. None of the above
3. **Role of teacher in the digital age is well described as:**
   a. Evolving role
   b. Facilitator
   c. Guide
   d. Philosopher
4. **MOOCs is an example of:**
   a. Fully online program
   b. Blended program
   c. Traditional program
   d. None of the above

5. Online program offers real time interaction between teacher and learners is called:
   a. Synchronous online teaching
   b. Asynchronous online teaching
   c. Interactive online teaching
   d. Linear online teaching
6. Sending recorded lectures is an example of:
   a. Linear online teaching
   b. Synchronous online teaching
   c. Asynchronous teaching
   d. None of the above
7. Flipped classroom is a combination of prerecorded lecture and:
   a. Discussion
   b. Role play
   c. Demonstration
   d. None of the above
8. WhatsApp group is mainly an example of:
   a. Communities of practice
   b. Peer group
   c. All of the above
   d. None of the above
9. Lecture conducted through video conferencing App is called:
   a. Webinar
   b. Linear teaching
   c. All of the above
   d. None of the above
10. Evidence-based teaching is mainly based on:
    a. Research
    b. Skills
    c. Attitude
    d. Knowledge

### ANSWER KEY

| 1. a | 2. b | 3. a | 4. a | 5. a | 6. a |
|------|------|------|------|------|------|
| 7. a | 8. a | 9. a | 10. a | | |

# CHAPTER 8

# Classroom Management

## LEARNING OBJECTIVES

After completing this chapter, reader will be able to:

- Define classroom management.
- Identify importance of classroom management.
- Explain goals of classroom management.
- List down components of classroom management.
- Identify factors influencing classroom management.
- Appreciate principles of classroom management.
- Follow strategies for effective classroom management.
- Realize practical guidelines for classroom management.
- Define classroom communication.
- List down types of classroom communication.
- Realize importance of classroom communication.
- Explain importance of communication competency in teaching.
- Identify facilitators of classroom communication.
- List down barriers of classroom communication.
- Overcome barriers of classroom communication.

An effective learning environment is very essential for attaining learning outcomes. Teacher can engage students actively in the teaching-learning process only through ensuring their proper conduct in the classroom. Implementing very strict or autocratic discipline is not advisable as it adversely affect the morale of students. At the same time too much relaxed atmosphere creates chaos in the classroom. Teachers need to know effective ways to create and maintain a positive learning environment through good class management in addition to content knowledge to become an expert teacher. Let us discuss briefly about effective classroom management.

## DEFINITION

Classroom management is the process of creating and maintaining a safe and effective learning environment essential for attaining learning outcomes by managing human resources and material resources in the most effective manner. The definition depicts the following:

- ❖ **Classroom management is a process:** Managing classroom is an integral part of the teaching-learning process. Classroom management consists of practices and procedures that teachers apply to keep students organized, orderly, focused, attentive and proactive in learning. Therefore, classroom management both as a process and as an approach has a great impact on students' learning by minimizing their inappropriate behavior.
- ❖ **Managing human resources:** Behavior of teacher as well as behavior of student has a great impact on classroom management. Classroom management is much more than implementing rules and regulations in a strict manner. It mainly involves specific

plans to utilize the abilities of teacher as well as students in the best possible manner. Most important aspect of classroom management is convincing students about teacher expectations for achieving learning outcomes by minimizing their undesirable behavior. Classroom management ensures teachers are providing rich and varied learning experiences for actively engaging students in classroom. At the same time classroom management also ensures learners are actively participating in the teaching–learning process. Teachers and students should develop a good interpersonal relationship and cooperate actively for effective classroom management.

- **Managing material resources:** Managing materials resources effectively by both teacher and students is an important aspect of classroom management. This is more significant in the use of media, technology and learning materials in the teaching–learning process. Material resources include lesson plans, textbooks, equipment, technology and other resources teachers use in the classroom. Using poorly designed lessons and uninterested learning materials by the teacher results in student disinterest and increased behavioral problems leading to poor classroom management. For example, using PowerPoint presentation without adequate explanation results in poor classroom management. Good material resources are more important in online classroom management than face to face teaching.
- **Safe and effective learning environment:** Good classroom management is essential for creating a safe and effective learning environment. This is applicable to both online and face to teaching. To a great extent, major goal of classroom management is the creation of an effective learning environment that promote student learning.

According to Charles D, "classroom management can be defined as a set of activities through which the teacher seeks to promote the desired behavior of students and works to limit or eliminate their inappropriate behavior in the classroom". This definition consider promoting desirable behavior among students as the goal of classroom management.

## GOALS OF CLASSROOM MANAGEMENT

The primary goal of effective classroom management is promoting student learning. Other goals listed below contribute to the achievement of this primary goal. Goals of classroom management are:

- Encouraging and establishing student self-control through a process of promoting positive student behavior and achievement.
- Improving academic achievement of students, teacher efficacy and student behavior.
- Maximize appropriate behavior that facilitate learning and minimize student misbehavior.
- Establishing positive teacher–student and peer relationship that help students to meet basic psychological needs. Students learn more effectively in an environment that meets their basic personal and psychological needs.
- Use group management methods that encourage student's engagement in curricular and cocurricular activities.
- Promote all–around development of students.
- Create a well-managed safe and positive learning environment that promote effective teaching and learning.
- Management of human resources as well as material resources in the best possible manner to achieve academic excellence.
- Enable teachers to influence student behavior in a desirable manner.
- Enabling students in attaining learning objectives or learning outcomes.

# PRINCIPLES OF CLASSROOM MANAGEMENT

Principles of classroom management are closely related to the teaching-learning process. Implementation of principles of classroom management largely depends on the teaching skills of the teacher. D Christian suggests following principles for better classroom management.

- **Principle of clarity and mastery over content:** Teacher should have a thorough knowledge about the subject she is teaching. Instead of blindly following textbooks and information from other sources she has to prepare her own teaching materials in accordance with the curriculum and level of students. Thorough knowledge in subject matter helps a teacher to teach effectively in a learner-friendly manner.
- **Principle of involvement:** Teacher needs to ensure active involvement of learners in the teaching-learning process. Meticulous preparation of content and effective use of teaching skills, especially skills of questioning, receiving and providing feedback will ensure active participation of students in the teaching-learning process. Active involvement of students ensures learning by minimizing student's inappropriate behavior in the classroom.
- **Principle of equal opportunity or democratic behavior:** The teacher needs to consider all students in the same manner. She should provide equal opportunity to every student to participate in the teaching-learning process. This behavior of teacher help student to participate in the teaching-learning process. This behavior of teacher helps students to develop a positive attitude towards learning. Democratic teachers encourage students to give their suggestions in smooth conduct of teaching-learning process. The democratic climate in the classroom allows the students to take initiative in the teaching-learning process and this will in turn lead to effective utilization of class time. No student feels neglected in the classroom.
- **Principle of teacher behavior:** While teaching the teachers' behavior should include various positive attribute like confidence, determination, will power, etc. This helps in creating a positive learning environment that promotes learning. This will also promote desirable behavior among students.
- **Principle of personal attributes or role modelling:** Teacher should be a role model to students. The personal attributes of the teacher such as warmth, sympathy, empathy, etc., have a strong influence on students' behavior in the classroom. Teacher should never judge a student with his or her past shortcomings. Respecting the dignity of students reduce undesirable behavior of the students. A good interpersonal relationship between teacher and student promote academic achievement of students. Effective teachers accept the feelings of their students and are sympathetic to academic and personal problems of students, The teacher can be a good friend, guide and philosopher to the students. The personal attributes of teacher is very important because they influence the feelings, interests, values and temperament of students.
- **Principle of self-control:** The teacher has to be firm and consistent in the classroom behavior. A deep commitment in teaching enables a teacher to manage instruction effectively. The self-control of a teacher enables her to control her behavior. This will motivate students to develop self-control in their behavior and promote their all-round development.
- **Principle of flexibility:** The principle of flexibility is not against to the principle of self-control. The teacher should be flexible in her behavior and consider students' valid suggestions and opinions. Depending upon the circumstances teacher should make appropriate changes in her behavior and in the teaching-learning activities. This will help her develop alternative strategies as needed and implement them to achieve the educational objectives.
- **Principle of communicating teacher expectations:** Teacher needs to communicate her expectations about academic achievement of students well in advance. Since teacher

expectations influence student behavior, teachers should always consider the need and level of students while communicating them to students.

## STRATEGIES FOR EFFECTIVE CLASSROOM MANAGEMENT

Research suggests that following strategies will assist teacher to maintain good classroom management.

- **Provide effective instruction at student appropriate level:** Effective instruction minimizes inappropriate behavior of students in the classroom. One goal of classroom management is to reduce in appropriate behavior of students. Hence, teachers must focus on effective instructional strategies that facilitate student achievement. Effective teaching promotes active participation of students in the teaching–learning process. When students are presented with information and material beyond their level, they became frustrated and may engage in behaviors that avoid participation in learning. On the other side, if the instruction level of the materials is too easy for students they may engage inappropriate behavior because of boredom and lack of challenge. Hence, it is important to provide instruction at student-appropriate level.

  Carnine suggest following measures to provide instruction at student-appropriate level:
  - Provide instructional materials that are educationally relevant for students.
  - Adopt a planned, sequential order of instruction that is logically related to the level of students.
  - Encourage active participation of students in the teaching–learning process.
  - Provide opportunities for guided practice.
  - Provide immediate feedback and positive reinforcement.

- **Following a comprehensive approach for effective classroom management:** Highly effective instruction reduces but does not fully eliminate classroom behavior problems. According to Emmer, effective classroom management requires a comprehensive approach that includes the following:
  - Structure the school and classroom environment.
  - Actively supervising student involvement in the teaching learning process.
  - Implementing classroom rules and routines.
  - Encouragement of appropriate behavior by positive reinforcement.
  - Discouraging inappropriate behaviors.
  - Collecting and using data to monitor student behavior and modifying classroom management procedures as needed.

- **Structuring a classroom that supports positive student behavior:** Highly effective teachers structure the classroom environment so that it decreases occurring of inappropriate student behavior, increases desirable student interactions and ensure success of students. Darch proposes following measures for effective classroom structuring:
  - Creating a physical arrangement that minimizes distractions and allow teachers to interact with students in order to respond to their questions and better control of behavior.
  - Making efficient use of classroom time, including transitions between various classroom activities.
  - Ensuring that the nature and quality of student interaction is positive.
  - Clearly communicate appropriate behavior for particular classroom activities. For example, students may be expected to interact with one another during cooperative learning activities but not during independent learning.

- **Effective use of classroom rules and routines:** The use of rules is a powerful, preventive component of classroom organization and management plan. Rules establish the behavioral context of the classroom by specifying what behaviors are expected from student, what behaviors will be reinforced and consequences of inappropriate behavior. Educators have identified following important guidelines for the construction of classroom rules.
    - Rules should be kept minimum to allow students to remember them.
    - Rules should contain language that is simple and appropriate to the level of students.
    - Rules should be stated positively.
    - Rules should be developed for various situations or contexts as needed. For example, rules are different for language classes and field trips.
    - Follow strategies promote student use of rules and regulations. After classroom rules and routine established, strategies to acknowledgment and encourage students appropriate use of these rules and routines must be included in the classroom management plan. Explaining about consequences of not following desired behavior is important to encourage desirable behaviors among students.
    - Implement techniques to decrease inappropriate behavior. Along with encouraging appropriate behavior of students teachers should also use effective techniques to decrease their inappropriate behaviors.
- **Provide professional development programs to teachers for improving classroom management skills:** Professional development programs help teachers to improve skills in classroom management. By improving skills in classroom management teachers can prevent undesirable behavior of students. It also enables teachers to detect undesirable behaviors at the beginning and take appropriate remedial measures.
- **Provide behavioral support to needy students at institutional level:** The goal of this type of behavioral support is to establish environment that are safe, predictable, consistent, and positive. When the institutional context is positive and predictable, implementing classroom-level behavior support becomes easier. Horner recommends following techniques that institution must adopt for achieving this goal:
    - Identify several positively stated behavioral expectations that apply to all students and staff in all settings (for example, be respectful).
    - Identify behavioral examples for each expectation that replace inappropriate behavior (for example "use polite language")
    - Teach and practice the expectations at the beginning of the academic year and periodically throughout the year (for example, beginning of academic year and after vacations).
    - Use efficient procedures that encourage and reinforce. Positive behavior (for example, praise positive behavior).
    - Monitor the effectiveness of the institution wide plan using data.
- **Seek help of the students support and guidance program as and when needed**: Every educational institution need to have an active students support and guidance program for providing guidance and counseling services to the needy students. When teacher feels that a student in her class need additional support for improving appropriate behavior or academic performance, she can seek help of the students support and guidance cell. This will help the needy student to improve appropriate behavior through proper guidance and support.

## IMPORTANCE OF CLASSROOM MANAGEMENT

Class management is the process by which teachers and educational institutions create and maintain appropriate behavior of students in the classroom. According to Emmer, the purpose of implementing classroom management strategies is to enhance prosocial behavior and increase student involvement in teaching–learning process. Thomas RK explains the importance of class management in the following manner:

- Establishes and maintains an orderly environment in the classroom
- Increases meaningful academic learning and facilitates social and emotional growth.
- Decreases negative behaviors and promote appropriate behaviors among students. This will in turn promote learning.
- Create a safe and positive environment for teaching and this will reduce stress of teachers as well as students.
- As a whole, classroom management enhances academic achievement, teacher efficiency and behavior of teachers and students.

## COMPONENTS OF CLASSROOM MANAGEMENT (THE THREE C'S OF CLASSROOM MANAGEMENT)

According to Froyen and Iverson, classroom management focuses on three major components: content management, conduct management and covenant management.

### Content Management

Content management includes both effectiveness of teaching and skills in organizing classroom organization. Effective teaching and consistent organizational skills reduce inappropriate behavior of students in the classroom. The most important aspect of content management is initiating and maintaining student cooperation in learning activities. According to Kounin, content management emphasis on effective teaching skills, providing additional or remedial instructional activities as needed and managing instruction-related discipline problems in a better manner.

### Conduct Management

Conduct management focuses on assisting students in developing appropriate behaviors. In planning classroom management, teachers should consider using an assertive communication style and behavior. In addition, teachers should always know what they want their students to do (teacher expectations) and involve them in the respective learning activities: According to Iverson, conduct management is essential to the creation of "an orderly, task-oriented approach to teaching and learning" which is essential for good classroom management.

Conduct management enable teacher to control student behavior in the following ways: acknowledging responsible behavior, correcting irresponsible and inappropriate behavior, gentle verbal reprimands, preferential seating arrangement in classroom, informing parents/guardians regarding inappropriate behaviors, written behavioral contract setting limits outside the classroom and positive reinforcement and feedback systems. Teachers should incorporate these ways in their teaching practice.

### Covenant Management

Covenant management focuses on creating a good social system in the classroom. Teacher and student roles and expectations should make classroom environment conducive for learning. Teachers and students should respect culture of others to create a good social system in the classroom. As teacher effectiveness and student achievement is greatly influenced by strong interpersonal relationship, teacher and student relationships are essential to create a positive classroom environment.

Classroom management discipline problems can be dealt with either on individual basis (between teacher and student) or by group problem solving (class meetings). As students develop a trust on teacher's efforts, they took responsibility of their own behavior. This will promote appropriate behavior in classroom and create a better classroom atmosphere. Through covenant management teachers and students become coparticipants in the teaching-learning process and this will result in achieving better learning outcomes.

## FACTORS INFLUENCING CLASSROOM MANAGEMENT

Major factors influencing classroom management can be summarized as follows:

- **Effective teaching:** Even though effective teaching alone cannot ensure good classroom management, it has a major role in promoting learning and discipline. Effective teaching with good learning materials, appropriate pacing, guided practice, attention to individual students, proper feedback, good interpersonal relationship with students, etc., help teachers to manage classroom in a better way and facilitate learning. If teaching is not effective, students may not get involved properly in the teaching-learning process and this may lead to ineffective classroom management.
- **Setting and implementing rules:** Proper implementation of rules helps to carryout instruction without much disruption. Teachers who are committed to achieve learning outcomes can manage classroom in a better manner. Hence, teachers should implement rules in a proper manner. Students should be made clear about the need of proper rules and how to follow rules in a proactive manner. The consequences of not obeying rule should also made clear to students in a non-threatening manner.
- **Proper intervention in a timely manner:** Ongoing monitoring of students' behavior and appropriate intervening as and when needed is every essential for better classroom management. A thoughtful implementation of rules with active participation of students will reduce the need of interventions. Frequent intervention for maintaining order while teaching adversely affects the teaching - learning process.
- **Good interpersonal relationship between teacher and students:** A teacher should be a friend, guide and philosopher to students. A teacher should be a role model to students in following rules. For example, teacher should not bring mobile phone to classroom when there is a restriction of mobile phone in the classroom. Good interpersonal relationship contributes to better classroom management as it always respect the dignity of students.
- **Proper and timely feedback and positive reinforcement of appropriate student behavior:** Feedback should focus on what students should do rather than what they are not supposed to do. The student expects feedback for his improvement so providing feedback influence classroom management in a better way.
- **Classroom environment:** Even though one goal of classroom management is the creation of good classroom environment, a good classroom environment also promotes good classroom management. Many factors such as proper guidance, individual attention to students, providing proper feedback, better classroom communication, better interpersonal relationship between students and teacher, etc., will assist in creating a good classroom environment.
- **Better classroom communication, especially communicating teacher expectations:** Better communication within the classroom facilitates better learning and influence classroom management in many ways. As said earlier, communicating teacher expectations minimize inappropriate behavior of students. This will in turn lead to better classroom management.

## PRACTICAL GUIDELINES FOR CLASSROOM MANAGEMENT

Following guidelines will help teacher in good classroom management:

- Consider each student as a teaching unit rather than the whole class. This is possible by giving individual attention to every student, give timely feedback, provide remedial teaching, etc.
- Introduce teacher guardian program, in teacher guardian program a particular number of students is assigned to a teacher. The teacher guardian regularly interact with students assigned to her and find out any learning or problems and report to the class teacher. In this way problems of students can be detected earlier and this will reduce inappropriate behavior in the classroom.
- Never punish the whole class for the mistake of a single student. This will further result in more issues.
- Never judge a student with his past mistake. While implementing discipline always consider the dignity of students.
- Communicate rules and regulations properly to student and implement them properly. It is better to include rules and regulation in the prospectus of the institution.
- Functioning of an effective parent teachers association helps in maintaining good classroom environment as it ensures appropriate behavior of students in the classroom.
- Provide a caring, stimulating and appropriate learning environment considering the needs and level of students.
- Use a variety of teaching methods with appropriate use of technology to ensure active involvement of students in the teaching-learning process.
- Proper management of individualized learning and group learning. For individualized learning, teacher can use technical devices like computers or use of self-learning materials and assignments depending on the availability of resources in the institution. Group learning, especially small group learning promotes achievement of learning outcomes. Group learning provides opportunity for interaction between students. During this interactive process, meanings are shared and information is exchanged. The classroom them becomes a social environment for increasing students' knowledge. Promoting individualized and group learning reduces inappropriate behaviors and results in better classroom management.
- Provide good learning materials. This will keep students engaged in the teaching-learning process and lead to better classroom management.
- Ensure effective communication between teacher and students in classroom. Effective communication removes barriers of communication and promotes desirable behaviors among children. This will in turn helps in achieving learning outcomes and results in better classroom management. Another advantage of effective communication is building good interpersonal relationship between teacher and students. This will also helps in good classroom management.

## CLASSROOM COMMUNICATION

### Definition

Classroom communication is defined as "effective communication between teacher and student or students in the classroom setting in a manner to achieve behavior modification of students and thereby attaining learning outcomes". This definition depicts the following about classroom communication:

❖ **Effective communication:** Teacher needs to know how to communicate effectively by overcoming barriers of communication and understanding facilitators of communication. As communication is the basis of teaching–learning process, teacher needs effective communication skills to manage the classroom.
Effective communication skills are crucial for being a good teacher. Effective communication skills that build a positive classroom environment are: (a) self-awareness, (b) sending direct, complete, relevant and congruent messages, (c) using feedback and (d) aware about what is communicating nonverbally.
❖ **Between teacher and student or students:** Classroom communication involves communicating effectively to both individual student as well as group of students. So teacher need to have skills in communicating individual student, small group of students and large group of students.
❖ **Achieving behavior modification of students:** All communication between teacher and students in the classroom should focus on building appropriate behavior among students. Communication should bring out behavior modification of students and this will ultimately results in attaining learning outcomes.

## Types of Classroom Communication

Communication within the classroom is essential for students to learn effectively. Classroom communication exists in three categories: verbal, nonverbal and written.
1. **Verbal communication** refers to sending or receiving a message through sounds and languages. Teacher can communicate to one student or the whole classroom through verbal communication.
2. **Nonverbal communication** refers to communicating without words through body language, gestures, facial expressions, the tone and pitch of the voice and posture. For example, if a teacher is nodding her head while a student is speaking, this can be encouraging or show that she agrees with the student.
3. **Written communication** is sending or receiving information through writing. For example, a teacher may arrange a written assignment for students to test their knowledge or conduct lecture with PowerPoint presentation or notes for transferring knowledge.

## Importance of Classroom Communication

❖ **Communication is an integral part of the teaching–learning process:** According to Sitihendon, teaching is a social activity that involves two-way communications between the teacher and learners. It is this two-way communication enables teachers to modify the behavior of learners and thereby attaining learning outcomes. In short, good teaching is not possible without understanding its relationship with communication process.
❖ **Improve self-esteem of students:** When teachers appreciate students' viewpoints in during communication, students will feel that their ideas are valuable. This promotes self-esteem and confidence among students. A self-confident student actively participates in the teaching–learning process. Active class participation leads to better learning outcomes.
❖ **Assist teacher in fulfilling various roles than a facilitator of learning:** 21st century learner have higher expectations about teachers. Teacher has to act as a counsellor, mentor, guide and a friend of student for his all-round development. Teacher also needs to fulfill many managerial functions and also use technology for achieving educational objectives. Through effective communication only teacher can fulfil all these roles or carryout all these activities.
❖ **Ensuring academic progress of students:** Providing timely feedback is an important aspect of teaching practice to ensure academic progress of students. Direct communication

between teacher and student provides immediate feedback to improve academic performance of students. Feedback takes place in both formal and informal situations. Thus, better communication facilitates maximum feedback and thereby learning also.

- **Promote teamwork:** Sometimes classroom communication occurs not only between teacher and students or students and students but also with other persons involving in the entire teaching-learning activity like principal, parents, nonteaching staff, related health and education professionals. Thus, proper classroom communication promotes teamwork essential for achieving the objectives of whole education program.
- **Ensure accessibility to teachers:** Proper classroom communication enable students to communicate with teacher individually and in groups. This will ensure access to teachers for all learners.
- **Assist in the professional growth of teachers:** Proper classroom communication enable students to provide feedback regarding performance of teachers. This will help teachers to improve their professional competence.

## Communication Competence in Teaching

According to Allen, communication competence involves selecting, adapting and implementing communication behaviors appropriate for the purpose, audience and context of the "situation". This definition reflects three basic assumptions of communication for teaching.

1. The major concern of communication in teaching is the development of the individual as a message strategist.
2. Communication competency is not restricted to competency in a particular language.
3. Communication behaviors can be modified.

### *Three Basic Skills for Communication Competence*

Del Polito identified three basic skills for communication effectiveness. These are: (1) social sensitivity, (2) active listening and (3) honest communication. These skills are important for the teacher to understand herself and students for communicating in a better manner.

### *Social Sensitivity*

Social sensitivity refers to one's ability to empathize with the other person: to see, feel and hear with the other person, to understand world from other person's perspective; to understand the thoughts needs and goals of the other person. Maximum understanding through social sensitivity occurs when the listener: (1) understands the speaker's perceptual world, including the speaker's attitudes, values, beliefs, knowledge, culture, social system, past experiences, and future expectations, (2) understands his/her own perceptual world and selectivity processes, (3) understands the content communicated and (4) understands the "feelings" communicated—how the message is expressed.

### *Active Listening*

To empathize with and become sensitive to the other person, one must listen actively. Active listening demands total commitment to the interaction. Active listening implies waiting until the other person completes his/her statement to understand the situation. To confirm an understanding and acceptance of the student during active listening, teacher should communicate "attention" during the interaction both verbally and nonverbally. Active listening helps in providing appropriate feedback to students.

### *Honest Communication*

Honest communication involves communicating honestly facts through ideas, feeling and attitudes. As we communicate honestly to students, we communicate trust in them, encouraging them to trust us and to share their feelings with us. Honest communication enhances understanding, acceptance, and more effective communication.

## Improving Classroom Communication Competencies

Del Polito recommends following measures for improving classroom communication competencies.

- **Establish realistic communication goals:** Recognizing her abilities and needs of students helps teacher to establish realistic communication goals. The classroom communication goals should be meaningful, relevant, challenging, attainable and clearly defined.
- **Conduct realistic, objective evaluation of communication behaviors:** Accurate, objective feedback which considers knowledge and abilities in communication as well as content expertise should be sought from competent sources to: (a) understand one's true strengths and weaknesses,(b) accept those strengths and weaknesses and (c) modify behaviors to achieve desired competence with the help of experts.
- **Concentrate on improving communication competencies, not perfection:** Striving for perfection increases the chance for failure in not achieving the "perfection" goal. So it is important to focus on strategies which would help to improve, not to become "perfect". This does not mean avoiding failures but rather to learn from mistakes and concentrate on modifying behaviors to improve classroom communication.
- **Identify, accept and promote personal communication strengths:** "Positive self-evaluation in the form of verbal reinforcement" is positively related to an enhanced self-concept. Once identified, strengths should be accepted and praised. This measure emphasis the need to evaluate continually the effectiveness of the strategies used in each communication transaction.

## Facilitators of Classroom Communication

Research shows that following factors facilitate classroom communication. Even though effectiveness of classroom communication depends mainly on efforts of teachers, it also depends on the communication skills of students and cooperation from higher authorities of the educational institution.

- **Teacher awarenesses:** In order to communicate effectively in the classroom teacher need to process information from various aspects related to teaching–learning process. Five awarenesses like (1) awareness of learners, (2) awareness of interaction between teacher, (3) awareness of self as a teacher, (4) awareness of teaching practice and (5) awareness of teaching context helps teacher to communicate effectively in the classroom. These awarenesses help teacher to adopt a learner-centered teaching which in turn facilitate better classroom communication.
- **Classroom communication need to be purposive, positive and pragmatic in nature:** Teacher needs to avoid unnecessary or irrelevant conversation while communicating with students in the classroom. Students have higher expectations from their teachers. So teacher need to communicate in a fruitful manner to students. Classroom communication involves speaking, lecturing, describing, explaining, discussion and nonverbal communication like eye contact, nodding head, etc. Teacher need to be purposive and positive while communicating to students irrespective of the mode of communication.
- **Facilitate maximum interaction between teacher and students:** To facilitate maximum interaction teacher should always try to create a learner-centered classroom even though the teaching method is a teacher-centered one. For example, if teacher is following lecture method, which is a teacher-centered one, teacher can convert lecture into a student-

centered teaching method by including discussion in between the lecture. In a learner-centered classroom, learners can easily ask questions, doubts and queries. This will facilitate promotion of effective classroom communication. Another method to facilitate interaction is facilitating maximum feedback. Timely and positive feedback is an essential component of classroom communication.

- **Classroom communication competencies of teacher:** Teacher should be proficient in communication skills, especially listening, speaking, reading and writing and should know how to utilize this proficiency effectively in a classroom setting. Self-awareness; sending direct, complete, relevant, congruent messages; using feedback and being aware of what is communication nonverbally are other communication skills that help to build a positive classroom environment. Among communication competencies, active listening deserves special mentioning. Even though teacher is aware that she cannot solve the problem of the student alone she should give enough time for the student to express her feelings and grievances. Research shows that active listening of students issues itself give them big relief and develop a security feeling that enables them to adopt appropriate behaviors.
- **Create a caring and conducive classroom environment that facilitates learning:** Students feel free to communicate in a caring and non-threatening environment. When teacher shows interest in a student's opinion, that student will feel that his thoughts or ideas are appreciated. This increases self-esteem of student and feel comfortable in the classroom. This will ultimately result in creating a caring and conducive classroom environment.
- **Ensure two-way communication in teaching–learning process:** Role of two-way communication is important in effective classroom communication. As discussed earlier, feedback plays an important role in two-way communication. Interpersonal communication allows a greater scope for feedback, which is essential for attaining learning outcomes.
- **Promote individual as well as group communication in classroom:** Some students require individual attention to meet their specific educational needs. Individual communication helps these kinds of students in learning by clarifying their doubts and misunderstandings. Teachers commonly use group teaching methods like lecture, seminars, discussion, etc., for group instruction.
- **Understanding role of teacher:** Teacher has a prominent role in ensuring effective classroom communication. Teacher need to develop academic and intellectual skills essential for conducting teaching in a student-centered manner. Abilities to communicate clearly and specifically, proper explanation, highlight important points, being a good listener, and good interaction skills are some of the behaviors needed for effective communication in the teaching practice.
- **Teacher preparation:** The first and foremost step in classroom communication is to define the objectives of communication clearly and realistically so that these can be met within the specified timeframe. Based on these objectives, message or content needs be designed which could be, verbal, written, pictorial or symbolic. The verbal message involves direct communication in the form of lectures, presentations, speeches, etc. Written message include published information in the form of books, research papers, PowerPoint presentation, handouts etc. Whatever be the chosen form, the message should be simple, clear, interesting and appropriate to the level of students. Nonverbal communication like maintaining eye contact, smiling, nodding, etc., also be used to communicate with students.
- **Developing an appropriate classroom climate for proper communication:** Teacher and students needs to follow certain rules and regulations for the effective functioning of the class. The class atmosphere should be democratic in nature with due respect to teachers. Inappropriate behaviors like talking loudly, shouting, etc., should be discouraged at once.

❖ **Assist students in developing communication skills:** Students need to be provided with assistance for developing communication skills such as verbal, writing, listening and questioning skills. This will also promote classroom communication.
❖ **Ensure better "teacher-student" and "student-student" relationship in the classroom:** Good human relationship in the classroom fosters classroom communication in a big manner. Teacher can create a learning friendly human environment by adopting following measures: (a) be understanding and sensitive to the emotional and academic needs of the students, (b) be always proactive to students' issues, (c) be sympathetic while dealing with problematic children in the classroom, (d) give equal opportunities to all students in co-curricular activities, (e) provide enough time for listening problem of students, (f) use pleasant words with firmness while handling indiscipline activities, (g) encourage cooperation and collaboration among students through group activities.
❖ **High-tech high-touch approach in teaching:** Teacher can use technology in teaching to a certain extent only. Technology alone only make teaching easier not better. Always give due consideration to human element while teaching. For example, while teaching with the help of PowerPoint presentation give adequate explanation with examples instead of simply scrolling slides.

## Barriers of Classroom Communication

Effective classroom communication occurs when messages are not distorted during communication process and communication serves the purpose for which it was planned or designed. However, when the desired effect is not achieved, factors which act as barriers need to be find out with the intention to discover why the communication has been ineffective. Let us discuss some of the barriers of classroom communication.

### *Teacher-centered Classroom Environment*

In a teacher-centered classroom environment students are not allowed to express their ideas or feelings in a proper manner. Most of the time, only one way communication is taking place instead of two-way communication. In a teacher-centered classroom, teacher fails to provide timely feedback to students based on the response of students. Providing timely and appropriate feedback is essential to achieve learning outcomes by guiding students properly. Thus, a teacher-centered classroom not only prevents proper communication but also hampers the effectiveness of the teaching–learning process.

Proper planning of lessons, defining role of teacher and students in the teaching–learning process, clearly communicating teacher expectations and encouraging student-teacher interactions in classroom will help in creating a learner-centered classroom. A learner-centered classroom environment definitely facilitates classroom communication.

### *Inappropriate Behavior of Teacher and Students*

Inappropriate behavior of teacher and students is a major barrier for effective classroom communication. Personality differences between students and teacher is one reason for this barrier. Another reason is psychosocial factors from the side of teacher as well as students. Peer pressure also contributes to inappropriate student behavior in classroom.

Personality difference leads to frustration, unhappiness and lack of communication between students and teachers. This personality differences discourage both teachers and students from developing and maintaining a good interpersonal relationship.

Psychological factors such as psychological state of mind, prejudice, disinterest, inattention, emotions, redundancy, confusion, unrewarding experience, feeling of anxiety, poor physical health or illness, lack of motivation, dissatisfaction, poor cognitive abilities and unfulfilled curiosity affect classroom communication.

Peer pressure forces a student to behave inappropriately in class by offering support to friends by responding to teachers through acting funny, cool or disengaging in class.

Professional conduct of teachers in a classroom, clearly communicating rules and regulations and explaining clearly the rights and responsibilities of students will minimize inappropriate behaviors in classroom. Teachers must also recognize and understand the personality differences and try to find a healthy balance, without showing partiality or favouritism. Rewarding positive behaviors also reduces the occurrence of inappropriate behavior due to peer pressure in classroom. Psychological barrier from the students side can be dealt through adopting appropriate teaching strategies and providing needed assistance such as guidance and counseling to facilitate learning.

### Semantic Barriers (Mainly Language Barriers)

The semantic barriers in communication can be defined as the misunderstanding and misinterpretation of meaning which restrict effective communication. It can be in the form of language, sign and symbol. The semantic barriers usually arise when the information is not in the simple language and contains those words or symbols that have multiple meanings. As a result misunderstanding occurs between sender and receiver regarding the meaning of the words. Language used the choice of word, pronunciation differences and spelling errors are the main causes of a semantic barrier. To avoid such semantic barriers, the teacher should use the precise and exact word that will convey the same meaning for the student in the given context.

The teacher must also make sure the students clearly understand the exact/ intended meaning of words.

Teachers use of excessive verbalism, verbosity and unclear symbols or graphics and improper body language along with students' language incompetence, poor receptive abilities, poor listening skill, lack of comprehension, difficulty of students in understanding teachers language and quality of media also adds to semantic barriers.

To overcome language barriers teachers need to follow some measures like: (a) teachers should assess the students' communication abilities, especially language receptive abilities and communicate according to the level of students, (b) use judicious mix of verbal and nonverbal means of communication, (c) promote active listening, (d) use simple language and less verbalism for explanation, (e) use graphic symbol for explanation as needed, (f) use audiovisual resources and media effectively and (g) take feedback from students and improve communication according.

### Physical Barriers

A conducive and safe classroom environment is essential for effective communication. Physical barriers include noise, invisibility, inaudibility, environmental and physical discomfort, distraction, lack of arrangement for proper lighting and lack of proper seating arrangement. Improper functioning of audiovisual aids is also a physical barrier.

Following measures will help teacher to overcome physical barriers: (a) arrange classroom environment by ensuring proper lighting, acoustics, etc. (b) make appropriate seating arrangements, (c) select appropriate audio-visual aids or media for ensuring effective communication, (d) ensure audibility and visibility in classroom, (e) minimize the visual and aural distractions and (f) provide environment comfort.

## Cultural Barriers

Cultural differences can be a barriers to effective communication in the classroom. It is possible for both a teacher and student to have predisposed idea about behavior based on what the other person's culture is. Messages are often misunderstanding if they are delivered in a way that is unfamiliar to the students culture. It is important to remove assumptions or biases based on cultural differences in a classroom.

## Perception Barriers

Perception is the process of selecting, organizing and interpreting information. This process affect classroom communication because students responds to message from teacher sometimes in a different manner than intended by the teacher. In simple terms, perception barriers in classroom are mental blocks that are result of internal biases students regarding teachers. These mental blocks disrupt effective classroom communication because they prevent students from proper interactions with teachers. Perceptional barriers also adversely affect interpersonal relationship between students and teachers. To avoid perceptional barriers teacher should give importance to both positive and negative aspects of conversation with students. She should also make sure that message is interpreted by the students in the right manner.

## Ineffective Teaching and Low Quality Learning Materials

Sometimes ineffective teaching may also create communication barrier. It is not possible to conduct classes very effectively in all days, but teachers should work hard to develop engaging lessons with interesting and relevant activities. Thought-provoking assignments, technology-enhanced lectures and creative projects enhance classroom communication and interaction.

Outdated, routine assignments and busywork create communication barriers-students don't want to interact with their teachers and just wait class to be over. Teachers can avoid this communication barrier by putting more energy, enthusiasm and creativity in the teaching practice.

## Curriculum-related Barriers

Sometimes curriculum-related aspects act as communication barrier in classroom communication. To overcome this barriers teacher should provide proper orientation regarding subjects on the beginning of the academic year. Before start teaching, teacher should explain how to learn and revise properly for gaining knowledge.

## SUMMARY

Classroom management is the process of creating and maintaining a safe and effective learning environment essential for attaining learning outcomes by managing human resources and material resources in the most effective classroom management is closely related to the teaching-learning process. Implementation of principles of classroom management largely depends on the teaching skills of the teacher.

Principles of classroom management are principles of clarity over content, principle of involvement, principle of equal opportunity or democratic behavior, principle of teacher behavior, principle of personal attitudes or role modelling, principle of self-control, principle of flexibility and principle of communicating teacher expectations.

Strategies like providing effective instruction at student appropriate level, following a comprehensive approach for effective classroom management, structuring a classroom that support positive student behavior, effective use of classroom rules and routines, providing professional development program for teachers, providing behavioral support to needy students and seek help of the students support and guidance program will help to maintain a good classroom environment.

Components of classroom management are content management, conduct management and covenant management. Factors influencing classroom management are effective teaching, setting and implementing rules, proper intervention in a timely manner, good interpersonal relationship between teachers and students, timely feedback and better classroom communication. Practical guidelines for classroom management help teachers to maintain good classroom environment.

Classroom communication is defined as effective communication between teacher and student or students in the classroom setting in a manner to achieve behavior modification of students and thereby attaining learning outcomes.

Communication within the classroom is essential for students to learn effectively. Classroom communication exists in three categories namely verbal, nonverbal and written. Communication competence in teaching is essential for good classroom communication. Three basic skills for communication competence are social sensitivity, active listening and honest communication.

Facilitators of classroom communication are teacher awareness, maximum interaction between teacher and students, classroom communication competencies of teacher, promoting individual as well as group communication in classroom, understanding role of teacher and following high-tech high-touch approach in teaching.

Barriers to classroom communication are teacher-centered classroom environment, inappropriate behavior of teacher and students, semantic barriers, physical barriers, cultural barriers, perception barriers and ineffective teaching.

## MULTIPLE CHOICE QUESTIONS

1. **Primary goal of effective classroom management:**
    a. Student-self control
    b. Management of human resources
    c. Management of material recourses
    d. Promote student learning
2. **Which is the most influencing factor in classroom management?**
    a. Teacher appearance
    b. Teacher expectations
    c. Student–teacher interaction
    d. Role modeling by teacher
3. **Covenant management component of classroom management is related to:**
    a. Creating a good social system in classroom
    b. Appropriate behavior
    c. Teaching skills
    d. Mastery of content
4. **In classroom management student behavior can be modified in a student friendly manner through:**
    a. Autocratic environment
    b. Reprimanding
    c. Giving assignments
    d. Providing appropriate feedback

5. Giving assignment to students is an example of:
   a. Verbal communication
   b. Nonverbal communication
   c. Written communication
   d. None of the above
6. One basic skill for communication effectiveness is:
   a. Role modeling
   b. Proper explanation
   c. Providing feedback
   d. Active listening
7. Maintaining eye contact during teaching is an example of:
   a. Verbal communication
   b. Showing interest in teaching
   c. Nonverbal communication
   d. None of the above
8. Semantic barrier is mainly related to:
   a. Language
   b. Interaction
   c. Teaching
   d. Learning
9. Inappropriate behavior resulting from peer pressure can be effectively dealt by:
   a. Giving punishment
   b. Seeking explanation
   c. Rewarding positive behavior
   d. None of the above
10. Difficulty in selecting, processing and interpreting information is example of:
    a. Cultural barriers
    b. Physical barrier
    c. Semantic barrier
    d. Perception barrier

## ANSWER KEY

| 1. d | 2. d | 3. a | 4. d | 5. c | 6. d |
|------|------|------|------|------|------|
| 7. c | 8. a | 9. c | 10. d | | |

# CHAPTER 9

# Introduction to Educational Technology

## LEARNING OBJECTIVES

**After completing this chapter, reader will be able to:**

- Define educational technology.
- Explain the evolution of educational technology.
- Describe the nature and scope of educational technology.
- Identify significance of educational technology.
- Explain role of technology in education.
- Realize impact of technology in teaching.
- Differentiate between technology and media.
- Select appropriate media.
- List down trends in educational technology.
- Differentiate between AV aids and educational technology.
- Define audiovisual aids.
- Classify audiovisual aids.
- Explain the purposes of audiovisual aids.
- Explain the principles in the use of AV aids.
- Identify the characteristics of a good teaching aid.
- Use chalkboard in an effective manner.
- Plan, prepare and use different types of charts.
- Design and use handouts effectively.
- Teach effectively by using models.
- Prepare and use transparencies.
- Teach effectively by using slide projector.
- Recognize the role of computers in nursing education.

Technology explosion' has yielded several new machines, materials and media, which have great potential for use in the educational enterprise. A judicious use of these together with new functions and roles of educational personnel in order to bring about more efficient and effective teaching-learning led to the development of a new branch of study, namely—educational technology. An adequate knowledge of theory and practices of educational technology and their proper use would enable the teacher to understand and effectively discharge his new roles in the present day education system.

## MEANING

The word technology is derived from the Greek word *'technic'* meaning art or skill and *logia* meaning science or study. As a matter of fact, techniques are reckoned as the software and the equipment as the hardware of technology. For example, overhead projector is the hardware and the overhead transparency is the corresponding software. Technology results in new designs and devices as also new ideas and process. Education, the act or process of acquiring and imparting knowledge, is crucial to the development of a learner with a view to his/her participation in the transformation of the world for a better tomorrow. Educational technology is more than the sum of the two interpretations namely technology in education and technology of education.

According to some educationists, educational technology is a system in education in which machines, materials, media, men and methods are interrelated and work together for the fulfillment of specific educational objectives. Educational technology is an applied or practical study, which aims at maximizing educational effects by 'controlling' such relevant factors as educational purposes, educational content, teaching materials, educational environment, conduct of students, behavior of teachers and interrelations between students and teachers. It is a branch of study in which the results of engineering techniques, information science, natural science and behavioral sciences are used together with the human skills in order to promote the efficiency of education. This phrase though coined and used three decades ago, first by the Brynmor Jones in UK has undergone vast changes in its connotation over all these years and is still flexible to accommodate each and every novel technique or process that concerns positive learning.

## DEFINITION

Definition for educational technology given by Commission on Instructional Technology, USA is that "it is a systematic way of designing, implementing and evaluating the total process of learning and teaching in terms of specific objectives, based on research in human learning and communication and employing a combination of human and non-human resources to bring about more effective instruction."

Unwin defined educational technology in the following manner, "Educational technology is considered with the application of modern skills and techniques to requirements of education and training. This includes the facilitation of learning by manipulation of media and methods and the control of environment in so far as this reflects on learning."

According to Council for Educational Technology, UK, "Educational technology is the development, application and evaluation of systems, techniques and aids to improve the process of human."

Above said definitions consider educational technology as a systematic way, a process or an application of the scientific knowledge to improve the efficiency of the process of learning and instruction. It is thus considered to be the technology of education more than technology in education.

## DEVELOPMENT OF EDUCATIONAL TECHNOLOGY

History of the educational technology starts from the stage when the subject matter becomes available in the form of printing materials and textbooks. It was soon supplemented by the use of teaching aids, such as blackboard, specimen, pictures, charts, models, maps, etc. In this way, the earlier concept of educational technology was limited to the use of simple audiovisual aids meant for direct teaching and learning.

Later with the industrial revolution and technical advancement, sophisticated scientific instruments, mass media and educational materials were being used. It brought the use of sophisticated hardware and software, such as radio, television, computers, etc., in the field of education. From this period onwards, educational technology has developed over three aspects, namely—mass communication, individual learning, and group learning strategies.

The concept of programmed instruction and theories of learning, later on added another dimension to the meaning and concept of educational technology. This was again broadened when the new approaches, such as micro-teaching, computer-assisted instruction, etc., came into existence.

Broadly speaking, education technology has passed through five stages.
1. The first stage of educational technology is linked with the use of audiovisual aids, such as charts, maps, models, specimen, etc. The term educational technology was used as synonym to audiovisual aids.

2. The second stage of educational technology is linked with the 'electronic revolution', which brought an era of sophisticated hardware and software. The projector, tape recorder, radio and television changed the educational scenario. Accordingly, educational technology was taken in terms of these sophisticated instruments and equipment for presenting instructional material.
3. The third stage of educational technology is linked with the mass media, which led to 'communication revolution' for instructional purposes. Computer-assisted instruction also became popular.
4. The fourth stage of educational technology is marked by the individualized process of instruction. The invention of programmed learning and programmed instruction gave a new dimension to educational technology. A system of self-learning based on self-instructional materials and teaching machines emerged.
5. The latest concept of educational technology is influenced by the concept of system engineering or system approach. According to this, educational technology is a systematic way of designing, carrying out, and evaluating the total process of teaching and learning in terms of specific objectives based on research.

## TYPES OF EDUCATIONAL TECHNOLOGY

A Lumsdeine classified educational technology into three distinct types or approaches as mentioned below:
1. **Educational technology (I) or hardware approach:** This type of educational technology has its origin in physical science and engineering. This includes charts, models, slides, film strips, audio cassettes, radio, television, films, projectors, tape recorder, video and computers. Mass media movement is a result of this approach.
2. **Educational technology (II) or software approach:** This has its origin in behavioral sciences, so it is referred as instructional technology, teaching technology or behavioral technology. This is a process oriented technique for the production of suitable teaching-learning material, teaching-learning strategies and educational techniques. Basically, this is the technique of developing and utilizing software.
3. **Educational technology (III) or systems approach:** This is related to the concept of systems engineering. This views education as a system having a set of inputs, which are subjected to a process designed to produce certain output. If the system meets the objectives, it is maintained, otherwise it is modified as desired.
4. According to the latest classification, there are exists five divisions of educational technology. They are:
    a. *Educational technology (I):* Here direct use of psychological principles is recommended. It deals with diagnostic assessment of pupils, educational objectives in behavioral terms, deciding for methods, devices for classroom instruction and stimulus control for self-instructional strategy.
    b. *Educational technology (II):* Here instructional materials and communication means are produced after designing and examining them carefully.
    c. *Educational technology (III):* The management aspects are considered here as planning, programming, budgeting, decision making operations, research, system analysis and organization of models for problem solving, computers and information system, and organization of a man-machine system.
    d. *Educational technology (IV):* It covers educational systems engineering, i.e., the planning, designs, construction and evaluation of instructional systems, administrative systems and operating systems.

e. *Educational technology (V):* Educational planning is considered here just like the manifestation of educational systems engineering. The economic aspects and finances are the main bases here.

## CHARACTERISTICS OF EDUCATIONAL TECHNOLOGY

From the above discussions, you can easily find out the following characteristics of educational technology:

- It is the application of scientific principles to education.
- It lays stress on the development of methods and techniques for effective teaching-learning.
- It stresses the organization of learning situations for effective realization of the goals of education.
- It emphasizes the designing and developing of evaluation methods for testing learning outcomes.
- It facilitates learning by controlling environment, media, and methods.
- It involves input, output and process aspect of education.
- It is not confined to the use of electronic media in education. It includes systems approach also.
- It is not to be taken as a synonym to audiovisual aids in education.
- It is a very comprehensive term and is not to be viewed in terms of its parts or processes. It includes instructional technology, teaching technology, programmed learning, systems analysis, etc.

## GENERAL OBJECTIVES OF EDUCATIONAL TECHNOLOGY

Hillard Jason has stated the following major objectives of education technology: (a) transmitting information, (b) serving as role models, (c) assisting the practice of specific skills, and (d) contributing to the provision of feedback. Mackenzie and others describe the following main objectives of educational technology: (a) the need to reach more students, (b) to reach them with an improved range of learning materials, (c) to offer greater opportunities for independent study, and (d) to permit at least a limited student response.

### Macro-level Objectives of Educational Technology

Macro-level objectives are objectives in terms of broad educational goals. They are: (a) Identification of educational needs and aspirations of the community. (b) determination of the aims of education, broad strategies and structure of education. (c) developing a suitable curriculum with interaction of arts, human values and sciences. (d) identification of man-material resources and strategies for achieving the desired aims of education, (e) developing certain models leading to improvement in the teaching-learning process, (f) identification of major constrains in the environment and the ways and means of tackling them, (g) assisting in extending vocational opportunities to masses, especially to the neglected sectors of society, and (h) managing the entire education system covering planning, implementation and evaluation phase.

### Micro-level Objectives of Educational Technology

Micro-level objectives are objectives in terms of specific classroom teaching activity. They are: (a) Identifying and analyzing the characteristics and educational needs of the students, (b) determining the specific classroom objectives and stating them in behavioral terms, (c) analyzing the contents of instruction and organizing them in proper sequence, (d) identifying the available teaching-learning material and resources, (e) identifying the nature of the interaction of the subsystems, such as students, teachers, teaching-learning material, content of instruction and methodologies, (f) evaluating the effectiveness of the classroom teaching in terms of the student's performance or change in behavior, (g) providing appropriate feedback to the students as well as teachers to bring about modification in the teaching-learning process.

## ADVANTAGES OF EDUCATIONAL TECHNOLOGY

The US commission on instructional technology has listed the following advantages of education technology: (a) it can make education more productive, (b) it can make education more individual, (c) it can give instruction a more scientific base, (d) it can make instruction more powerful, (e) it can make access to education more immediate, (f) it can make access to education more equal.

## SCOPE OF EDUCATIONAL TECHNOLOGY

Scope of educational technology is as wide as education itself. Its scope ranges from the concrete educational process to the most abstract and subtle ones. It includes the use of hardware and software and systems analysis in various educational operations. The possibility of using educational technology in almost all areas of education has been and is being explored. There are three major areas in education in which its scope is very wide. These are: (a) technology related to general educational administration and management, (b) technology related to general educational testing, and (c) technology related to the instructional process.

Rowntra has stated the following as the province of educational technologists: (a) identifying the aims and objectives of learning, (b) planning the learning environment, (c) exploring and structuring the subject matter, (d) selecting appropriate teaching strategies and learning media, (e) evaluating the effectiveness of learning system, and (f) using the insights gained from evaluation to improve their effectiveness for the future.

According to JC Aggarwal, important areas which should comprise educational technology are (a) concept and various facets of educational technology, (b) teaching-learning process, (c) individualized instructional technology, (d) programmed learning, (e) teaching models, (f) learning theories, (g) multimedia approach to teaching, (h) mathetics, (i) cybernetics, (j) task analysis, (k) modules, and (l) systems approach.

*Mathetics* is the newest and most controversial approach to programmed instruction. Mathetics came from the Greek word 'mathein', which means to learn. Thomas F Gillbert is the originator of the concept of mathetics and he described the systematic procedures of mathetics in 1962. Mathetics is more suited to teaching of skills. It is considered as a complete training system that gives the programmer: (a) a guide for determining what to teach, (b) a basis for making teaching strategy decisions, and (c) a detailed procedure for construction of a program. Mathetics can be described as clinical in its purpose. It analyzes the deficiency and tries to make it up. Mathetics is elective in nature but is unique in application if not in principles. All inclusively mathetics is a step towards technology of education.

The word *'cybernetics'* was first used by Norbert Wener to define the field of automatic control systems. Wiener defined cybernetics as the science of control and communication in animals, men and machines. The notion of being "machine like" or what we sometimes call an algorithm or a decision procedure is essential to cybernetics. A decision procedure is a set of rules, which allows you to solve some particular problem without any understanding of the details of the problem or knowledge of why the problem is should be solved. It is in this sense, we think of it as machine-like. The concept of machine-like was directly related to the use of the computer. The modern cyberneticians feel that this definition of machine-like is too limited and we must extend it to include creative ability, concept and hypotheses formation and similar creative abilities on the part of mathematicians and scientists. The word 'machine' means something more than a computer use in the conventional routine way. According to the new concept, it is a flexible self-adapting mechanism, which is capable of changing its responses according to the changing environment in which it is placed. When we come to build cybernetic machines, we intentionally copy human intelligence and behavior. Models are constructed for perception, memory, learning, thinking, language and all the functions of which man is capable. We are still far away from constructing such a machine or programming a digital computer to fulfil the role of human behavior. Applied cybernetics is automatic and something more, since we can apply cybernetics to problems of human intelligence. Indeed, artificial intelligence is the central theme of current cybernetic thinking.

Self-instructional module is a learning package planned and prepared from the beginning till end with an aim to facilitate self-learning. It is self-explanatory, self-sufficient, self-directed, self-motivating and self-evaluating. Above all, it should facilitate self-learning. In the strict sense, module is an organized collection of learning experiences assembled in order to achieve a specified group of related objectives or a self-contained section of a course or program of instruction.

## SIGNIFICANCE OF EDUCATIONAL TECHNOLOGY

The significance of educational technology in education can be summarized as follows:
- Helps teachers to impart knowledge in a meaningful manner
- Provide visual and sensory experience that can effectively substitute direct experience
- Assist in developing methods and techniques for effective learning
- Creation of a learner-centered multimedia learning environment in classroom
- Make education more accessible by overcoming barriers of time, distance and shortage of resources
- Helps in attaining goals of education by organizing effective teaching-learning situations
- Assist in developing measuring instruments for assessing learning outcomes
- Promotes learning by controlling environment, media and method
- When carefully designed and thoughtfully applied, technology can improve effectiveness of teaching practice
- Provide access to huge informational background. The internet connects individuals, thereby it can be used as an effective tool for gaining knowledge. Web users can access huge informational background through search engines, such as Google
- Help teachers in saving time by providing assistance in preparing and organizing study material in an effective manner.

## ROLE OF TECHNOLOGY IN EDUCATION

Role of technology can be discussed under: (a) providing easy access to information, (b) learning with technology, (c) teaching with technology, (d) assessment of learning, (e) assessment of teacher performance and (f) offering affordable good quality educational programs.

### Providing Access to information

Distinctive feature of modern technology is the possibility to make data accessible from various locations. Internet can be used as an effective tool for gaining knowledge. Students can use the internet to get all the additional information they need to expand their knowledge base. Information is available irrespective of geographical and political boundaries.

## Learning with Technology

Technology helps in providing, engaging and empowering learning experience in both formal and informal settings. Following are the ways technology can improve and enhance learning:

- ❖ Technology can enable personalized learning or experiences that are more engaging and relevant.
- ❖ Technology helps to learn complex concepts and content with the help of a wide variety of digital learning devices and resources.
- ❖ Technology can help learning more beyond the classroom and take advantage of learning opportunities available out of school settings.
- ❖ Technology can help learners pursue passions and personal interests.
- ❖ Equitable access to technology can help close the digital divide and make transformative learning opportunities available to all learners.

## Teaching with Technology

Technology empowers teachers to provide more effective teaching for all learners. Technology helps teachers in the following ways to improve teaching practice:

- ❖ With technology teachers can connect with other teachers and experts around the world to expand their knowledge base. Tools, such as video conference, online chats and social media sites help teachers to connect and collaborate with experts.
- ❖ Teachers can design highly engaging and relevant learning experiences by using technology.
- ❖ Teachers get more time to function as guide or facilitators than more content experts with the effective use of technology. As information is available through high speed internet, by helping students' access online information and engage in simulations teachers get more time to function as a facilitator of learning.
- ❖ Effective use of technology helps teachers to confront challenges in a proper manner. Knowing how to use technology effectively to realize learner's expectations is essential to become a inspiring teacher.
- ❖ Effective use of technology also fosters ongoing professional learning of teachers which is essential to maintain competency in teaching practice (see also impact of technology on teaching).

## Assessment of Learning

Measuring learning is an integral part of teaching practice. Technology enabled assessments can help reduce the time, resources and disruption to learning while administering paper tests. Technology enabled assessment also can provide a more complete picture of student needs, interest and abilities than traditional assessments. Technology can help assessment in the following ways:

- ❖ **Preparing-enhanced question types:** Technology-based assessment allows for a variety of question types beyond the traditional types. Examples of enhanced question types are graphic response, simulations, performance based assessment, etc.
- ❖ **Measure complex competencies:** Technology helps in the assessment of non-cognitive competencies in a fruitful manner. Technology also helps in measuring knowledge and skill in a more meaningful manner.
- ❖ **Provide real-time feedback:** Technology-based formative assessment can offer real-time reporting of results. This will help teachers to evaluate and respond to student performance more quickly than traditional assessment.

❖ **Adapt to learner ability and knowledge:** Computer-based adaptive testing has facilitated the assessment in a more accurate manner. This assessment estimates accurately what students know and can do in a shorter testing session than traditional tests.
❖ **Embedded with the learning process:** Technology-based assessment is closely linked to the learning process. It is simply a part of effective instruction and useful for identifying learning problems and offering support.

## Assessment of Teacher Performance

Educational technology not only helps to assess student learning but also in evaluating teacher performance. In general, teacher evaluation refers to the formal process an educational institution uses to review and rate teachers' performance and effectiveness in the classroom. Educational technology provides tools for teacher evaluation and guide teachers in professional development by using feedback from evaluation.

## Offering Affordable Good Quality Programs

Educational technology offers affordable good quality educational programs. Best example is MOOCs. MOOCs (massive open online courses) is a course of study made available through internet with or without a reasonable fee to a very large number of people.

## IMPACT OF TECHNOLOGY IN TEACHING

According to Tony Bates impact of technology in modern education is evident from the following facts:

## Fully Online Education

Fully online learning is now becoming a major and central activity of most academic departments in universities and colleges. In India now online education is growing at a swift pace due to: (a) growth in internet and smart phone usage. The internet offers huge accessibility to join for distance education program for the young people, (b) cost of online education is low, (c) digital friendly government policies and (d) demand among working professionals and job seekers.

## Blended or Hybrid Learning

Blended learning is a combination of online learning and traditional classroom methods. Online learning is gradually blended with face-to-face teaching, but without changing the basic classroom teaching model. Here online learning is used as a supplement to traditional teaching.

## Flipped Classroom

A flipped classroom consists of students completing direct instruction, such as viewing a lecture online prior to the in-class discussion of the material. The intent is for students to familiarize with the learning content before hand, so they can learn the concepts at their own pace. By doing so students can participate better in classroom teaching. This help students to engage in active learning through debates and small group discussions.

## Open Educational Resources

Open educational resources are another recent development due to the advancement of technology. These are digital educational materials freely available in internet that can be downloaded by teachers or students without any charge. Open textbooks and internet video lectures recorded with lecture capture as well as supporting materials, such as slides are best examples of open educational resources. Open textbooks are digital textbooks that can be downloaded in a digital format by students for free of cost.

## MOOCs

MOOCs are the latest example of the rapid evolution of technology in education. In 2008, the University of Manitoba in Canada offered the first MOOC with an enrollment of 2000 students. Since then there has been a rapid growth of MOOCs around the world. Although the format of MOOCs can vary in general they have the following characteristics, such as: (a) open to anyone to enroll and simple enrollment, (b) very large number of enrollment, (c) free access to video-recorded lectures, often from the most elite universities, and (d) computer-based assessment, usually using multiple-choice questions and immediate feedback, combined sometimes with peer assessment.

## TECHNOLOGY AND MEDIA

Tony Bates explains the relationship between technology and media as follows in his open textbook, namely—'Teaching in the Digital Age'. Technology in education can be considered as things or tools used to support teaching and learning. Thus, computers, software programs, such as learning management system or a transmission or communication network are all technologies. Technology often includes a combination of tools with particular technical links that enable them to work as technology system, such as the telephone network or the internet.

The word 'medium' comes from the Latin, meaning in the middle and also that which intermediates or interprets. Media require an active act of creation of content and /or communication and someone who receives and understand the communication as well as the technology that carry the medium. Medium is useful only when there are two types of interventional takes place, such as (a) the creator who constructs information and communicate it and (b) the 'receiver' who interpret the meaning of communication.

In simple words by creating learning content, communicating learning content and enabling interpretation of meaning of the content we are turning a technology into medium. For example, internet in technical sense is a technology but when we add learning content in the form of audios, videos, graphics and words internet become a media for learning and teaching in education.

We use our senses to interpret media. In this sense, we can consider text, graphics, audio and video as media because they convey meaning through ideas and images. Computing can also be considered as a medium in this context. Computing as a medium would include animations, online social networking, using a search engine or designing and using simulators. Thus, in terms of representing knowledge Tony Bates suggests following media for educational purposes:

- **Text:** Textbooks, novels, poems
- **Graphics:** Diagrams, photographs, drawings, poster, graffiti.
- **Audio:** Sounds, speech.
- **Video:** Television program, YouTube clips, "talking heads".
- **Computing:** Animation, simulation, online discussion forum, virtual world.

## SELECTING APPROPRIATE MEDIA

The choice of single media or combination of media will need to be determined by the following factors:
- The overall teaching philosophy behind the teaching.

- The presentational and structural requirement of the subject matter or content.
- The knowledge that need to be transferred to learners.
- The attitude and skills need to be developed in learners.
- Possible role of different media as identified by teacher and learners.

## TRENDS IN EDUCATIONAL TECHNOLOGY

Trends in educational technology can be summarized as follows:
- **Artificial intelligence:** The role of artificial intelligence in the education sector is no longer limited to aspects, such as speech recognition, problem solving and planning. Rather AI facilitates automation of administrative tasks, such as students' grading, the addition of smart content in the curriculum and personalisation of learning content.
- **Virtual reality in education:** The high adoption of VR in education is partly due to the rise in demand for experiential learning. By taking the learning process beyond the classrooms, VR has facilitated the growing trend towards independent learning route.
- **Gamification:** Gamification is an education approach for motivating students to learn by using video game designing and game elements in learning process. The adoption of gamification is perhaps one of the biggest trends in educational technology that turns the learning process lot more fun by bringing video game designs into the learning process.
- **Learning analytics:** Learning analytics is the measurement, collection, analysis and reporting of data about learners and their context. The purpose of LA is understanding and optimizing learning and learning environment.
- **Immersive learning:** Immersive learning is the process of learning with the usage of simulated environment. The environment enables the learner to completely get immersed in the learning.
- **Smart learning environment:** SLES are one of the best ways in which the hybrid learning approach can be put into action. This IOT (internet of things) based learning solution encourages personalised education system leading to better engagement and skill enhancement.
- **Digital course materials:** Educational technology helps to create digital content that have a positive impact on education.
- **Mobile technology and IOT:** The abilities of IOT to track the staff and students along with connecting devices across the campus has helped to improve the safety standards of institutions. The improvements in mobile technology have further enabled the use of IOT as a major educational technology.

## AUDIOVISUAL AIDS

### Definition

- According to Kinder, "Audio-visual aids are any device which can be used to make the learning experience more concrete, more realistic and more dynamic."
- Mckown and Roberts believe that audiovisual aids are supplementary devices by which the teacher, through the utilization of more than one sensory channels is able to clarify, establish and correlate concepts, interpretations and appreciations.

From the above definitions, it is clear that audiovisual aids are the different types of tools that appeal to the sense of hearing and vision and are used in classrooms, especially for presenting abstract information.

### Educational Technology and Audiovisual Aids

Educational technology is a vast subject concerned with the application of scientific knowledge about learning and conditions of learning in order to improve the effectiveness of teaching, learning and evaluation, whereas audiovisuals are merely the aids or resources, i.e., materials which are employed to improve the quality of the message. Audiovisual aids are part of the subject of educational technology. KL Kumar differentiates educational technology from audiovisual aids as shown in **Table 9.1**.

**TABLE 9.1:** Educational technology and audiovisual aids.

| Audiovisual aids | Educational technology |
|---|---|
| Audiovisual aids are physical objects. | Educational technology is a vast subject. |
| Audiovisuals consist of print matter, projected and electronics resources, such as slides, video and computer | The subject of education technology encompasses learning psychology, communication and advances in science and technology |
| Audiovisuals are material products, which may be used or misused | Educational technology connotes processes and products of instructional design |
| Audiovisuals improve the quality of the message; they impart audio and visual dimensions to it | Educational technology aims at improving all aspects of communication, i.e., encoding, message, channel, barriers, decoding, retention and application |
| Audiovisual aids exist without regard to group dynamics and individual differences | Educational technology deals with the process of implementing methods and resources with regard to group dynamics and individual differences |
| Audiovisuals are products of technology alone. They are technical gadgets | Educational technology is a great deal more than technology; it is based on psychology, social anthropology, etc. |
| Audiovisuals stand alone. These are unrelated articles | Educational technology is a system with a number of interconnected and interdependent components |
| Audiovisual aids are different for different topics and subjects. They fit in a curriculum | Educational technology principles are applicable to all topics and subjects and hence related to basic total curriculum development |

KL Kumar believes that visuals with/without aural components are called audiovisual resources, aids, media or simply audiovisual aids. Audiovisual resources consist of hardware and software components. For every hardware, there is a corresponding software as shown in **Table 9.2**.

**TABLE 9.2:** Educational hardware and corresponding software.

| Hardware | Software |
|---|---|
| Chalkboard | Chalkwork |
| Overhead projector | Overhead transparencies |
| Slide projector | Slides |
| VCR and monitor | Video program |
| Computer | Computer program, apps |
| Blank paper | Written matter |
| Audio-recorder | Recorded audio |
| Mobile phone | Apps |

## Learning Experience

A discussion on learning experience is needed for the judicious use of AV aids. The aim of using audiovisual aids is for providing effective learning experience. Research shows that learning experiences can be at three levels, namely, direct, vicarious and symbol (**Fig. 9.1**).
1. **Direct experience:** Direct experience is one that is obtained through the immediate sensory contact with real objects. It is the rich and purposeful experience gained by seeing, hearing, handling, fasting, touching and smelling.
2. **Vicarious experience:** Vicarious experiences are indirect ones. Whenever direct experience is either impossible or undesirable due to hazards we represent the real situation in the form of models or images. This may become necessary when real object is too small like an atom or too large like the solar system, too fast like the electromagnetic waves, too slow like this growth of a plant or too danger like harmful rays. Experience gained by observing models, pictures, charts films, etc., are said to be vicarious in nature.
3. **Symbolic experience:** Symbolic experience are offered through verbal symbols oral or written. Here the experience occurs at the conceptual level. The teacher codes the original item into symbols and passes it on to the student. To have the experience the students decode the symbols back into the original image.

From the discussion, it is clear that the symbolic experience is the least effective from the point of learning.

## Edgar Dale's Cone of Experience

Edgar Dale has classified and arranged audiovisual experiences in the form of a pinnacle which he called cone of experience (**Fig. 9.2**). The cone of experience is a visual aid that explains the interrelationship of the various types of experiences provided by the different audiovisual aids as well as learning hierarchical placement in the learning process. The ones considered by Dale as the most effective are placed at the bottom of the cone and those considered least effective at the top. As per the **Figure 9.2**, the first experience is most effective and is placed at the base of the cone.

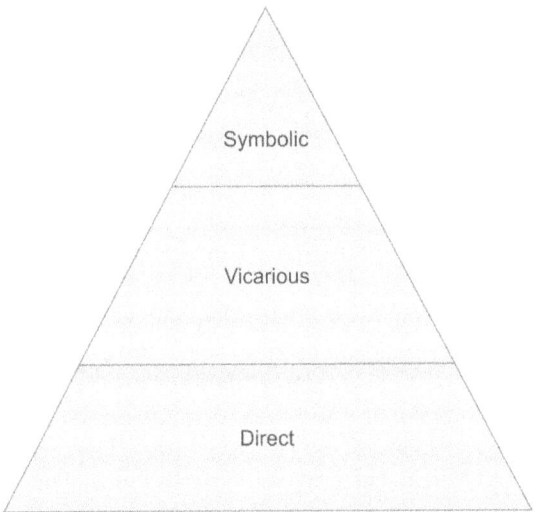

**Fig. 9.1:** Learning experience.

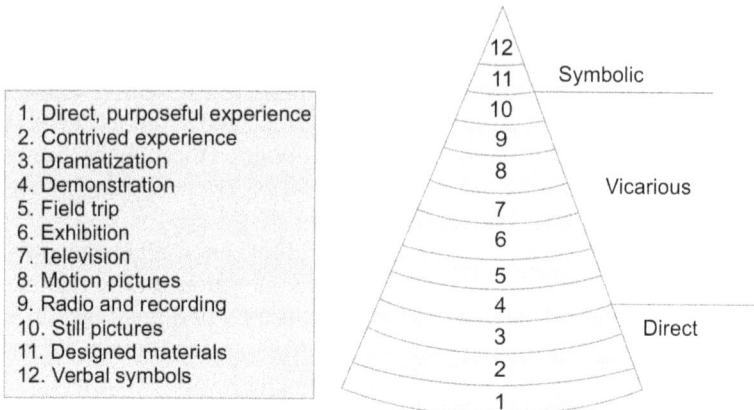

**Fig. 9.2:** Edgar Dale's cone of experience.
*Source:* Dale E. Audiovisual methods in teaching. New York: Dryden; 1969.

## Classification of Audiovisual Aids

The audio component may be added to any one of the resources. It may either be with recorded voice on cassettes, tapes and discs, or it may be live oral messages by the presenter.

Audiovisual aids can be classified in different ways like: (a) simple and sophisticated aids **(Table 9.3)**, (b) audio materials, visual materials and audiovisual materials **(Table 9.4)**, (c) projected aids, nonprojected aids and activity aids.

## Purposes of Audiovisual Aids

Purposes of audiovisual aids are: (a) to provide a basis for more effective perceptual and conceptual learning, (b) to initiate and sustain attention, concentration and personal involvement of the students in learning, (c) to provide concreteness, realism and life likeness in the teaching-learning situation, (d) to bring the remote events of either space or time into the classroom, (e) to increase the meaningfulness of abstract concepts, (f) to gain practical skill, and (g) to introduce opportunity for situational or field types of learning as contrasted with linear-order verbal and written communication.

## Principles in the Use of Audiovisual Aids

### Principle of Selection

Teaching aids prove effective only when they suit the teaching objectives and unique characteristics of the special group of learners. The aids must be adapted to the intellectual maturity of the pupils and to the nature and extent of their previous experience. There is no best aid which has all the advantages, so the teacher should be familiar with the advantages and disadvantages of the different aids in order to select the appropriate one. In all cases, the time and effort on the use of a particular aid in preference to others must be justified. Teaching aids should have specific educational value besides being interesting and motivating. Above all, they should be the true representatives of the real things. For example, a chart showing the picture of gas exchange between alveoli and capillaries is the vital one among visual aids used for teaching respiration and without this particular chart the purposes of visual aids cannot be achieved fully while teaching respiration.

## Chapter 9: Introduction to Educational Technology

**TABLE 9.3:** Classification number 1: Simple aids and sophisticated aids (audiovisual aids)

| Simple (S) | Sophisticate (SO) |
|---|---|
| Chalkboard/blackboard | Slides-slide projector |
| Whiteboard/glass board | Sound films-8 mm/16 mm film projectors |
| Wallboard | Video films (cassettes) |
| Bulletin board | Television |
| Charts | Film strips |
| Posters | Film strip projector |
| Drawings | Overhead transparencies/overhead projector |
| Graphs | Audio cassettes/tape recorder |
| Album | Radio |
| Pamphlets | Computer |
| Booklets | LCD |
| Leaflets | |
| Handouts | |
| Flip charts | |
| Flash cards | |
| Flannel graphs | |
| Puppets | |
| Objects | |
| Models | |
| Specimens | |
| Exhibits | |

### *Audiovisual Aids are Means to an End, not the End in Themselves*

Teaching aids should not be considered as substitutes for oral and written methods of acquiring knowledge, instead, they should be used to supplement the classroom teaching.

### *Principle of Preparation*

This principle deals with the cost-effective ways of preparing aids. In addition to purchasing commercially available teaching aids, whenever possible teacher should try to prepare teaching aids by using locally available materials with the help of students.

### *Principle of Proper Presentation*

This principle suggests the following points for the effective use of an aid: (a) the instructional program should be so organized and administered that the audiovisual aid material must function as an integral part of the teaching activity, i.e., teacher has to plan well in advance, (b) visual instruction in the classroom should not be confused with entertainment, (c) teacher should check the adequacy or working condition of an aid before using it so that she can conduct teaching properly, (d) teacher should be confident in handling the aid, (e) adequate care should be taken while handling the aid in order to prevent any damage, (f) the aid should be displayed properly so that all the students are able to see it, observe it and derive maximum benefit out of it, (g) as far as possible, distraction of all kinds should be avoided so that full attention may be paid to the aid.

## TABLE 9.4: Classification number 2: Audio materials, visual materials and audiovisual materials.

| Audio materials | Visual materials | Audiovisual materials |
|---|---|---|
| Language laboratories | Bulletin boards | Demonstrations |
| Radio | Chalkboards | Films |
| Sound distribution system sets | Charts | Printed materials with recorded sound |
| Tape recordings | Drawings | Sound filmstrips |
| | Exhibits | Study trips |
| | Filmstrips | Television |
| | Flash cards | Video-tapes |
| | Flannel boards | Computers |
| | Flip books | LCD |
| | Illustrated books | |
| | Magnetic boards | |
| | Maps | |
| | Models | |
| | Pictures | |
| | Posters | |
| | Photographs | |
| | Silent films | |
| | Slides | |

### Principle of Physical Control

This principle is related to the arrangement of keeping aids safely and also to facilitate their lending to the teachers for use.

### Principle of Response

This principle demands that the teachers have to guide the students to respond actively to the audiovisual stimuli so that they can achieve learning objectives in a better way.

### Principle of Evaluation

This principle stipulates that there should be continuous evaluation of both the audiovisual aids and accompanying techniques in the light of the realization of the desired objectives.

## Aspects of the Use of Audiovisual Aids

The teacher who is contemplating the use of audiovisual aid should have in mind certain questions. They are: (a) does the attainment of my lesson objectives really require the employment of any audiovisual aid?, (b) what is the precise matter to be learned and how may the probability of learning may be heightened by the use of audiovisual aid?, (c) what are the specific properties of the audiovisual aids which will enable me to utilize them so as to attain the required lesson objectives?, (d) what particular responses do I require from the use of audiovisual aid—for example, comprehending, remembering?, (e) what prerequisite knowledge is required from the class if they are to benefit from the audiovisual aid?, (f) how is the class likely to respond to the audiovisual aid? and (g) how shall I evaluate the effectiveness of the audiovisual aid?

## Advantages of Audiovisual Aids

Advantages of the audiovisual aids can be stated as follows:

- By using audiovisual materials, inaccessible processes, materials, events, objects, changes in time, speed and space could easily be brought to the class. Teachers often face difficulties in making information available to students in certain cases. Students in a large classroom may not be able to see the demonstrations, small models, objects and small pictures shown by the teacher. Further, the teacher may not be able to show the microscopic things to the whole class. Audiovisual aids can help the imaginative teacher to solve all these communication problems.
- Use of audiovisual aids results in greater acquisition of knowledge and ensures longer retention of the information gained. Audiovisual materials provide first hand experiences in a variety of ways and motivate the pupils to participate actively. Hence, they not only help to develop meaningful vocabulary but also enable the pupils remember facts for a pretty long time. Audiovisual technology provides pupils with meaningful sources of experiences.
- Use of audiovisual materials in the classroom can provide effective substitutes for direct contact of students with environment, both physical and social. Audiovisual materials enable us to cut through the physical limits of time and space. A teacher may 'take' his students by means of an appropriate motion picture to any distant place and 'to meet' the people who live there and to observe places and things. Such media may serve as a 'magic carpet' for providing needed experiences. Motion pictures, television, and carefully prepared slide sequences would be particularly valuable.
- By using suitable audiovisual materials, any expected change in behavior and attitude could be facilitated. Audiovisual materials generally add an interest and involvement to the lesson. Students learn more, if they are engaged in significant and appealing activities. Active participation maintains interest and increases learning whether they are participating in individual or group activities. The entire gamut of audiovisual technology offers much scope for making models and exhibits, writing and producing plays, and making charts, diagrams, maps, posters, etc.
- Proper audiovisual materials can provide integrated experiences varying from abstract to concrete. Audiovisual materials supply a concrete basis for conceptual thinking and conceptual thinking is essential for developing meaningful concepts. Audiovisual technology presents abstract information to the learners in various forms. On many occasions, teacher can prepare the students for experiences which are normally beyond their comprehension with the help of audiovisual aids. Teachers in this complex age should be able to guide students to the vast reservoir of knowledge by making use of additional resources, such as television, films, diagrams, charts, etc. All these resources enhance clarity of communication and increase the speed of comprehension.
- While using audiovisual aids, the approach is through more than one sense, i.e., multisensory approach; hence, they will be able to secure and retain the attention of pupils as well as to develop the communication skills of pupils.
- Audiovisual materials could be used to motivate and stimulate interest of pupils to gain further knowledge. Interest is not an end in itself. Interest that has been created by means of an audiovisual aid must act as a spring board for launching the students into a wide variety of learning activities. Audiovisual media can develop an awareness about problems, open

up possibilities for exploration, present meaningful preliminary information and thereby open avenues to new activity.
- ❖ Audiovisual materials could be used for any age or ability groups. In a conventional teaching method, the teacher is the center of attention and the primary source of information. Audiovisual media may be used as supplements to illustrate, to clarify and to focus attention. When properly programmed, media alone can teach. For example, the computer assisted instruction can provide individualized instruction. The particular student using the program receives immediate confirmation or correction of responses made by him. In brief, proper use of audiovisual aids helps to multiply teacher efficiency and helps in remedial teaching too. When the audiovisual aids are used, it is necessary to make sure that the entire class pupils are able to perceive any specific aspect pointed by the teacher at the same instant.
- ❖ **Saving of energy and time:** A good deal of energy and time of both the teachers and students can be saved on account of the use of audiovisual aids as most of the concepts and phenomena may be easily clarified, understood and assimilated through their use.
- ❖ **Meeting individual differences:** Different types of instruction and guidance may be needed for individual students. Some are ear oriented, some can be helped through visual demonstrations, while others learn better by doing. The use of a variety of audiovisual aids helps in meeting the needs of different types of students.
- ❖ **Development of higher abilities**: Use of audiovisual aids stirs the imagination, thinking process and reasoning power of the students. They also promote creativity, inventiveness and other higher mental activities on the part of students. Thus, helps the development of higher abilities of students.
- ❖ **Provides positive environment for creative discipline**: A balanced, rational and scientific use of audiovisual aids develops motivation, attracts the attention and interests of the students and provides a variety of creative outlets for the utilization of their tremendous energy and thus keeps them busy in the classroom work. In this way, the overall classroom environment becomes conducive to creative discipline.

## Characteristics of Good Audiovisual Aids

JG Aggarwal outlines the following qualities for good audiovisual aids: (a) the aid must be adapted to the intellectual maturity of the pupils and to the nature and extent of their previous experience, (b) they should be meaningful and purposeful, (c) as far as possible, they should be improvised, i.e. locally available materials should be used in the preparation of audiovisual aids by the teacher, (d) they should be simple, (e) they should be cost-effective as well as cheap, (f) they should be large enough to be properly seen by the whole students in the class, (g) they should be up to date, (h) they should be easily portable. Above all, they should supplement the instruction properly and motivate the learners.

## Description of Different Audiovisual Aids

### Chalkboard

Chalkboards and the newer white felt-tip pen boards are universally used in education and may never be replaced. It is the oldest and the best friend of the teacher. It is a mirror through which students visualize all about the teacher's mind, his way of explaining, illustrating and teaching as a whole. It is the cheapest and the most valuable teaching device. The modern chalkboard is not black but made in different colors mostly in pleasing green. Whiteboards are becoming more common because colorful figures stand out much better on them than on chalkboards. Whiteboards may also be used as screen for overhead projection and slide projection.

To be used properly, a chalkboard must be placed where the entire class can see it easily and where glare is minimal. The height of the chalkboard is fixed with reference to the height of the human beings. The lower edge of the board is placed at half the human height. A one meter height of the board is generally manageable by a human being extending his/her hands above and below the mid level of the board. A rectangular box is fixed at the bottom of the board to hold the chalk piece and duster. Concealed tube lights should be installed over the chalkboard for adequate lighting.

## Use of Chalkboard

The chalkboard is an excellent supplement to other aids. The lesson can be summarized in the right manner with the help of the board. The teacher can illustrate his lesson on the blackboard and draw attention of the class to salient features in the lesson. Facts, ideas and processes can often be illustrated with the help of drawing, sketches and other visual symbols. The outstanding feature of chalkboard is that it allows for spontaneity in the classroom. New ideas or solutions to problems can be jotted down as they are mentioned. If students are suddenly confused about something, the point can be illustrated on the board. When students cannot visualize an object, it can be quickly sketched. Chalkboards are especially useful for working out the mathematical problems, for outlining the materials to be taught in the class and for having several students placing their ideas on the board at the same time.

## Guidelines for the Effective Use of Chalkboard

- Plan the use of chalkboard and everything needed for using the chalkboard should be kept ready before the class begins, i.e., collection of chalk, duster, etc.
- It should be ensured that chalkboard is well lit by natural or artificial means.
- Clean the chalkboard completely before starting the class. A clean board reflects the clarity of teacher's mind and avoids distractions to students. Also ensure glare free visibility of the written word to all the students.
- Write on the board according to a pre-decided plan. You can divide the board into two or three parts by drawing vertical lines. Writing should be started from the top left corner. The right part is good for writing the headings so that a revision can be held towards the end. If there is a chequered part of the board, use it for drawing graphs. Decide to write less and mean more. Keywords written legibly may convey more than illegible verbalisms. Never use abbreviation which is not standard. Always use running handwriting with the keywords in capital letters. Do not over write on the letters. Writing should be in straight rows. Write only on the upper two-thirds of the board because students often have difficulty in seeing the bottom of the board.
- Diagrams and pictures can be sketched before class. Doing so not only saves time but also permits the teacher to draw a neater sketch than might be produced under pressure and eyes of the students. If the teacher wishes to draw the picture while the students are watching, she can at least put in some faint chalk lines before class to guide her during the actual drawing. Colored chalks helps make drawing more interesting and can be used to highlight important points. Teacher need not apologize for lack of drawing skills, students do not expect teachers to be artists and such apologies only draw attention to the teacher rather than the subject matter.
- Do not speak to the chalkboard. Keep turning back and forth; speak to the students while writing on the board.
- Do not crowd the chalkboard with too much matter. A few important points make a vivid impression. Stand clear of the written word. Do not hide what you write. Allow the students to see the board uninterrupted.

- Plan your rubbing off sequence. Rub off a section of the board and write there. Then rub the rest of it, duster and not hand or hand kerchief should be used for rubbing.
- Hold the chalk between thumb and fingers. Break off a little piece to avoid squeaking while writing. Use colored chalks in order to distinguish some parts and to highlight some components of the visuals on the board.
- Occasionally, students may be asked to write or draw diagrams on the chalkboard.
- It should be ensured that the blackboard is periodically serviced.

### *Merits of Chalkboard*
Chalkboard offers a number of merits over other audiovisual aids. Its affordability, versatility, usability and common availability are highly appreciated. Other merits are:
- It is simple to use with little practice.
- Electricity is not a must for using the blackboard.
- It is economic and reusable.
- It can be put to wide and varied uses.
- Sequential development of the content can be done effectively.
- Pupils interest in class work can be stimulated.
- Can be used indoor and outdoor.
- Provides a lot of space for decorative and creative work.
- Allows note taking.
- Teacher can make students to write on the board.
- Teacher can review the whole lesson for the benefit of students with the help of the chalkboard.
- Mistakes can be rubbed off and corrected instantly.
- Charts can be hung on the board.
- It allows for spontaneity in the classroom.

### *Demerits of Chalkboard*
Among the drawbacks of using the chalkboard are that it cannot be used with large groups and that the material usually cannot be saved until the next class. The fact that teacher's back is to the students while writing on the board is a disadvantage because teacher lose eye contact with the students and may interrupts communication. Advanced preparation of the material is not possible and cannot illustrate moving parts. Finally, this method is poor for the teacher who has poor hand writing, since the information may be lost because students cannot read what is written.

## *Overhead Projector*

Overhead projector (OHP) is a device for projecting a matter, which is written or drawn on transparent sheet of acetate on to a screen. It is the cheapest projecting aid currently available.

### *Preparation of OHP Transparencies*
- Use a standard size of acetate sheet measuring 18 cm × 22.5 cm.
- OHP markers are available in two types—temporary and permanent. Temporary markers have soluble ink and written matters can be wiped off with the help of a damp cloth. Permanent markers are oil, spirit or wax based and their writing is preserved for long time. One may prepare reusable transparencies with permanent OHP markers. Additions and alterations during teaching should be made with water soluble OHP markers so that the same are wiped off after use. If you want to reuse the transparency sheet later for another purpose, be sure to use a marker with soluble ink.

- Transparencies must be clearly written with at least 8 mm size letters either free hand or by transfer letters or templets, etc. A transparency which can be clearly read from a distance of 2 m should project well for a classroom 6 m deep. Transparencies should be patiently prepared with bright harmonizing or contrasting colors, legibly and systematically. There should be no more than six words in each line and no more than eight lines in each transparency. Put margins appropriately. Of the various types of visuals, diagrams, schematics, cue words, cartoons and graphs make better visuals for the OHP.
- The best colors to use to write on transparencies are black, blue and green. Use red sparingly. It is not a color that project well.
- Whether you are drawing the image on the transparency or copying it from a printed page, keep the amount of information on the sheet to a minimum and make the image large enough so that students in the back of the room will be able to see it.
- Avoid copying information from a printed book or journal page or a type written sheet. Such pages present too much information for the students to take in and the print is usually too small for them to see easily. If you want to type some information on to a transparency, type it on paper first, enlarge the type on a copier with an enlarging function and then make a transparency by taking photocopy of the material.
- Transparencies can be very creative, especially, if you have artistic help. If you have produced a transparency worth saving for future classes you may want to mount it in a cardboard frame that gives it some protection, enables you to handle it without touching the acetates and reduces glare around the image.

### *Effective Use of Transparencies*
- The overhead projector and the screen should be positioned in such a way that every student in the class can see every part of the projected image with ease.
- OHP should be on, with the transparency in position as and when required.
- The fan switch if provided should not be switched off until the light source cools down. The main plug and switch should not be turned off soon after using the projector. One should not transport an overhead projector while the lamp is still hot. A spare lamp may, however kept ready.
- Transparent color Perspex arrow heads or pointed objects, such as pencils placed on the transparency at the platform are recommended for pointing. Pointer should not roll down. Never hold pointer in hand to avoid silhouetting effect. It is better to laid the pointer flat on the transparency than waving around.
- Human silhouettes are irritating, so one should not interrupt the beam of light by movement and gesticulation.
- It is best not to project the entire transparency at the very beginning. Optimal progressive disclosure of information achieves the same objective as the sequential presentation of information on the blackboard. Progressive disclosure of information can be achieved by unmasking the information at a controlled rate. A paper or carboard may be used as a mask. This technique is called *revelation technique.*
- Never leave a visual on the screen after a point has been discussed. Turn off the projector by keeping the fan on when you are not actually projecting the transparency.
- Many radiographs can be projected successfully with the overhead projector. For this purpose, the classroom must be darkened. Dense photographs are not suitable for use with overhead projector.
- Transparencies can also be made with overlays-additional acetate sheets can be placed over the base transparency to add new features or colors. For example, the base sheet may show the gross anatomy of the heart chambers and a hinged overlay placed on the top of the base

sheet can show, with arrows the direction of blood flow. Another overlay may indicate areas where various heart sounds originate.

- ❖ By using silhouetting effect, opaque objects can be projected.
- ❖ While you are showing a transparency, be careful that you are not blocking the students' view. You may be in the direct visual path of students sitting near the projector, so once you have turned the projector on, move around occasionally or move back close to the screen. Leave the transparency on screen long enough for students to read and absorb all the information.
- ❖ Transparencies can be used similarly to a chalkboard for writing down spontaneous ideas, outlining class content or doing math problems.

### *Advantages of Overhead Projector*

Transparencies can be prepared before hand to save class time and to help organize and illustrate content. Diagrams and drawings can be drawn or copied on to transparencies. Concepts can be illustrated. Lectures can be outlined. Cartoons can be projected for interest and illustration. Teachers can face the students while using it, thus, eye contact with students can be maintained. The room does not have to be dark, although it is often helpful to dim the lights around the screen. The projector is easy to use, requiring only manipulation of an on-off switch and a focus knob. It is the cheapest of all projected audiovisuals. Photocopies of transparencies may be handed to the students if desired. Transparencies can be made in different colors and used in a variety of ways, such as revealing gradually, overlaying, etc. Transparencies may be reused by employing washable color markers or can be preserved for future use by employing permanent markers. Using transparencies is less pollutant and less strenuous than using a chalkboard. Transparencies may be referred to back and forth in the same or in different sessions.

### *Charts*

Charts are visual displays arranged on thick sheets, poster paper, newsprint or cardboard. Visual display could be a pictorial, graphic, numerical or written material. Charts may be arranged as single sheet charts or as a series of sheets. In either case, one chart is designed to convey one idea. A single sheet chart can be displayed or removed at will; shown single or together with other charts placed alongside it and other teaching aids. For example, two single-sheet charts can be shown in parallel to differentiate between two types of joints, two concepts or two interpretations of the same thing. Single sheet charts can be arranged in different combinations to suit different lesson plans. *Flip charts* are a series of charts arranged sequentially by holding them together at the top edge. The material is arranged in order of progress of the session. Some charts may be left blank with a view to writing while presentation in a set of flip charts. Some techniques, for example, revelation, masking and overlaying are usually employed with flip charts.

### *Purposes of Charts*

Charts serve the following purposes: (a) for presenting material symbolically, (b) for summarizing information, (c) for showing continuity in process, (d) for presenting abstract ideas in visual form, (e) for showing development of structure, (f) for stimulating critical thinking, (g) for encouraging Introduction to the utilization of other media of communication. (g) For motivating the students.

### *Types of Charts*

The following is a list of basic types of charts in terms of arrangements and the kinds of ideas which they may express:

- **The narrative chart,** an extended left to right arrangement of facts and ideas for expressing: (a) the events in a process, such as water purification, (b) the events in the development of a significant issue to its point of resolution or to present status. For example, development of consumer protection act and its impact on the present day health care system, (c) technological improvement over a period of years, such as innovations in cardiac monitoring.
- **The tabulation chart,** a left to right top to bottom arrangement of facts and ideas for expressing: (a) numerical data for making comparisons, (b) list of antenatal mothers, under fives or other specific groups in a selected area.
- **The cause and effect chart,** usually a limited left to right arrangement of facts and ideas for expressing: (a) relationship between lifestyle and predisposing factors of various diseases, (b) relationship between pathology and clinical features and the like.
- **The chain chart,** a circular or semicircular arrangement of facts and ideas for expressing: (a) transitions, such as transition from raw materials to finished products, (b) cycles, such as citric acid cycle.
- **The evolution chart,** a left to right arrangement of facts and ideas for expressing changes in specific items from beginning to date, perhaps with projections into the future. For example, origin of mental health nursing and its subsequent development and present trends.

## Preparation of Charts

Usual materials required to prepare charts are sheets of thick white or light colored paper, fiber tipped round-point and chisel-point color markers, graphic materials, scissors, drawing aids and adhesives. Before making a chart, one should plan the content in terms of the objectives and decide the layout. The layout should be 'balanced' and should use the space effectively. One should draft the plan on a small sheet of paper with the aspect ratio, i.e., as is required for the chart. Having done so, one may start directly on the chart fixed on a drawing table by looking at the draft. The following points may be observed while preparing a chart:

- The size of the chart, the size of the letters and the contrast of the display material should be such that it is readable by the farthest viewer, standard chart paper in sizes 90 × 60 cm and 70 × 55 cm is suitable for most purposes. The size of letters for the captions, labels and keywords written on a chart should be between 2 and 3 cm for a classroom of depth 6 m. The thickness of the lines should be between 2 and 3 mm. The display material should be contrasted with the background so that it stands out. Light-colored chart paper, e.g., yellow, light green and white are better suited for dark colored pens, e.g., black, blue, red and orange. Flat pictures and other material from books should be enlarged sufficiently before placing on charts.
- Simple hand-drawn charts with non-decorative lettering are more effective than elaborately drawn or machine-made charts.
- One chart should convey just one idea or one principle. Charts crowded with information are less effective.
- Charts can be arranged to create one or more of the following visual effects:
    - *Revelation:* The whole chart can be covered with three or more paper strips from top to bottom. During display, the strip may be removed one by one in the desired sequence. Alternatively, one may mask off some information when it is no more required. Such techniques catch the attention of the students and maintain their interest.
    - *Overlay effect:* A part of the chart may be overlaid by another chart or by a cellophane paper chart. The former is useful for filling in details and the latter for shading the desired area of a diagram or for labelling the components.

- *Flow effect:* Single charts can be displayed one by one and so arranged on the board as to make a pattern, a flow diagram on the sequence of steps. For this, the charts should be shown in quick succession.
- *Magical effects:* A teacher may prepare the outlines of a complicated diagram in advance by using monochromatic harmony. He can then trace the diagram quickly with bright colors during the class.

❖ Numerical data should be presented in the form of tables. Relationships between two or more variables are better demonstrated by drawing graphs.
❖ Classifications, organizations and processes are better represented by means of flow diagrams.
❖ Colors should be used meaningfully, i.e. to simulate real colors, to highlight some items, etc.

### *Effective Use of Charts*

Single sheet charts must be shown when necessary. It should not be displayed before it is needed for teaching. It has an impact on presentation if it is shown while explaining about its content. Flip charts are mounted on a wooden or metallic easel at a convenient height. The top edge should be provided with one or other device, e.g., ring clips, long wooden strips or flat clips in order to secure the charts on the easel and to enable flipping-over easily.

Single sheet charts can be displayed one by one and so on arranged on the board to make a pattern, a flow diagram or the sequence of steps. For this, the charts should be shown in quick succession.

Sometimes, a teacher may prepare the outlines of a complicated diagram in advance by using monochromatic harmony. He can then trace the diagram quickly with bright colors during the class. It is very effective to show some movement on a chart.

Sometimes, a part of the chart may be overlaid by another chart or by a cellophane paper chart. The former is useful for filling in details and the latter for shading the desired area of a diagram or for labeling the components. When a chart is to be used in the classroom, the teacher should make sure that there is a provision for hanging the chart at a vantage point. Teacher should use a pointer to point out specific facts in the chart. Charts should be carefully stored and preserved for use in future.

### *Handouts*

A handout is a well-planned document prepared by a teacher for his students in order to promote their participation in the teaching-learning process. Handouts are useful in supplying information unavailable in textbooks or by other media. Handouts also ensure that all students have access to the same information and can review that information whenever necessary. Well-structured handouts can be very valuable in terms of interest, motivation and records of information. Handouts can be classified as follows:

1. **Summary type:** To reinforce the keywords, key statements and principles.
2. **Completion type:** To enable students to complete the information during the progress of a lecture: Introduction to: (a) In blank spaces, (b) on unlabeled or semi drawn sketches and (c) in response to some questions.
3. **Notes type:** To enable the students to read through them, particularly in the absence of textbooks.
4. **Assignment type:** To assign work, home-task, library work or field jobs
5. **Laboratory sheets:** For a practical class to provide some motivational information, to suggest format of data sheets, tables of analysis, questions for discussion, etc.
6. **Work sheets:** To state a problem and to give some hints to enable the student to start off and to complete a design or an analysis.

7. **Question sheets:** To pose objective questions, generally multiple-choice type items, together with response sheets if considered appropriate.

## Preparation of Handouts

Handouts should never be repetitious of the material provided in the textbook or given in live lectures. To be used effectively, handouts should be carefully planned. Necessary information should be typed neatly and concisely. KL Kumar suggests the following points for the preparation of handouts: (a) decide on the type of the handout. The type and purpose can be different for different lectures in order to create variety, (b) record only those items which are directly relevant to the subject of the lesson and for the desired objectives, (c) recognize the key-words and catch-words and emphasize them in the handout by underlying them, (d) use simple and clear language. Make short sentences, (e) draw sketches and graphs labelled or unlabeled. Remember 'one sketch may be worth a thousand words', (f) draw graphs. Write point-wise, wherever possible, (g) give titles and subtitles suitably, (h) use visual symbol and easy to recognize nomenclature, (i) use colors appropriately, if possible. Alternatively ask the students to color the black and white handouts. (j) underline some words and place some key-equations and statements in boxes to emphasize them, (k) if possible, prepare enlarged transparencies to match the handouts. The teacher can project the transparencies to aid filling in the blanks, labeling the parts, etc. This is a very effective method.

## Giving out Handouts

Teacher should explain the purpose of the handout and how it should be used. Handouts may be given out to the learners at one of the following points of time: (a) much in advance of the presentation, (b) just before the start of the session, (c) during the progress of the session, as necessary, (d) just after the completion of the session.

Giving out handouts much in advance is only, such as textbooks. It is advantageous to do so if books are not available or if prior reading/working is necessary before attending the class. Handouts given out at the commencement of a lesson draw attention of the class to the objectives and the contents of the lesson. This is generally satisfactory.

Handouts provided at appropriate timings; either just before a discussion, sometimes just after a series of points have been raised or just after viewing a video and at more than one point of time, maintain high level of attention, motivation, and interaction.

Giving out handouts just after the completion of a lesson leaves a record for the lesson, which the student may or may not read depending upon the follow-up by the teacher. Handouts given out much too late for the requirements have no academic purpose. It is a mere formality and may well be avoided.

## Slides

Slides are small transparent visual aids which can be viewed with the help of a slide projector or slide viewer. Slides can be effective promoters of discussions, can help make abstractions concrete and can lend realism to an otherwise academic discussion.

Based on the method of preparation they can be classified into: (a) slides made by photographic process, (b) computer made slides, and (c) handmade slides. Based on the content they are classified into live slides and flat copy slides. Live slides give three dimensional image of specimens, organs, life events and environmental conditions. Flat copy slides are made by taking pictures of graphics, artwork and visuals drawn on sheets.

Slides are prepared in sets of ten, twenty or more for selected topics. If slides are using, at least five to six slides should be there for a presentation. Based on the objectives of instruction, content may include written words, sketches, cartoons, graphs, pictures of objects, etc. By combining different types of slides made by different techniques we can create a variety of projected visuals in a set of slides. As a rule, only one concept or one sketch or one graph is adequate for one slide. Descriptions accompanying the visuals should be legible, simple and correct without any spelling mistakes. Preferably use key words to convey the message. The size of the letter should not be less than 6 mm. Six to nine lines can be included in a slide.

It is often helpful to number the slides to keep them in order; the number itself can then be used as an indicator of how slides should be positioned in the tray. Take care to position the slides correctly in the tray, to avoid the surprise of upside-down or sideways shots or backward lettering. Before showing a set of slides to a class, teacher should carefully organize the slides to fit into the lecture or discussion. The easiest way to organize a large group of slides is to place them on a table top slide previewer. This will enable the teacher to see all the slides at once and select the order in which she wants to show them. Switch off lights while showing slides. Slides must be shown, one by one, at a slow rate taking care of the slow learners. A long pointer, i. e., a stick or a radioaerial or a light pointer should be used to point at appropriate places on the screen. After the slide show, teacher has to summarize the presentation or ask questions or request someone to summarize.

The advantages of slides are that they are compact, easy to carry, easy to store and can be preserved for a long period of time, less eye soring and increased visual impact. Speed of slide presentation can be controlled by the teacher so that each slide can be discussed for the desired length of time. A remote-control extension allows the teacher to walk around or stand in front of the class and still control the slides; it is also easy to back up the previous slides if a question arises pertaining to them. Slide projectors are light weight and easy to carry.

The disadvantages of slides are that they are expensive and can easily get dirty and smudged with finger prints. Projector bulbs do not last very long and are expensive to replace. Reduced room light is necessary to get a clear image on the screen, which makes it difficult for students to take notes. Also, the size of slide trays is not standardized, so a teacher's personal slide tray may not fit the projector used in a particular institution.

## *Models*

Models are concrete objects, some considerably larger than the real object, some small replicas of objects which are too large to be seen as a whole, mostly three dimensional or sectional to explain clearly the structure or functions of the original. In many cases, working scale models of the original are used where the specific action of the original is duplicated and could be explained easily. Models offer a kind of short cut or substitute for the real things. It is just a recognizable three-dimensional representation of a real object. Model will help if the real objects cannot be used Introduction to for teaching due to one or more of the following reasons, such as: (a) too small to be observable, (b) too large to be available, (c) too concealed to be observable, and (d) too fast to be perceived.

The very purpose of a model is to incorporate observability, to aid perception and to be easily available. A model is the best aid if it is desired to proceed 'from concrete to abstract' while teaching. Models simplify reality and as they are three dimensional, they evoke greater interest.

### *Teaching with Models*

A model may either be carried into a classroom or be kept in a laboratory depending upon its size and appropriateness. A model kept on view for a long time, often goes unnoticed and loses its educational value. It should, therefore, be stocked away until needed. While using it, the teacher may employ the inquiry method; question/answering technique, group discussion or a demonstration. The value of a model is enhanced if the students are permitted to handle it. It is well and good if teaching with the model is supplemented with the use of other audiovisual aids, such as chalkboard, OHP transparencies, etc. This will enhance the learning.

## Posters

Posters are graphic representation of a theme through a combination of graphic materials, such as pictures, cartoons, lettering and others. Posters are very effective in holding attention of learners and maintaining their interests in the teaching-learning process. Posters can be used for introducing a topic in a motivating manner. Posters are effective into reinforce desirable attitudes and values. They also provide opportunities for creative expression. A poster on account of its quality of reminding and making one aware of something, always become a constant source of inspiration. Hence, posters can be very effectively used in encouraging health practices, goods habits and moulding behavior.

## Flash Cards

Flash cards are small compact cards and contain some picture, photographs, sketch, diagram and reading material neatly and boldly drawn and written. The display of these cards can be at their own or on the flannel board is done for a very short period of time, just, such as a flash. Hence, it is called flash cards. Flash cards are arranged in the sequence for presenting subject matter, flash cards can be effectively used in teaching almost all themes and topics.

## Cartoons

The cartoon is a visual graphic aid in the form of pictorial representation of an object, person, organization, idea or situation which uses symbolism, humor, satire, etc., to convey a message or point of view as quickly as possible. Cartoon is a good attention capture device and a source of motivation to the learners. It helps in the desirable modification of behavior and development of character. A good cartoon clarifies many concepts in a very interesting and humorous manner. Cartoons provide an opportunity for expressing talents of students.

## LCD Projector

LCD (Liquid Crystal Display) Projector is the most advanced and sophisticated projecting aid. It is used to present a topic in the classroom or in front of a large audience. In the area of educational technology, we can replace all other projected and non-projected aids with a single LCD projector and a computer system. We can present a topic by using computer made slides, graphics, pictures, video clips, movies and special effects. The LCD projector has connection jacks to interface with the computer and other video equipment.

# COMPUTERS IN NURSING EDUCATION

Computers can teach at any level of learning, from knowledge and comprehension up through application, analysis and synthesis. They can be programmed to teach problem solving and decision making.

One of the biggest advantages of computers over most of other audiovisual technologies is that the student is an active participant in the learning process, able to manipulate information, take action in vicarious situations and use trail and error. In addition to their teaching role, computers can be used to monitor student progress, evaluate student responses and tailor student remedial work. The teacher can obtain a record of the kinds of responses that students make to questions in the computer program and can see the paths into which the students thinking is taking them. Errors in reasoning or calculations can be identified so that appropriate help can be given to the student.

The primary computer application for students in a nursing program is computer-assisted instruction or learning by means of computer programs. Computer-managed instruction is also important in education; in this mode, the computer is primarily used by the instructor to organize and keep records of student learning. Finally, learning to use the computer as a tool is an important general aspect of the student's education, as the knowledge will have many future applications. Graduates of nursing programs will be expected to learn how to use computers in providing patient care and they must obtain the necessary basic computer education in college so that they can apply their learning in the work place.

### Computer-assisted Instruction

Computer-assisted instruction, also known as CAI, occurs in several formats or modes. The simplest level is the "drill and practice" mode. In this format, students have already learned certain information, either through computer programs or other teaching methods and are now presented with repetition and application of the information. This mode particularly lends itself to teaching mathematical calculations. The students may have received a lecture/demonstration on solving math problems in pharmacology. They are then send to the computer, which presents problem after problem to be solved. The computer program tells the student whether the answers are correct and may go so far as to diagnose the problem if the answers are incorrect. Drill and practice can also be used in learning drug names and actions, in learning medical terminology or in any situation requiring memorization of facts and concepts. It is probably the mode in which the least amount of software has been written, because of the low level of learning that it represents.

The second mode in which educational computer software may be written is the "tutorial mode". The program "tutors" or "teaches" the student a body of knowledge by presenting information and asking questions, giving hints if the student gets stuck. Tutorials are most useful in teaching material at the rule and concept level. Tutorial software can free faculty members from teaching some of the routine basic material, which becomes tedious after lecturing on it the first few times and allows them to use their time more productively and creatively on higher-level learning. At the same time, students may find that tutorials on basic information are more interesting and fun than an instructor's lectures.

Any information taught by means of lecture could potentially be written as a computer tutorial program. That does not mean that all basic classroom lectures should be turned into computer instruction, but it is possible to do so.

The "simulation and problem-solving" mode is one of the most exciting forms of computer software. Simulations of real-world experiences provide students with all the details about a particular introduction to patient situation and then ask them to assess the patient, arrive at diagnoses, plan interventions and evaluate care. Simulations can demand decisions in emergency situations and can show the results of good or poor decisions.

The advantage of providing these learning experiences via computer is that all students can be exposed to the same learning situation, which is not the case in a clinical setting. Students can take risks and make mistakes with no danger to the patient. In a computer simulation, the student is functioning in a controlled world where unexpected variables and pressures characteristic of the clinical area do not occur. Of course, the disadvantage of computer simulations is that instructors find out only what students might do or are capable of doing in a situation, not how they would actually perform in reality.

Finally, computer programs can be written in the "examination" mode. Questions, with/without situations, can be written in multiple-choice, true/false or fill-in-the-blank format. Rationales can be given following the answers, if desired. There are also programs that teachers can use to construct tests used for grading purposes.

## Computer-managed Instruction

Teachers can use computers to manage, prepare and organize educational experiences and to conduct examinations. Any system of record keeping can be included in this category as well, such as calculating and recording grades, ordering class ranks and recording student profiles. Nursing faculty may use computers to schedule clinical postings, assignments and maintain record of students.

## Using Computers as a Tool

Today's students will probably at sometime in their nursing career use computers as part of a hospital information system. Nurses using such systems have to develop proficiency in computer language in order to enter physicians orders and to order lab tests, diets, and drugs. They will be required to send messages to other departments and other nursing units and they will have to learn how to chart medications and nursing care as well as formulate nursing care plans. Many hospitals have computer terminals at the nurses stations, where all these data are loaded in and accessed.

The best way to prepare students to use the computer as a professional tool is to teach it to them in a hospital that has a computerized information system. However, many clinical facilities where teaching is done do not yet have computers at the nurses stations. The next best approach is to introduce students to computers by means of CAI so that they become familiar with general computer commands, with menu-driven programs and with types of information that computers can handle.

## Advantages of Computer Instruction

The primary advantage of computers is that they allow the student to interact in the learning situation; he/she can respond to questions, manipulate variables or select appropriate items from a menu, all of which provide activity for the student and make learning more interesting, memorable and valuable.

Computers can also individualize learning to an extraordinary degree. Not only does the student usually work alone at the computer and have the freedom to use whichever programs are available at the preferred rate of speed, but he/she also can receive individual help by means of branching within the programs. In a well-written program, if a student is already familiar with a certain portion of the material, he or she can skip ahead or move into a more advanced side track. On the other hand, if a student is having difficulty, branching may permit him/her to review certain segments of the program or branch into a tutorial lesson. Individual learning needs can truly be met if a variety of high quality software is available. Computer-assisted instruction can also enhance a student's self-esteem in several ways. The student is in control of the computer, especially in relation to the pace of learning. Between the controlled pace and the step-by-step increments of learning, the student is quite likely to be successful, a phenomenon that is rare for some students.

The feedback from computer programs can also be rewarding. The computer can reply to the student's answers with statements, such as "good job Saju" or "Jinsu, you have really learned that well". Such instant positive feedback is not always given by teachers, but the computer never forgets to reward the student, if it is so programmed. Wrong answers trigger nonpunitive feedback. The computer screen may say, "sorry, that is incorrect, try again, Joe"or "you need a little more review of this material before proceeding". The immediate feedback, whether positive or negative is invaluable. The use of the student's name gives the impression of a human teacher providing the feedback.

The nonjudgmental nature and endless patience of the computer are also important advantages. If the student takes four tries to get the right answer, the computer will still never make him/her feel worthless or stupid. Students thus become less afraid of making mistakes and less embarrassed about taking more time to learn the material.

Records of students performances on simulations or practice tests can be kept on the computer. The teacher can keep track of the ease or difficulty with which students are moving through the programs and then provide individual counselling where needed or spend more instructional time on an area that is perplexing more students. Computer can also be available to students for more hours than the instructor. This flexibility of computer learning may make educational experience more available to students.

## Disadvantages of Computer Instruction

The initial and sometimes overwhelming disadvantage is cost. Unless a nursing institute can afford large capital outlays, the large scale purchase of computers may be impossible. Even if hardware is affordable, the costs of software can be prohibitive. Another problem with both hardware and software is lack of compatibility and transferability between companies. An institute with an investment in one company's hardware may find that it cannot use some desirable software from another company. The limited choice of high-quality software is a problem at present, but at the rate that nurses are becoming computer literate and collaborating with expert programmers, this should become less of a problem in the near future.

Computer use also has some disadvantages from a student's standpoint. Many institutes have a few computers but not enough for the number of students in the program. Therefore, students have to wait their turn to get a computer and the computers may not be available when the students have free time to use them.

The fact that computer assignments usually require-on-campus time can be a drawback. Textbook and programmed instruction can be taken home and studied, but many students do not have computers at home. The time it takes for a student to use an educational program may also be a drawback in some situations. An average student using a program as it was designed to be used may learn the material in less time than it would take to learn it in a traditional classroom. But sometimes, the time variable backfires. Students may stop to take notes on the computer tutorials and lack of typing skill may slow some students down on programs that require a lot of answers to be keyboarded.

## SUMMARY

Technology results in new designs and devices as also new ideas and process. Educational technology is the application of the scientific knowledge in a systematic way to improve the efficiency of the process of learning and instruction. It is considered as the technology of education more than technology in education.

Audiovisual aids are a part of the subject of educational technology. Audiovisual resources consist of hardware and software components. Knowledge regarding the hardware and corresponding software is essential for the optimum utilization of them. Audiovisual materials can be classified in different ways. They must suit to the teaching objectives as well as to the unique characteristics of the learner, such as intellectual maturity, extent of previous experience, etc. Teaching aids should be used as a supplement to the classroom teaching and not as a substitute for teaching methods.

Teacher has to plan in advance so that she can incorporate audiovisual materials effectively in the teaching-learning process. This will help to convert a usually teacher-centered classroom into a more desirable student-centered one. There is no best audiovisual aid which has all the advantages, so the teacher has to be familiar with the advantages and disadvantages of different teaching aids. Moreover, awareness regarding advantages and disadvantages will help the teacher to minimize the disadvantages to the possible extent by employing proper techniques. Chalkboards, charts, models, overhead projectors, slide projectors, handouts and computers are some of the commonly used audiovisual aids.

## MULTIPLE CHOICE QUESTIONS

1. **Tools used for supporting teaching and learning is better known as:**
   a. Technology
   b. Media
   c. Devices
   d. None of the above

2. **Video is an example of:**
   a. Technology
   b. Media
   c. Devices
   d. None of the above

3. **Animation is an example of:**
   a. Computing
   b. Graphics
   c. Text
   d. Video

4. **Diagram is an example of:**
   a. Graphics
   b. Computing
   c. Text
   d. Video

5. **Cone of experience is developed by:**
   a. Edgar dale
   b. Tony Bakes
   c. Skinner
   d. KL Kumar

6. **Blackboard is an example of:**
   a. Simple aid
   b. Sophisticated aid
   c. Projected aid
   d. None of the above

7. **Exhibits is an example of:**
   a. Simple aid
   b. Audio aid
   c. Visual aid
   d. Audiovisual aid

8. "Revelation" is a technique related to the use:
   a. Chart
   b. Blackboard
   c. Slide
   d. Video
9. Computes is an example of:
   a. Sophisticated aid
   b. Simple aid
   c. Visual aid
   d. None of the above
10. Educational technology (I) is otherwise known as:
    a. Hardware approach
    b. Software approach
    c. Systems approach
    d. None of the above

## ANSWER KEY

| 1. a | 2. b | 3. a | 4. a | 5. a | 6. a |
|------|------|------|------|------|------|
| 7. c | 8. a | 9. a | 10. a | | |

# CHAPTER 10

# Evaluation

## LEARNING OBJECTIVES

After completing this chapter, reader will be able to:

- Define evaluation.
- Differentiate between evaluation and measurement.
- Explain the principles of evaluation.
- Describe the characteristics of evaluation.
- Explain objective-based evaluation.
- Describe the functions of evaluation.
- Enumerate the purposes of evaluation.
- Describe the types of evaluation.
- Explain the techniques of evaluation.
- Explain the tools of evaluation.
- Describe the qualities of a good evaluation tool.
- Construct achievement test.
- Recognize the importance of internal assessment.
- Explain clinical evaluation methods.

Education is considered to be a planned developmental endeavor meant for effective strengthening of the human resource. Since education has adopted the technological outlook in its planning and actions, the scope of educational evaluation has become so broad that it embraces each specific aspect of education as well as the system in its totality. It is much more than conducting few tests and examinations. Let us have a look into the trends and practices in evaluation with special reference to classroom evaluation.

## MEANING AND DEFINITION

The term evaluation is derived from the word *'valoir,'* which means 'to be worth'. Thus, evaluation is the process of judging the value or worth of an individual's achievements or characteristics. In broad sense, educational evaluation is concerned with judging the value or worth of the goals attained by the education system.

Ralph Tyler defines evaluation as "the process of determining to what extent the educational objectives are being realized." This definition highlights the relationship between educational objectives and evaluation.

Encyclopedia of educational research explains the concept of evaluation as, "evaluation in education signifies describing something, in terms of selected attributes and judging the degree of acceptability or suitability of that which has been described. The 'something' that is to be described and judged may be any aspect of the educational scene, but it is typically: (a) a total school program, (b) a curricular procedure, (c) an individual or a group of individuals. The process of evaluation involves three distinct aspects: (1) selecting the attributes that are important for judging the worth of the specimen to be evaluated, (2) developing and applying procedures that will describe these attributes truly, and (3) synthesizing the evidence yielded by these procedures into a final judgment of worth."

According to Howard, "Evaluation refers to a periodic process of gathering data and then analyzing it for determining the effectiveness of teaching or educational program and the extent to which it is achieving its stated objectives".

## COMPONENTS OF EVALUATION

According to Howard, evaluation is comparing a student's achievement with other students or with a set of standards. The emphasis of evaluation is based upon broad behavioral modification of learner and the major objectives of the educational program. In Kislik's opinions evaluation is a process that includes five basic components.
1. Articulating the purpose of the educational system.
2. Identifying and collecting relevant information.
3. Having ideas that are valuable and useful to learners in their lives and careers.
4. Analyzing and interpreting information for learners.
5. Classroom management or classroom decision making.

## ASSESSMENT

### Definition

According to Brown, "assessment refers to a related series of measures used to determine a complex attribute of an individual or group of individuals". This involves gathering and interpreting information about students' level of attainment of learning goals. Assessments are also used to identify individual students' weaknesses and strengths so that educators can provide specialized academic support.

### Components of Assessment

Assessment is a process that includes four basic components.
1. Measuring improvement over time.
2. Motivating student to study.
3. Assessing the effectiveness of teaching methods.
4. Assessing the effectiveness of students support and guidance program (SSGP).

## EVALUATION, MEASUREMENT, ASSESSMENT, AND TESTING

The dictionary of education explains the concept of evaluation and assessment as, "evaluation is often used interchangeably with assessment. This is because there is a considerable overlap in their meanings. Both involve measurements designed to describe the amount of certain attributes. Both involve procedures for obtaining these measurements which can involve tests as well as less objective instruments, such as rating scales. There is a tendency, however, for evaluation to be used in a more general way, involving a wide range of measures with a great acceptance of subjective judgments. There is also a tendency for evaluation to be used more when the subject of evaluation is not a person (or group of persons) but is the success of a course of teaching or method of teaching. Assessment is, therefore, used more usually in situations where the procedures involve more objective instruments and when these instruments are measuring personal attributes." In other words, we can say that the term assessment is used when a numerical value is not involving, e.g., checklists of behaviors.

NE Grounlund defines the terms test, measurement and evaluation in the following manner:

- *Test:* An instrument or systematic procedure for measuring a sample of behavior (Answers the question, "How well does the individual perform either in comparison with others or in comparison with a domain of performance tasks"?).
- *Measurement:* "The process of obtaining numerical description of the degree to which an individual possesses a particular characteristic (answer the question, "How much").
- *Evaluation:* "From the stand point of classroom evaluation, it is the systematic process of collecting, analyzing and interpreting information to determine the extent to which pupils are achieving instructional objectives (answers the question, "How good"?)

Aggarwal differentiates measurement and evaluation in the following manner

Evaluation is integrated with the entire task of education and not only with examinations, tests and measurement. It encompasses tests and measurement but also goes beyond them. Evaluation depends upon measurement but is not synonymous with it. Measurement is a quantitative determination of how much an individual's performance has been, while evaluation is a qualitative judgment of how good or how satisfactory an individual's performance has been.

Measurement describes a situation; evaluation judges its worth or value. Measurement is only a tool to be used in evaluation. By itself, it is meaningless, but without it evaluation is likely to be of little significance.

Sound evaluation is based upon the results of accurate and relevant measurement. It is also to be remembered that not all uses of a test or measurement in education can be considered as evaluation. Evaluation is always carried out in the light of some particular goal, purpose or value.

Evaluation is not only quantitative but also qualitative and includes value judgment about students' achievements and abilities. The difference between evaluation and measurement may be explained with the help of the following examples:

1. A teacher measures Sajan's height to be 170 cm. He evaluates his height when he says that he is 'tall'.
2. A teacher measures Anil's achievement in anatomy is 60%. He evaluates his achievement when he says that Anil's achievement in Anatomy is 'satisfactory'.
3. Measurement helps in evaluation. For example, Anil and Sajan are studying in the same class. In the first test, they scored 50 and 70 marks respectively in microbiology. In the second test, both of them obtained 80 marks. Now, in the second measurement (test scores), achievement in microbiology is the same, yet the evaluation will differ, when the teacher states that the rate of progress of Anil is better than that of Sajan.

## DIFFERENCE BETWEEN ASSESSMENT AND EVALUATION

Howard identifies following difference between assessment and evaluation.

1. The process of collecting, reviewing and using data for the purpose of improvement in the current performance is called assessment. A process of passing judgment, on the basis of defined criteria and evidence is called evaluation.
2. Assessment is diagnostic in nature as it tends to identify areas of improvement. On the other hand, evaluation is judgmental, because it aims at providing an overall grade.
3. The assessment provides feedback on performance and ways to improve performance in future. As against this, evaluation ascertains whether the standard or criteria are met or not.
4. The purpose of assessment is to improve quality whereas purpose of evaluation is to judging quality.
5. Assessment is concerned with process, while evaluation focuses on product.

6. In an assessment, the feedback is based on observation and positive and negative points. In evaluation feedback relies on the level of quality as per predetermined standards.
7. The criteria for assessment is well known to both students and teachers. In evaluation the criteria are mainly set by evaluator.

## GENERAL PRINCIPLES OF EVALUATION

The following principles proposed by Groundlund will form a general framework within which the ongoing process of evaluation may be viewed.

- **Determining and clarifying what is to be evaluated always has priority in the evaluation process:** No evaluation device should be selected or developed until the purposes of evaluation have been carefully defined. In evaluating pupil progress, this means that the first step is to identify and clearly specify the learning outcomes to be measured.
- **Evaluation techniques should be selected according to the purposes to be served:** When the particular aspect of pupil performance to be evaluated has been precisely defined, the evaluation technique that is most appropriate for evaluating that performance should be selected. All too frequently, evaluation techniques are chosen on the basis of how accurately they measure? how objective the results are? or how convenient they are to use? All of these criteria are important but secondary to the main criterion—whether this evaluation technique is the most effective method for determining what we want to know about the pupil? Each evaluation technique is appropriate for some purposes and inappropriate for others. The appropriateness of the technique for the intended purpose should be the first consideration in its selection.
- **Comprehensive evaluation requires a variety of evaluation techniques:** No single evaluation technique is adequate for appraising pupil progress toward all of the important outcomes of instruction. In fact, most evaluation techniques are rather limited in scope. To obtain a complete picture of pupil achievement, we typically need to combine the results from a variety of techniques.
- **Proper use of evaluation techniques requires an awareness of both their limitations and strengths:** Evaluation techniques vary from fairly well developed measuring instruments to rather crude observational methods. Even our best educational measuring instruments, however, fall far short of the precision we would like them to have, as all are subject to one or more types of error.

  First, there is sampling error. Because we can measure only a small sample of an individual's response at one time, there is always the question of the sample's adequacy. Is this test of anatomy a representative sample of what the pupils should know about anatomy? Are these observations of the pupils' social behavior typical of their general social adjustment? Such questions make clear the problem of obtaining an adequate sample and the possibility of sampling errors.

  A second source of error is found in evaluation instrument itself or in the process of using the instrument. A major source of error arises from improper interpretation of evaluation results. A healthy awareness of the limitations of evaluation instruments makes it possible to use them most effectively. Many of the errors that commonly occur in the evaluation process can be eliminated by carefully constructing and selecting evaluation techniques. Others can be controlled by developing skill in their use. The remainder can be dealt with when interpreting the results.
- **Evaluation is a means to an end, not an end in itself:** The use of evaluation techniques implies that some useful purpose will be served and that the user is clearly aware of it. Most of the misuses of tests and other evaluation techniques can be avoided by viewing

evaluation as a process of obtaining information on which to base educational decisions. This implies that the types of decisions to be made will be identified before the evaluation procedures are selected so that the evaluation procedures will be selected according to the decisions to be made and that no evaluation procedure will be used unless it improves instructional, guidance or administrative decisions.

Kellaghan proposes following principles for effective evaluation.

- *Effective evaluation is a continuous, ongoing process*: Much more than determining the outcome of learning, it is a way of assisting learning. Learning and evaluation are never completed. They are always evolving and developing.
- *A variety of evaluative tools is necessary to provide the most accurate assessment of students learning and progress*. Using only one type of tool results in poor evaluation.
- *Evaluation must be a collaborative activity between teachers and students*: Students must be able to assume an active role in evaluation so they can develop individual responsibilities for learning and self-monitoring.
- *Evaluation needs to be authentic*: It must be based on natural activities and processes students do both in the classroom and in their everyday lives.

## CHARACTERISTICS OF EVALUATION

From an analysis of the above said principles, we can make out the following characteristics of evaluation:

- **Evaluation is a continuous process:** Evaluation is a continuous process, it forms an integral part of the total system of education and is intimately related to educational objectives. It exercises a great influence on the pupils' study habits and the teachers' method of instruction and helps not only measure educational achievement but also improve it.
- **Evaluation includes academic and nonacademic subjects:** Evaluation in its broader concept includes evaluation of academic and nonacademic aspects of education. In examination and measurement the emphasis is upon the academic subjects only, whereas evaluation covers all the changes that take place in the development of a balanced personality.
- **Evaluation is a procedure for improving the product:** According to Wiles, "evaluation is a process of making judgments that are to be used as a basis for planning. It consists of establishing goals, collecting devices concerning growth or lack of growth towards goals, making judgment about the evidence and revising procedure and goals in the light of the judgments. It is a procedure for improving the product, the process and even the goals themselves."
- **Discovering the needs of an individual and designing learning experiences:** Chester observes that the purpose of any program of evaluation is to discover the needs of individuals being evaluated and then to design learning experiences that will solve these needs. Evaluation is an important and delicate process not only from the standpoint of determining the needs and growth of programs and individuals but also from the standpoint of what it does to the individuals being evaluated.
- **Evaluation is purpose oriented:** Evaluation should be conceived primarily in terms of purposes which the process of evaluation is intended to serve.
- **Evaluation emphasizes the broad behavioral changes and objectives of an educational program:** Evaluation includes not only subject-matter achievements but also attitudes, interests and ideals, ways of thinking, work habits and personal and social adaptability. Evaluation always assumes that educational objectives have previously been identified and defined. Hence, teachers always need to formulate educational objectives during

the teaching–learning process. In other words, evaluation is the determination of the congruence between the objectives and performance.
* **Comprehensive evaluation requires a variety of evaluation techniques:** No single evaluation technique is adequate for appraising pupil progress toward all of the important outcomes of instruction. Evaluation involves use of a great variety of tests and other techniques.

## PURPOSES OF EVALUATION

Properly used, evaluation procedures can contribute to improved pupil learning by: (a) clarifying the intended learning outcomes, (b) providing short-term goals to work toward, (c) offering feedback concerning learning progress, and (d) providing information for overcoming learning difficulties and selecting future learning experiences. Although these purposes are probably best served by periodic evaluation during instruction, the final evaluation of intended outcomes should also contribute to these ends.

Information from carefully developed evaluation techniques can also be used to assess and improve instruction. Such information can aid in judging (a) the appropriateness and attainability of the instructional objectives, (b) the usefulness of the instructional materials, and (c) the effectiveness of the instructional methods. Thus, evaluation procedures can contribute to both improvements in teaching–learning process itself and pupil learning. Groundlund observes that the main purpose of evaluation is to improve learning and instruction, whereas uses in curriculum development, reporting pupil progress to parents, guidance and counseling, school administration and research are secondary or supplementary.

## PURPOSES IN NURSING EDUCATION

Heidgerken lists down the following functions of evaluation in nursing education: (a) to determine the level of knowledge and understanding of students, (b) to determine the level of student's clinical performance, (c) to become aware of the specific difficulties of individual students or of an entire class, as a basis for further teaching, (d) To diagnose each student's strengths and weaknesses and to suggest remedial measures which may be needed, (e) to encourage students' learning by measuring their achievements and informing them of their success, (f) to help students acquire that attitude of and skills in self-evaluation, (g) to help students become increasingly self-directing in their study, (h) to provide the additional motivation of examinations that provide opportunity to practice critical thinking, the application of principles, the making of judgments, etc., (i) to estimate the effectiveness of teaching and learning techniques, of subject content and of instructional media in attaining the goals of the program, (j) to gather information needed for administrative purposes.

## OBJECTIVE-BASED EVALUATION

Objective-based evaluation is a widely accepted concept among teachers. It depicts the relationship between instructional objectives, instruction or learning experiences and evaluation as shown in **Figure 10.1**.

## FUNCTIONS OF EVALUATION

According to K Soman, functions of evaluation can be divided into two major categories:
1. Functions associated with the instructional process (which involves both learning and teaching).
2. Functions associated with the education system as a whole.

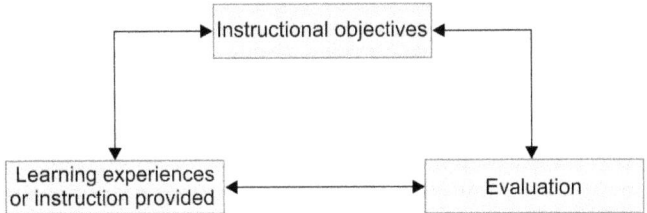

**Fig. 10.1:** Interrelationship of objectives, instruction, and evaluation.

## Functions Related to Instructional Process

- **Measurement function:** As said earlier, accurate and reliable measures of a variety of attributes associated with the physical and psychological development of the learner act as the basis for evaluation. Of these, for the ordinary classroom teacher, measuring the attainment of instructional objectives is of primary concern and importance.
- **Diagnostic function:** The results obtained through evaluation helps in determining the causes of persistent learning difficulties related to intellectual, physical, emotional and environmental reasons. The main aim of diagnostic evaluation is to determine the causes of learning problems and to formulate a plan for remedial action.
- **Guidance and remediation:** This function of educational evaluation is a natural extension of the diagnostic function. Once the causes of learning difficulties are diagnosed, the teacher can help the student by adopting appropriate remedial measures.
- **Motivating function:** The knowledge that one is going to be evaluated itself creates a feeling of mild anxiety. This will in turn act as a motivating force that promotes systematic learning. It is harmful only when the anxiety grows to undesirable levels. In the case of achievers, the thrill of success and the resulting self-esteem further contributes to systematic learning.
- **Assessment of the final output:** The functions of evaluation discussed till now have been those aiming at leading the learner towards this ultimate goal. Hence evaluation will ultimately have to assess the final performance of the learner also, the value judgment being made in terms of the quantity and quality of the total attainment with respect to a specific curricular area–say a unit, a set of units or a complete course.
- **Classification and placement:** For many purposes, students of a particular group will have to be classified on the basis of their level of attainment and other abilities. At other times, it has to be determined whether a particular student can promote to a further stage, based on the realization of the expected level. This function of the final evaluation is said to be the placement function.
- **Prognosis, prediction and selection:** This aims at determining the prerequisites possessed by a student, which are essential to succeed in a course of study that he is intended to take up. This predictive function of evaluation helps in conducting educational and vocational guidance in a more scientific manner.

## Functions Related to Total Education System

While discussing the broader scope of educational evaluation, it was pointed out that it covers program evaluation, institutional evaluation, evaluation of the performance of the personnel concerned, etc., in addition to the evaluation of pupil performance. Education in its totality is a system with a well defined output, a set of appropriate inputs leading to the output and process linking these two. Educational evaluation has to take up functions for the betterment of this system as a whole.

- **Improvement of inputs and process of education:** The inputs of an education system include items like the curriculum, textbooks, teaching aids, infrastructure facilities, environmental conditions, expertise of the teachers, societal support, etc. All these are to be utilized for the development of the raw material—the learner. If the anticipated output, i.e., student development has to be achieved to the maximum level possible, the inputs should be pooled and processed systematically. This could be done only on the basis of input analysis and process analysis to be followed by their proper evaluation on the basis of the objectives formulated as well as the feedback obtained from the final evaluation of pupil performance.
- **Maximization of the output (that is student development):** This function of educational evaluation is a natural extension of the previous one. By improving inputs and process, by setting high but realistic targets and by ensuring progress through diagnosis, remediation and reinforcement, educational evaluation contributes to the student development.

## TYPES OF EVALUATION

We can classify evaluation in the following ways: (a) based on the frequency of conducting, evaluation can be classified into summative evaluation and formative evaluation, (b) based on the nature of measurement, evaluation can be classified into maximum performance evaluation and typical performance evaluation, (c) based on the method of interpreting results, evaluation can be classified into criterion-referenced evaluation and norm-referenced evaluation.

### Formative Evaluation

Formative evaluation is used to monitor learning progress during instruction and to provide continuous feedback to both pupil and teacher regarding learning success and failures. Feedback to pupil reinforces successful learning and identifies the learning errors that need correction. Feedback to the teacher provides information for modifying instruction and prescribing group and individual remedial work. Formative evaluation depends heavily on especially prepared tests for each segment of instruction like unit or chapter. Tests used for formative evaluation are most frequently prepared by the teacher, but published tests are also available. Since formative evaluation is directed toward improving learning and instruction, the results are typically not used for assigning course grades.

Formative evaluation helps a teacher to ascertain the pupil progress from time to time. At the end of a topic or unit or a chapter the teacher can evaluate the learning outcomes. Then based on these outcomes teacher can modify his methods and techniques of teaching to provide better learning experiences.

Examples of formative evaluation include monthly tests, class tests, unit tests, periodical assessment, teacher's observation, etc.

### Characteristics of Formative Evaluation

- It is mainly instruction based and helps the teacher to know the learning progress of students.
- It works along with the perspectives of evaluation for learning.
- It helps students to focus on learning goals.
- It use continuous and multiple techniques of evaluation.
- It ensures more student participation in evaluation by motivating students to attain learning goals.

- It occurs frequently during the course of instruction and is an integral part of the learning process.
- Its results are made immediately known to students through feedback.
- It helps to solve learning difficulties of students and thereby assisting students in the learning process.
- It consider role of evaluation as a process.
- Its results cannot be used for grading or placement purpose.

## Summative Evaluation

Summative evaluation typically comes at the end of a course or unit of instruction. It is designed to determine the extent to which the instructional objectives have been achieved and is used primarily for assigning course grades or certifying pupil mastery of the intended learning outcomes. The techniques used in summative evaluation are determined by the instructional objectives, but they usually include teacher-made achievement tests, ratings on various types of performance (e.g., laboratory, oral report) and evaluations of products (e.g., themes, drawings, research reports). Although the main purpose of summative evaluation is grading or the certification of pupil achievement, it also provides information for judging the appropriateness of the course objectives and effectiveness of the instruction.

Summative evaluation focuses on the outcome of a program or a course. The primary goal of summative evaluation is to measure a student's achievement at the end of a particular instructional period typically at the end of a course, semester or a academic year. Standardized tests are used for summative evaluation. Summative evaluation results are used for grading and placement purpose.

Summative evaluation helps to judge the appropriateness of instructional objectives. It indicates the degree to which the students have mastered the course content. Generally summative evaluation assesses change in knowledge, perceptions, attitudes, skills and behaviors of students after attending a particulars educational program. In short, summative evaluation comprehensively assesses student learning and the effectiveness of an instructional method or an educational program. Examples of summative evaluation are traditional school and university examination, standardized tests, university practical examination, etc.

## Characteristics of Summative Evaluation

- It works along with the perspectives of evaluation of learning.
- It is terminal in nature as it takes place at the end of a program or course.
- It is judgmental in character—in the sense that it judge the achievement of students.
- It views evaluation "as a product" because it focuses on attainment of learning outcomes.
- Its results can be used for grading or placement purpose.
- It may or may not motivate a learner. Sometimes, it may have negative effect.
- It does not provide immediate feedback to students.

## Differences between Formative and Summative Evaluation

The key differences between formative and summative evaluation (**Table 10.1**) are the following:
- Formative evaluation is an ongoing activity and takes places during the teaching–learning process. Summative evaluation is not regular and is done after the completion of a unit or course.
- Goal of formative evaluation is to monitor student's learning in order to provide ongoing feedback. Ongoing feedback will in turn improve learning. Goal of summative evaluation is to evaluate learning at the end of the course against some standards for assigning grades or evaluate student's achievement.

**TABLE 10.1:** Difference between formative and summative evaluation.

| Formative evaluation | Summative evaluation |
|---|---|
| Assessment for learning | Assessment of learning |
| Frequent and is planned at the same time as teaching | Looks at post achievement. Not frequent |
| Provides instant feedback and is forward looking | Involves only marking and feedback grades to student |
| More scope for feedback and self-monitoring | Less scope for feedback and self-monitoring |

- Formative evaluation considers evaluation as a process, whereas summative evaluation considers evaluation as a product.
- Formative evaluation includes little content areas, whereas summative evaluation includes more content areas.
- In definite sense, formative evaluation is for learning and summative evaluation is of learning.

### Maximum Performance Evaluation

Maximum performance evaluation determines what individuals can do when performing at their best. Evaluation of this type is concerned with determining a person's abilities and how well an individual performs when motivated to obtain as high a score as possible. Aptitude and achievement tests are useful in measuring maximum performance.

### Typical Performance Evaluation

Typical performance evaluation determines what individuals will do under natural conditions, i.e., their typical behavior. How does the individual usually behave in normal or routine situations? Results in this area, then will indicate what individuals will do rather than what they can do. The importance of this distinction between ability and typical behavior is easily illustrated. A student with considerable aptitude for community health nursing may, however, show little interest in its pursuit. A student who knows the rules of good sportsmanship may refuse to abide by them. Attitude tests, personality inventories and observational techniques will help measure typical behavior.

### Criterion-referenced Evaluation

This describes pupil performance according to a specified domain of clearly defined learning tasks. For example, formulates the nursing diagnosis of patients with typhoid fever. Thus, criterion-referenced evaluation directly describes the specific performance that was demonstrated. Criterion-referenced interpretations enable us to describe what an individual can do, without reference to others' performances. Evaluation instruments include teacher made tests, published tests and observational techniques. Criterion-referenced test is a test designed to provide a measure of performance that is interpretable in terms of a clearly defined and delimited domain of learning tasks.

### Norm-referenced Evaluation

Norm-referenced evaluation describes pupil performance according to relative position in some known group; for example, ranks tenth in a classroom group of 30. Norm-referenced interpretations enable us to determine how an individual's performance compares with that of others. This might be local, state or national group, depending on how the results are to be used. Evaluation instruments include standardized aptitude and achievement tests, teacher made tests, interest inventories and adjustment inventories. A norm-referenced test is a test designed to provide a measure of performance that is interpretable in terms of an individual's relative standing in some known group.

## CONTINUOUS COMPREHENSIVE EVALUATION

Continuous comprehensive evaluation is an attempt to limit the shortcomings of evaluation process **(Figure 10.2)**.

- *C: Continuous:* Regular and continuous activities conducted throughout the year to achieve all round developments.
- *C: Comprehensive:* Mental, emotional and physical aspects of the student's progress, i.e., all round development of the student.
- *E: Evaluation:* Variety of tools and techniques are used to assess and evaluate the student's progress.

Continuous evaluation involves regular assessment of students by the institution. The characteristics of continuous evaluation are:

- Formative and institutional based
- Carried out by classroom teacher
- Aims at improvement of learning
- Largely informal
- Use multiple techniques
- Involves continuous feedback
- Completely integrated with the learning and teaching process

As growth, development and learning is a continuous process evaluation should also be a continuous process **(Fig. 10.3)**.

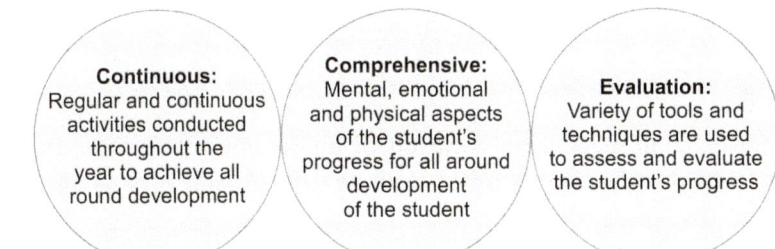

**Fig. 10.2:** Continuous comprehensive evaluation.

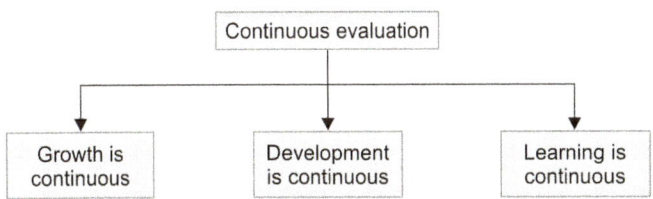

**Fig. 10.3:** Importance of continuous evaluation.

## STEPS IN EVALUATION

Guilber identified four steps in evaluation they are:
1. Defining the acceptable level of performance by way of stating educational objectives.
2. Development and use of appropriate measuring instruments to measure learning outcomes.
3. Interpretation of the collected data
4. Formation of judgment regarding the findings and taking appropriate actions.

## TECHNIQUES AND TOOLS OF EVALUATION

### Techniques

- Written examination
- Oral examination
- Practical examination
- Interviews
- Observation
- Projective techniques
- Sociometric techniques

### Tools

- Tests: These include: (i) Achievement tests like written test, oral test and practical or performance test. Achievement tests may be teacher made test or standardized test. (ii) Diagnostic tests. (iii) Intelligence tests. (iv) Aptitude tests, etc.
- Anecdotal records
- Checklists
- Cumulative records
- Interview schedules
- Inventories
- Questionnaires
- Rating scales

## OBSERVATION

Teachers' daily observation gives them a wealth of information concerning the learning and development of students. Observation has been defined as a measurement without instruments.

In education, observation is the most commonly employed of all measurement techniques. In the present as well as in the past, students have been labeled as good, fair or poor in achievement and lazy or diligent in study, etc., on the basis of observation.

On the basis of evidence drawn from observations of behavior and listening to oral contributions, teachers will draw inferences about a student's attitudes, personal qualities, abilities, motivation and commitment, learning speed and style, intelligence, attainments and progress. These inferences in turn will help the teachers make certain judgments and decisions about students.

### Merits of Direct Observation

- Being a record of the actual behavior of the student, it is more reliable and objective.
- It is a study of an individual in a natural situation and is therefore more useful than the restricted study in a test situation.

- This method can be employed to all sections of students.
- It can be used with some training and experience and almost all teachers can use it. It does not require any special tool or equipment.
- It can be used in every situation.
- It is adaptable both to individuals and groups.
- Frequent observations of a student's behavior can provide a continuous check on his progress.
- The problems can be detected immediately as they arise and remedial measures can be taken accordingly.
- Observational data provide teachers with valuable supplementary information.

## Limitations and Demerits
- There is a great scope for personal prejudices and bias of the observer.
- Observations may not be recorded with 100% accuracy.
- The observer may get only a small sample of student behavior. It is very difficult to observe everything that a student does or says.
- It reveals the overt behavior only—behavior that is expressed and not that is within.

## Principles to be Followed in Making Observations
- Observe the whole situation.
- Select one student to observe at a time.
- Students should be observed in their regular activities, such as in classroom and in the clinical area.
- Observation should be made over a period of days.
- As far as possible, observations from several teachers should be combined.

## Requisites of Good Observation
Good observation should be based on: (a) proper planning, (b) proper execution, (c) proper recording, and (d) proper interpretation.

### Proper Planning of Observation
- Areas of behavior to be observed must be clearly defined.
- Scope of observation—whether individual or group—should be decided.
- The duration of each observation period and the number of recordings and tools for observation should be decided.

### Proper Execution of Observation
Proper carrying out of observation demands skill and resourcefulness on the part of the investigator. Observation can be meticulously conducted by implementing the plan properly, like, focusing attention on the selected areas of behavior, following the decided pattern of observation, etc.

### Recording of Observation
Depending upon the nature of the activity or behavior to be observed and the skill of the observer, observation can be recorded simultaneously or after completing the observation.

### Interpretation
Results should be interpreted cautiously and judiciously after taking into account the various limitations of planning, sampling or procedure.

## Devices Used in Observation

Anecdotal records, checklists and rating scales are the devices commonly used for observation.

### ANECDOTAL RECORDS

Anecdotal records are factual description of the meaningful incidents and events that the teacher has observed in the pupils' lives. Each incident should be written down shortly after it happens.

The descriptions may be recorded on separate cards or as running accounts, one for each pupil, on separate pages in a notebook. A good anecdotal record keeps the objective description of an incident separate from any interpretation of the behavior's meaning. For some purposes, it is also useful to keep an additional space for recommendations concerning ways to improve the pupil's learning or adjustment.

#### Uses of Anecdotal Records

The use of anecdotal records has frequently been limited to the area of social adjustment. Although they are especially appropriate for this type of reporting, this is a needless limitation. Anecdotal records can be used for obtaining data pertinent to a variety of learning outcomes and to many aspects of personal and social development like skills, work habits, social attitudes, interests, appreciations, adjustments, scientific attitudes, etc. It is obvious that we cannot observe and report on all aspects of pupil behavior, no matter how useful such records might be. Thus, we must be selective in our observations.

### RATING SCALES

Rating scales consists of a set of characteristics or qualities to be judged and some type of scale for indicating the degree up to which attribute is present.

As with other evaluating instruments, it should be constructed in accordance with the learning outcomes to be evaluated and its use should be confined to those areas in which there is a sufficient opportunity to make the necessary observations. If these two principles are properly applied, a rating scale will serve several important evaluative functions like: (a) It will direct observation toward specific aspects of behavior. (b) It will provide a common frame of reference for comparing all pupils on the same set of characteristics. (c) It will provide a convenient method for recording the observers' judgments.

#### Types of Rating Scales

Numerical rating scale, graphic rating scale and descriptive graphic rating scale are the commonly used ones for educational evaluation.

#### *Numerical Rating Scale*

One of the simplest types of rating scales is that in which the rater puts a check (×) or circles a number to indicate the degree to which a characteristic is present. Typically, each of a series of numbers is given a verbal description that remains constant from one characteristic to another. The numerical rating scale is useful when the characteristics or qualities to be rated can be classified into a limited number of categories and when there is general agreement concerning the category represented by each number.

## Example

*Directions:* Indicate the degree to which this student contributes to care plan discussion by circling the appropriate number. The numbers represent the following values: 5—outstanding, 4—above average, 3—average, 2—below average and 1—unsatisfactory.
1. To what extent does the student participate in discussion?
   1 2 3 4 5
2. To what extent are the opinions related to the patient's condition?
   1 2 3 4 5

## Graphic Rating Scale

In graphic rating scale, each characteristic is followed by a horizontal line. The rating is made by placing a check on the line. A set of categories identifies specific positions along the line, but the rater is free to check between these points.

## Example

*Directions:* Indicate the degree to which this student contributes to care plan discussion by placing a check (×) anywhere along the horizontal line under each item.
1. To what extent does the student participate in discussion?

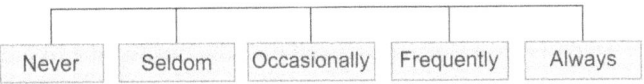

2. To what extent are the opinions related to the patient's condition?

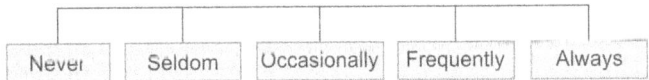

The scale shown in this example uses the same set of categories for each characteristic and is commonly referred to as a *constant-alternative scale*. When these categories vary from one characteristic to another, the scale is called a *changing alternative* scale. Below mentioned graphic scale for indicating the social attitude of the student is an example of changing alternative scale.

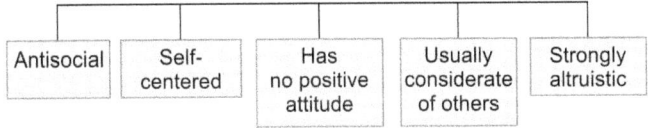

## Descriptive Graphic Rating Scale

The descriptive graphic rating scale uses descriptive phrases to identify the points on a graphic scale. The descriptions are brief details that convey in behavioral terms how pupils behave at different steps along the scale. In some scales, only the center and end positions are defined. In others, a descriptive phrase is placed beneath each point. A space for comments is also frequently provided to enable the rater to clarify the rating or to record behavioral incidents pertinent to the rating or to record behavioral incidents pertinent to the characteristics being rated.

## Example

*Directions:* Make your ratings on each of the following characteristics by placing an × anywhere along the horizontal line, under each item. In the space for comments, include anything that helps clarify your rating.

1. To what extent does the student participate in discussions?

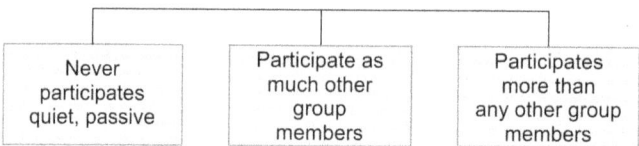

*Comment:* The descriptive graphic rating scale is generally the most satisfactory for educational evaluation. The more specific behavior descriptions also contribute to greater objectivity and accuracy during the rating process.

## Uses of Rating Scales

The uses may be classified into three evaluation areas:

1. **Procedure evaluation:** In many areas, achievement is expressed specifically through student's performance. Examples include ability to give a health education, work effectively in a group, performing various procedure, etc. Such activities do not result in a product that can be evaluated and paper and pencil tests are generally inadequate. Consequently, the procedures used in the performance itself must be observed and judged. Rating scales are especially useful in evaluating procedures because they focus on the same aspects of performance in all pupils and have a common scale on which to record judgments.
2. **Product evaluation:** When pupil performance results in some type of product, it is frequently more desirable to judge the product rather than the performance. The ability to make a model of sanitary well, for example, is best evaluated by judging the quality of the product itself. Little is to be evaluated by observing the student's performance.
3. **Evaluating personal-social development:** One of the most common uses of rating scales in the schools is rating various aspects of personal-social development. Rating personal social characteristics is quite different from procedure and product evaluation. When judging procedures and products, the ratings are usually made during or immediately after a period of observation. In contrast, ratings of personal-social development are typically obtained at periodic intervals and represent a kind of summing up of teacher's general impressions.

## Common Errors in Rating

Certain types of errors occur so often in ratings that special efforts are needed to counteract them. These include errors due to:

* **Personal bias** errors are indicated by a general tendency to rate all individuals at approximately the same position on the scale. Some raters tend to use the high end of the scale only, which is probably the most common type of bias and is referred to as *generosity error*. Occurring much less frequently but persistently for some raters is the *severity error*, in which the lower end of the scale is favored. Still a third type of constant response is shown by the rater who avoids both extremes of the scale and tends to rate every one as average. This is called the *central tendency error*.
* **The halo effect** is an error that occurs when a rater's general impression of a person influences the rating of individual characteristics. If the rater has a favorable attitude toward

the person being rated, there will be a tendency to give high ratings on all traits, but if the rater's attitude is unfavorable the ratings will be low. This differs from the generosity and severity errors in which the rater tends to rate everyone high or everyone low.
* **A logical error** results when two characteristics are rated as more alike than they actually are because of the rater's beliefs concerning their relationship.

## Principles Governing Rating Scales

The principles governing effective use of rating scales are: (a) characteristics should be educationally significant, (b) characteristics should be directly observable, (c) characteristics and points on the scale should be clearly defined, (d) between three and seven ratings positions should be provided and raters should be permitted to mark at intermediate points, (e) raters should be instructed to omit ratings when they feel unqualified to judge, (f) ratings from several observers should be combined whenever possible.

# CHECKLISTS

Checklist is basically a method of recording whether a characteristic is present or absent or whether an action had or had not taken place. Thus, it provides a simple yes-no judgment.

In nursing, checklists are useful in evaluating performance skills that can be divided into a series of specific actions. The following steps summarize the development of a checklist for evaluating a procedure consisting of series of sequential steps.
1. Identify each of the specific actions desired in the performance.
2. Add to the list those actions that represent common errors (if they are useful in the evaluation, are limited in number and can be clearly stated).
3. Arrange the desired actions (and likely errors if used) in the approximate order in which they are expected to occur.
4. Provide a simple procedure for checking each action as it occurs (or for numbering the actions in sequence if appropriate).

In addition to its use in procedure evaluation, the checklist can also be used to evaluate products. For this purpose, the form usually contains a list of characteristics that the finished product should possess. In evaluating the product, the teacher simply checks whether each characteristic is present or absent. Before using a checklist for product evaluation, teacher should decide whether the quality of the product can be adequately described by merely noting the presence or absence of each characteristic. In the area of personal-social development, the checklist can be a convenient method of recording evidence of growth toward specific learning outcomes. Typically, the form lists the behaviors that have been identified as representative of the outcomes to be evaluated.

## Example

Checklist for evaluating student's performance during surgical dressing, directions: mark yes or no to indicate whether skills have been demonstrated.

| Sl. No. | Behaviors | Yes | No | Remarks |
|---|---|---|---|---|
| 1. | Explains procedure | | | |
| 2. | Collects necessary equipment | | | |
| 3. | Arranges equipment for convenient use | | | |

| Sl. No. | Behaviors | Yes | No | Remarks |
|---|---|---|---|---|
| 4. | Prepares patient | | | |
| 5. | Washes hands | | | |
| 6. | Follows aseptic technique | | | |
| 7. | Removes previous dressing | | | |
| 8. | Inspects condition of wound | | | |
| 9. | Cleans wound | | | |
| 10. | Applies dressing | | | |
| 11. | Removes equipment | | | |
| 12. | Makes patient comfortable | | | |
| 13. | Completes charting | | | |
| 14. | After care of equipment | | | |

## CUMULATIVE RECORD

In all nursing institutes, the progress in the personal and academic development of each student is recorded cumulatively in an orderly fashion, usually on an yearly basis, in a comprehensive record designed for the purpose. Such a record is known as cumulative record.

Cumulative record will have provision for recording the results of a variety of dimensions. Physical development, relevant details of health condition, conditions of home environment, levels of attainment in the various subjects of study, special interests and attitudes, personality traits, participation in cocurricular activities like sports, etc., will have to be recorded year after year. There is also a provision for recording the general overall remarks about the student. It will give a very comprehensive picture of a student and hence will help in providing vocational guidance. Compared to other educational institutes, nursing institutes are very particular in maintaining cumulative records.

In Jane Warters opinion, "it aids teachers in the study of the individual student by making it possible for them to understand his present through an analysis of his past, by furnishing clues regarding the cause of his behavior, difficulties and failures and by disclosing his strengths and weakness".

## ACHIEVEMENT TESTS

Teachers depend upon the achievement tests for measuring the progress of students. Groundlund defines an achievement test as "a systematic procedure for determining the amount a student has learned through instruction." Popham believes that "the achievement test focuses upon an examinee's attainment at a given point of time".

## SELECTION OF APPROPRIATE TEST ITEM

Achievement tests employed in nursing education can be classified as in **Flowchart 10.1**

## OBJECTIVE TEST

Objective test item can be classified into those that require student to *supply* the answer and those that require the student to *select* the answer from a given number of alternatives. These two general classes are further divided into various types as shown in **Flowchart 10.1**. Thus,

**Flowchart 10.1:** Classification of achievement tests used in nursing education.

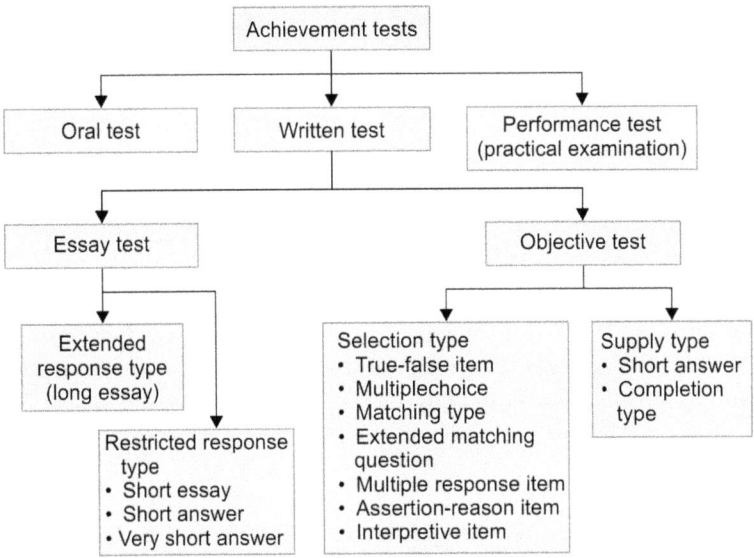

objective items are highly structured and requires the student to supply a word or two or to select the correct answer from a number of alternatives.

The various types of objective test items have one feature in common that distinguishes them from the essay test. They present the students with a highly structured task that limits the type of response they can make. To obtain the correct answer, the students must demonstrate the specific knowledge, understanding or skill called for in the item; they are not free to redefine the problem or to organize and present the answer in their own words. They must select one of several alternative answers or supply the correct word, number or symbol. This structuring of the problem and restriction on the method of responding contribute to objective scoring that is quick, easy and accurate. On the negative side, this same structuring makes the objective test item inappropriate for measuring the ability to select, organize and integrate ideas. To measure such outcomes we must depend on the essay question.

## SHORT ANSWER ITEMS

The short answer item and completion item are supply type test items that can be answered by a word, phrase, number or symbol. They are essentially the same, differing only in the method of presenting the problem. The short answer item uses a direct question, whereas the completion item consists of an incomplete statement.

*Examples*
Short-answer: What is the name of the man who discovered penicillin? (Alexander Fleming)
*Completion*: The name of the person who discovered penicillin is (Alexander Fleming)

## Uses of Short-answer Item

The short-answer item is suitable for measuring a wide variety of relatively simple learning outcomes such as knowledge of terminology, knowledge of specific facts, knowledge of principles, knowledge of method or procedure and simple interpretations of data.

## Suggestions for Constructing Short-answer Item

The following suggestions will help the teacher to avoid possible pitfalls and will provide greater assurance that the items will function as intended: (a) word the item so that the required answer is both brief and specific, (b) do not take statements directly from textbooks to use as a basis for short-answer items, (c) blanks for answers should be equal in length and in a column to the right of the question, (d) When completion items are used, do not include too many blanks.

## TRUE-FALSE OR ALTERNATIVE-RESPONSE ITEMS

The alternative-response test item consists of a declarative statement that the student is asked to mark true or false, right or wrong, correct or incorrect, yes or no, fact or opinion, agree or disagree and the like. In each case, there are only two possible answers. Because the true-false option is the most common, this item type is most frequently referred to as the true-false test item.

### Uses of True-False Item

Probably the most common use of the true-false item is in measuring the ability to identify the correctness of statements of facts, definition of terms, statements of principles, differentiating facts from opinions and the like. For measuring such relatively simple learning outcomes, a single declarative statement is used with any one of several methods of responding.

### Suggestions for Constructing True-False Items

The following Suggestions will help in constructing true-false items in a better way: (a) avoid broad general statements if they are to be judged true or false, (b) avoid trivial statements, (c) avoid the use of negative statements, especially double negatives, (d) avoid long, complex sentences, (e) avoid including two ideas in one statement, unless cause-effect relationships are being measured, (f) if opinion is used, attribute it to some source, unless the ability to identify opinion is being specifically measured, (g) true statements and false statements should be approximately equal in length, (h) the number of true statements and false statements should be approximately equal: This will prevent students from guessing and answering all questions 'true' or 'false'. The best procedure seems to be to vary the percentage of true statements somewhere between 40 and 60%. Under no circumstance should the statements be all true or all false.

## MULTIPLE CHOICE ITEM

Multiple choice item is the most widely used and useful type of objective test item. In addition to measuring simple learning outcomes, it can measure a variety of more complex outcomes in the knowledge, understanding and application areas.

### Characteristics of Multiple Choice Item

A multiple choice item consists of a problem and a list of suggested solutions. The problem may be stated as a direct question or an incomplete statement and is called the *'stem of the item.'* The list of suggested solutions may include words, numbers, symbols or phrases and are called *alternatives (also called 'choices or options')*. The student is typically requested to read the stem and the list of alternatives and to select the one correct or best alternative. The correct alternative in each item is called *the answer or key and the remaining alternatives are called distractors*. These incorrect alternatives receive their name from their intended function—to distract those students who are in doubt about the correct answer.

*Example*

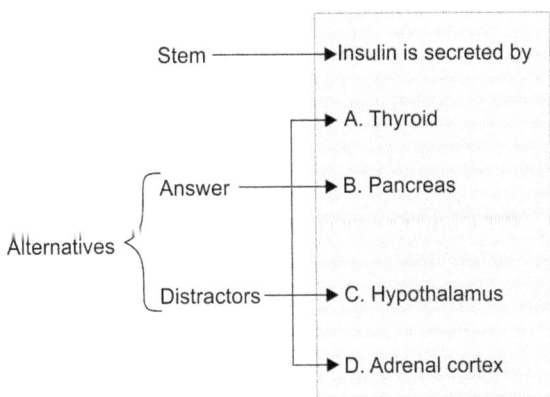

Whether to use a direct question or incomplete statement in the stem depends on several factors. The direct question form is easier to write, is more natural for students and is more likely to present a clearly formulated problem. On the other hand, the incomplete statement is more concise and if skillfully phrased, it too can present a well-defined problem.

**Examples**
*Direct—Question Form*
    **Which one of the following glands produces growth hormone?**
    A. Thyroid
    **B. Anterior pituitary**
    C. Adrenal cortex
    D. Pancreas

*Incomplete—Statement Form*
    **Growth hormone is produced by:**
    A. Thyroid
    **B. Anterior pituitary**
    C. Adrenal cortex
    D. Pancreas

In these examples, there is only one correct answer. Growth hormone is produced by anterior pituitary. All other alternatives are wrong. Thus, this is known as the *correct-answer* type of multiple choice items. Not all knowledge can be stated so precisely that there is only one absolutely correct response. In fact, when we go beyond the simple aspects of knowledge, represented by questions of the whom, what, when and where variety, answers of varying degrees of acceptability are the rule rather than the exception. Questions of the why variety, for example, tend to reveal a number of possible reasons, some of which are better than the others. Likewise, questions of the how variety usually reveal several possible procedures, some of which are more desirable than others. Measures of achievement in these areas, then become a matter of selecting the *best answer*, as the following illustrates.

**Example**
*Best Answer Type*
    **Which one of the following factors contributed most to the selection of mannitol for reducing cerebral edema?**

A. Osmotic diuretic
**B. Site of action**
C. Easy to administer
D. Quick action

## Uses of Multiple Choice Items

The multiple choice item is the most versatile type of test item available. It can measure a variety of learning outcomes from simple to complex and it is adaptable to most types of subject matter content. Measuring knowledge outcomes and measuring outcomes at the understanding and application levels are the main uses of multiple choice items.

### Measuring Knowledge Outcomes

Learning outcomes in the knowledge area are so prominent in all subjects and multiple choice items can measure such a variety of these outcomes.

- **Knowledge of terminology:** A simple but basic learning outcome measured by the multiple choice item is knowledge of terminology. For this purpose, students can be requested to show their knowledge of a particular term by selecting a word that has the same meaning as the given term or by choosing a definition of the term.
  *Example*
  **Which one of the following terms has the same meaning as the word newborn?**
  A. Infant
  B. Toddler
  **C. Neonate**
  D. Pubescent

- **Knowledge of specific facts:** Another learning outcome basic to all subjects is the knowledge of specific facts. It provides a necessary basis for developing understanding, thinking skills and other complex learning outcomes. Multiple choice items designed to measure specific facts can take many different forms, but questions of the who, what, when and where variety are the most common.
  *Example*
  **When did Florence Nightingale start her first nursing school?**
  A. 1901
  **B. 1862**
  C. 1865
  D. 1904

- **Knowledge of principles:** Multiple choice items can be constructed to measure knowledge of principles as easily as those designed to measure knowledge of specific facts.
  *Example*
  **The principle of capillary action explains how fluids:**
  A. Enter solutions of lower concentration
  B. Escape through small openings
  C. Pass through semi permeable membranes
  D. Rise in fine tubes

- **Knowledge of methods and procedures:** Another common learning outcome readily adaptable to the multiple choice form is knowledge of methods and procedures. This include such diverse areas of knowledge of laboratory procedures; knowledge of methods underlying communication; computational and performance skills; knowledge of methods used in problem solving and knowledge of common social practices.

*Example*
**If you were making a scientific study of a problem, your first step should be to:**
**A. Collect information about the problem**
B. Develop hypotheses to be tested
C. Design the experiment to be conducted
D. Select scientific equipment

## Measuring Outcomes at the Understanding and Application Levels

❖ **Ability to identify application of facts and principles:** A common method of determining whether students' learning has gone beyond the mere memorization of a fact or principle is to ask them to identify its correct application in a situation that is new to the student.
*Example*
**Which one of the following is an example of an osmotic diuretic?**
A. Frusemide
B. Triamtarine
**C. Mannitol**
D. Aldactone

*Directions:* In the following statement circle the appropriate drug.
Aldactone
Frusemide is the drug of choice to reduce cerebral edema.
**Mannitol**

❖ **Ability to interpret cause and effect relationship:** Understanding can frequently be measured by asking students to interpret various relationships among facts.
*Example*
**Bread will not become mouldy as rapidly if placed in a refrigerator because:**
**A. Cooling retards the growth of fungi.**
B. Darkness retards the growth of mould.
C. Cooling prevents the bread from dryingout rapidly.
D. Mould requires both heat and light for best growth.

❖ **Ability to justify methods and procedures:** This can be measured with multiple choice items by asking the student to select the best of several possible explanation of a method or procedure.
*Example*
**While administering test dose most important thing is to:**
A. Explain to the patient.
B. Circle the area after administration.
**C. Keep a syringe loaded with adrenaline.**
D. Ensuring cooperation of relatives.

## Advantages and Limitations of Multiple Choice Items

The multiple choices item is one of the most widely applicable test items for measuring achievement. It can effectively measure various types of knowledge and complex learning outcomes. In addition to this flexibility, it is free from some of the shortcomings characteristic of other item types. The ambiguity and vagueness that frequently present in the short-answer item are avoided because of the alternatives better structure the situation. One advantage of the multiple choice item over the true-false item is that students cannot receive credit for simply knowing that a statement is incorrect; they must also know what is correct. Another advantage of the multiple choice item over the true-false item is the greater reliability per item.

Because the number of alternatives is increased from two to four or five, the opportunity for guessing the correct answer is reduced and the reliability is correspondingly increased. Using the best answer type of multiple choice item makes it possible to measure learning outcomes in the numerous subject matter areas in which solutions to problems are not absolutely true or false but vary in degree of appropriateness. Another advantage of the multiple choice item over the matching exercise is that the need for homogeneous material is avoided. Two other desirable characteristics of the multiple choice item are worthy of mention. First, it is relatively free from response sets. That is, students generally do not favor a particular alternative when they do not know the answer. Second, using a number of plausible alternatives makes the result amenable to diagnosis. The kind of the incorrect alternatives students select provides clues to factual errors and misunderstandings that need correction. The wide applicability of the multiple choice item, plus its advantages makes it easier to construct high-quality test items in this form than in any of the other forms.

Despite its superiority, the multiple choice item does have limitations. First, as with all other paper and pencil tests, it is limited to learning outcomes at the verbal level. The problems presented to students are verbal problems, free from the many relevant factors present in natural situations. Second, as with other types of selection items, the multiple choice item requires selection of the correct answer and therefore is not well adapted to measuring problem solving skills. It measures whether the student knows or understands what to do when confronted with a problem situation, but it cannot determine how the student actually will perform in that situation. Third, the multiple choices item has a disadvantage not shared by the other items: the difficulty of finding a sufficient number of incorrect but plausible distractors.

## Suggestions for Constructing Multiple Choice Items

Advantages of multiple choice items can be maintained by constructing good quality multiple choice items. This involves formulating a clearly stated problem, identifying plausible alternatives and removing clues to the answer. The following suggestions will help to achieve this purpose: (a) the stem of the item should be meaningful by itself and should present a definite problem, (b) the item stem should include as much of the item as possible and should be free of irrelevant material, (c) use a negatively stated item stem only when significant learning outcomes require it, (d) all of the alternatives should be grammatically consistent with the stem of the item, (e) an item should contain only one correct or clearly best answer, (f) items used to measure understanding should contain some novelty but beware of too much, (g) all distracters should be plausible: to the student who has not achieved the learning outcomes being tested, the distractors should be at least as attractive as the correct answer, and preferably more so, (h) verbal associations between the stem and the correct answer should be avoided, (i) the relative length of the alternatives should not provide a clue to the answer, (j) the correct answer should appear in each of the alternative positions an approximately equal number of items, but in random order, (k) use sparingly special alternatives such as "none of the above" or "all of the above", (l) do not use multiple choice items when other item types are more appropriate, (m) break any of these rules when you have a good reason for doing so: Although these rules provide valuable guidelines for constructing multiple choice items, you may encounter instances where an exception to the rule may improve them.

## MULTIPLE-RESPONSE ITEM

In multiple-response or multiple-completion item, more than one of the given alternatives is correct; but there is only one correct answer to the precise question stated in the first sentence of the item. This is a versatile type of objective test, lending itself to the testing of recall, reasoning and the exercise of judgment.

## Example

**Which of the following would be included among the group of potassium sparing diuretics?**
I. Diamox and bumet
II. Chlorthalidone and chlorthiazide
III. Spironolactone and triamterene
IV. Frusemide and ethacrynic acid
**A. III only**
B. II only
C. I and IV
D. II and III

## MATCHING ITEM

In its traditional form, the matching exercise consists of two parallel columns, with each word, number of symbol in one column being matched to a word, sentence or phrase in the other column. The items in the column for which a match is sought are called *premises* and the items in the column from which the selection is made are called *responses*. The basis for matching responses to premises is sometimes self-evident but more often must be explained in the directions. Matching item is useful in testing lower level intellectual skills such as recall.

## Merits of Objective Type Tests

From the above discussion, you can make out the following merits of objective type tests:
1. As the name indicates, they are more objective in their scoring, since the responses of the students are controlled, and since there can be no doubt regarding correctness or incorrectness of their responses.
2. They may be very comprehensive and can be constructed in a way to cover more subject matter. Since student does very little writing, he can devote his time to thinking process and can thereby answer a more number of questions compared to essay tests.
3. They are very easy to score as compared to essay tests. Even though they are more comprehensive, they may be scored in less time and with less effort. A key of the objective questions may be prepared so that anybody can evaluate them. Introduction of computers in evaluating objective type tests by employing optical mark recognition (OMR) technique again increased the scope of objective tests.
4. Students like them. There is no question regarding the accuracy of marks they receive. There is no chance for the teacher to show favoritism or personal bias. The students, relieved of much writing, find these tests less tiring.
5. They are more educative for the students. After the tests they can easily decide whether they need further study or preparation.
6. They are more reliable. Same results will be secured whoever may be the examiner. An essay type test cannot give the same results, if it is evaluated by different examiners.

## Limitations of Objective Type Tests

1. The student does not have an opportunity to show his ability to organize his thought. He has nothing to do except check over the truth and falsity of statements or fill in the missing words or incomplete sentences. Students miss the valuable experience of making

comparisons, giving explanations or giving definitions. They are not asked to summarize the material or to make applications of principles and of course, these are valuable abilities which we do not want to neglect.
2. Objective tests are not diagnostic in that they do not tell where the students reasoning process goes wrong or where he stops reasoning altogether and starts guessing.
3. Like the essay tests, objective tests also fail to test the character building aspects.

## ESSAY TESTS

Essay test is one of the oldest type of tests and have a long history that dates back to more than four thousand years. Gilbert Sax believes that "essay test is a test containing questions requiring the student to respond in writing. Essay tests emphasize recall rather than recognition of the correct alternative. Essay tests may require relatively brief responses or extended responses". They have been used so widely that it is assumed that everybody understands their meaning.

### Forms and Uses of Essay Questions

The distinctive feature of essay questions is the freedom of response. Students are free to select, relate and present ideas in their own words. Although this freedom enhances the value of essay questions as a measure of complex achievement, the associated scoring difficulty makes them inefficient as a measure of factual knowledge. For most purposes, knowledge of factual information can be more efficiently measured by some type of objective item. They should be primarily used to measure those learning outcomes concerned with the abilities to select, organize, integrate, relate and evaluate ideas that require the freedom of response and originality provided by essay questions.

Essay questions allow varying degree of freedom of response. At one extreme, the response is almost as restricted as that in the short-answer objective item, in which a sentence or two may be all that is required. At the other extreme, the students are given almost complete freedom in making their responses and their answers may require several pages. Although variations in freedom of response tend to fall along a continuum between these extremes, essay questions can be conveniently classified into two types, *the restricted response type and the extended response type.*

### Restricted Response Questions

The restricted response question usually limits both the content and the response. The content is usually restricted by the topic to be discussed. Limitations on the form of response are generally indicated in the question.

*Examples*
 a. State the main differences between kwashiorkor and marasmus.
 b. How good nutrition prevents pressure sore?
 c. Describe two health problems arising out of poor environmental sanitation.

Another way of restricting responses in essay tests is to base the questions on specific problems. For this purpose introductory material has to be given.

*Example*
Some teachers suggest that integrating discussion and questioning with the traditional lecture will help minimize its disadvantages. However, many teachers disagree with the suggestion *by pointing out the time consuming nature of questioning and discussion.*
 a. Indicate whether you agree or disagree with the italicized part of the last statement.
 b. List reasons that support your position.

Because the restricted response question is more structured, it is most useful for measuring learning outcomes requiring the interpretation and application of data in a specific area. Unfortunately, the same restrictions make them less valuable as a measure of those learning outcomes emphasizing integration, organization and originality.

## Extended Response Questions

The extended response question allows pupils to select any factual information that they think is pertinent, to organize the answer in accordance with their best judgment and to integrate and evaluate ideas as they deem to appropriate. This freedom enables them to demonstrate their ability to select, organize, integrate and evaluate ideas. On the other hand, this same freedom makes the extended response question inefficient for measuring more specific learning outcomes and introduces scoring difficulties that severely restrict its use as a measuring instrument.

### Examples
a. Explain the role of a nurse in the health care team.
b. Describe the contributions of Florence Nightingale towards the development of nursing.

## Advantages and Limitations of Essay Questions

The main advantage of the essay question is that it measures complex learning outcomes that cannot be measured by other means. A second advantage of the extended response question is its emphasis on the integration and application of thinking and problem solving skills. Because the students must present their answers in their own handwriting, the essay test is often regarded as a device for improving writing skills. Another commonly cited advantage of the essay question is its ease of construction. This apparent advantage can be very misleading, however constructing essay questions that require the specific behaviors emphasized in a particular set of learning outcomes take considerable time and effort.

The most serious limitation of the essay question is the unreliability of the scoring. Another limitation of essay questions is the amount of time required for scoring the answers. Another shortcoming of essay questions is the limited sampling they provide. Only few questions can be included in a given test so that some areas are measured thoroughly, but many others are neglected.

## SUGGESTIONS FOR THE ESSAY TESTS

According to Grounlund, the improvement of the essay question as a measure of complex learning outcomes requires attention to two problems: (1) How to construct essay questions that call forth the desired behavior? and (2) How to score the answers so that achievement is reliably measured? Grounlund recommends the following ways to improve construction and scoring of essay tests.

## Suggestions for Constructing Essay Questions

- Restrict the use of essay questions to those learning outcomes that cannot be satisfactorily measured by objective items.
- Formulate questions that will call forth the behavior specified in the learning outcomes (**Box 10.1**).
- Phrase each question so that the student's task is clearly indicated.
- The expected length of the answer of each question should be indicated on the test form.

**Box 10.1:** Some types of thought questions and sample item stems.

1. Comparing
   - Describe the similarities and differences between.....
   - Compare the following two methods for. ...
2. Relating cause and effect
   - What are major causes of...?
   - What would be the most likely effects of...?
3. Justifying
   - Which of the following alternatives would you favor, and why?
   - Explain why you agree or disagree with the following statement.
4. Summarizing
   - State the main points included in...
   - Briefly summarize the content of...
5. Generalizing
   - Formulate several valid generalizations from the following data.
   - State a set of principles that can explain the following events.
6. Inferring
   - In light of the facts presented, what is most likely to happen when...?
7. Classifying
   - Group the following items according to...
   - What do the following items have in common?
8. Creating
   - List as many ways as you can think of for...
9. Applying
   - Using the principle of...as a guide, describe how you would solve the following problem situation.
   - Describe a situation that illustrates the principle of...
10. Analyzing
    - Describe the reasoning errors in the following paragraph
    - List and describe the main characteristics of...
11. Synthesizing
    - Describe a plan for proving that...
    - Write a well-organized report that shows...
12. Evaluating
    - Describe the strengths and weaknesses of the following...
    - Using the criteria developed in class, write an evaluation of...

*Source:* Grounlund

- ❖ While preparing questions, it should be kept in mind that the maximum subject matter content is covered.
- ❖ The question should clearly indicate the significance of each part so that students may determine the time to be devoted to each part: this can be done by dividing the question into component parts and offering marks according to the significance. For example, a 15 marks essay question on nursing management of cirrhosis can be stated as: (i) Define cirrhosis of liver (2 m). (ii) Briefly explain the medical management (5 m). (iii) Explain the nursing management of a patient with cirrhosis of liver (8 m).
- ❖ Avoid the use of optional questions: Except for the desirable effect on pupil morale, however, there is little to recommend the use of optional questions. If students answer different questions, it is obvious that they are taking different tests and so the common basis for evaluating their achievement is lost. Each student is demonstrating the achievement of different learning outcomes. The use of optional questions might also influence the validity of the test results. When students anticipate the use of optional questions, they can prepare

answers on several topics in advance, commit them to memory and then select questions to which the answers are most appropriate.

## Suggestions for Scoring Essay Questions

1. **Prepare an outline of the expected answer in advance:** This should contain the major points to be included, the characteristics of the answer to be evaluated and the amount of marks to be allotted to each. Preparing a scoring key provides a common basis for evaluating the students' answers and keeps the standard stable throughout the scoring.
2. **Use the scoring method that is most appropriate:** There are two common methods of scoring essay questions. *One is called the point method and the other the rating method.* With the point method, each answer is compared with the ideal answer in the scoring key and a given number of points is assigned according to the adequacy of the answer. With the rating method, each paper is placed in one of a number of piles as the answer is read. These piles represent degrees of quality and determine the marks assigned to each answer. If eight points are allotted to the question, for example, nine piles might be used ranging in value from eight points to none questions can generally be satisfactorily scored by the point method. The extended response question, however, usually requires the rating method.
3. **Decide how to handle factors that are irrelevant to the learning outcomes being measured:** Several factors influence our evaluations of answers to essay questions that are not directly pertinent to the purposes of measurement. Prominent among these are legibility of handwriting, spelling, sentence structure, punctuation and neatness. We should make an effort to keep such factors from influencing our judgment when evaluating the content of the answers. In some instances, such factors may, of course, be evaluated for their own sake. When this is done, you should obtain a separate score for written expression or for each of the specific factors. As far as possible, however, we should not let such factors contaminate the extent to which our test scores reflect the achievement of other learning outcomes. Another decision concerns the presence of irrelevant and inaccurate factual information in the answer. Probably the best way to deal with irrelevant factors is to decide in advance approximately how much the score on each question is to be lowered when the inclusion of irrelevant material is excessive.
4. **Evaluate all answers to one question before going to the next one:** One factor that contributes to unreliable scoring of essay questions is a shifting of standards from one paper to the next. A paper with average answers may appear to be of much higher quality when it follows a failing paper than when it follows one with near-perfect answers. One way to minimize this is to score all answers to the first question, shuffle the papers, then score all answers to the second question and so on, until all of the answers have been scored. A more uniform standard can be maintained with this procedure, because it is easier to remember the basis for judging each answer and answers of various degrees of correctness can be more easily compared.
5. **Evaluating all answers to one question at a time helps counteract another type of error that creeps into the scoring of essay questions.** When we evaluate all of the answers on a single paper at one time, the first few answers create a general impression of the student's achievement that influence our judgment concerning the remaining answers. Thus, if the first answers are of high quality, we tend to overrate the following answers; whereas if they are of low quality, we tend to underrate them. This "halo effect" is less likely when the answers for a given student are not evaluated in continuous sequence.
6. **Evaluate the answers without looking at the student's name:** The general impression we form about each student during our teaching is also a source of bias in evaluating essay

questions. When possible, the identity of the students should be concealed until all answers are scored.

7. **If especially important decisions are to be based on the results, obtain two or more independent ratings:** Sometimes essay questions are included in tests used to select students for awards, scholarships, special training and the like. In such cases, two or more competent persons should score the papers independently and their ratings should be compared. After any large differences have been satisfactorily arbitrated the independent ratings may be averaged for more reliable results.

### Bluffing—A Special Scoring Problem

It is possible for students to obtain higher scores on essay questions than they deserve by means of clever bluffing. This is usually a combination of writing skill, general knowledge and the use of common "tricks of the trade". Following are some ways that students might attempt to influence the teacher and thus, increase their marks.

- **Writing something for every question**—even if it is only a restatement of the question (students think that they might get some marks if they fill the space).
- **Stressing the importance of the topic covered by the question**, especially when short of facts (e.g., "This disease is a major health problem in India").
- **Agreeing with the teacher's views whenever it seems appropriate** (e.g., "The recovery of the patient depends upon the quality of the nursing care rendered").
- **Being a name dropper** (e.g., "The above said points are supported by the viewpoints of Florence Nightingale." The teacher assumes that student knows about the viewpoints of Florence Nightingale).
- **Writing on a related topic and fitting it to the question** (e.g. prepared to write on congestive cardiac failure but asked to write about myocardial infarction, the student might start with: "Myocardial infarction occurs due to cessation of blood supply to myocardium—from here on there is more about congestive cardiac failure").
- **Writing in general terms that can fit many situations** (e.g. when writing nursing diagnosis, students always include knowledge deficit, anxiety, etc.).

Although bluffing cannot be completely eradicated, carefully phrasing the questions and following clearly defined scoring procedures can reduce it.

## ORAL EXAMINATIONS

Oral examination is a face-to-face question answer activity between the examiner and the examinee. The examiner ask questions and the examinee attempts to answer them. Finally, the examiner judges the quality of the answers and grades the examinee accordingly.

### Forms of Oral Examination

Important forms of oral examinations are interview, viva voce, quiz contest, panel discussion or group discussion. Each of these can be used as a teaching-learning technique and as an evaluation technique.

In nursing, oral examination can be conducted either as a theoretical oral examination or as a part of the practical examination. Theoretical oral examination is conducted to evaluate students' knowledge on certain subjects like physiology, microbiology, etc., while conducting as a part of the practical examination; oral examination is conducted in two phases. The first phase, which is scheduled during the nursing care delivery by the student, is known as the bedside viva. It is very brief and mainly aims to evaluate students' knowledge regarding the patient assigned to her. Bedside viva is conducted at the bedside and the examiner may or may not interact with the patient besides asking questions to the student. The second phase is conducted after the nursing care delivery by the student. During this phase examiner may go through the care plan prepared by the student. This phase is detail in nature and concentrates more on complex learning outcomes.

The oral examination has for centuries been the predominant method used to assess nursing students. The traditional oral, which gives considerable freedom to the examiner to vary the questions asked from student to student and to exercise personal bias has consistently been shown to be very unreliable.

## PRACTICAL EXAMINATIONS

Practical examinations are integral part of nursing examinations. The aim of practical examination is to evaluate the nursing competence or practical skills. Practical examination is essentially a combination of test methods like rating scales, checklists, etc. An oral examination also accompanies the practical test in order to supplement the information obtained through it. The students proceed through a series of 'steps' and undertake a variety of practical tasks like assessing the patient, formulating nursing diagnosis according to priority, planning the care, implementing the care and evaluating the care. Marking sheets, checklists and rating scales are prepared in advance to improve the reliability of scoring. All students are thus evaluated on the same criteria by the same examiners.

## QUALITIES OF AN EVALUATION TOOL/CHARACTERISTICS OF A GOOD ACHIEVEMENT TEST

The most essential characteristics of a good achievement test are *'validity,' 'reliability'* and *usability or practicability.*

### Validity

Validity refers to the appropriateness of the interpretations made from test scores and other evaluation results, with regard to a particular use. In other words, a test is said to be valid if it measures what it intends to measure. Objective-basedness, comprehensiveness and objectivity of a test will contribute to validity.

### *Types of Validity*

The most important types of validity are content validity, predictive validity or criterion related validity and construct validity.

#### *Content Validity*

It is a measure of the degree to which the test contains a representative sample of the material taught in the course. Thus, content validity is determined against the course content. Content validity demands that the requirements of the course content in terms of the subject matter as well as the objectives should be tested completely and without going beyond the scope. If the test content agrees with the course content with regard to both the dimensions, the test may be said to possess content validity.

#### *Criterion-related Validity or Predictive Validity*

The criterion-related validation may be defined as the process of determining the extent to which test performance is related to some other valued measure of performance. This validation adds authenticity to the predictive function of the test. Because of this dependence on the external criterion for establishing the validity of the test, it is said to be criterion related validity.

**Construct Validity**
Construct validity is concerned with how well test performance can be interpreted as a meaningful measure of some characteristic or quality. In the first two types of validity, our concern was how well a test represents achievement or how well it predicts some desired aspect. But while measuring some psychological phenomena, say a few personality traits like integrity, sociability, etc. our concern will be to know "what the scores obtained by the test signify". Such a question becomes necessary, as such traits are not directly observable or measurable. Therefore, what an examiner has to do is to operationally define the traits by associating them with certain observable behaviors that might project the trait. In other words, the trait is associated with something constructed by the tester to represent the traits that is a *'construct'*. Such a test is critically examined by asking the question how well the test score corresponds to the construct and hence such validity is known as construct validity. From the above discussion, it is evident that for an achievement test, content validity is more important than others, because it is especially relevant for such tests. Hence, every teacher who is more concerned with the measurement of achievement rather than the other aspects has to master the ways and means of maintaining content validity.

**Measures to Improve Validity**
Validity can be improved by: (a) carefully matching the test with learning objectives, content and teaching methods, (b) increasing the sample of objectives and content areas included in any given test, (c) using methods that are appropriate for the objectives specified, (d) employing a range of methods, (e) ensuring adequate security and supervision to avoid cheating in examinations, (f) improving the reliability of the tests.

## Reliability

Reliability of a test refers to the degree of consistency and accuracy with which it measures what it is intended to measure. Theoretically, a reliable test should produce the same result if administered to the same student on two separate occasions. Various methods like test-retest method, equivalent-forms method, split-half method and Kuder–Richardson method are available to provide statistical indices of reliability.

*Measures to Improve Reliability*

Reliability can be improved by: (a) limiting subjectivity of all kinds, (b) ensuring that questions are clear, suitable for the level of students and based on predetermined behaviors, (c) ensuring that the expected answers are definite and objective, (d) developing a scoring scheme of high quality, (e) checking to make sure time limits are realistic, (f) giving simple, clear and unambiguous instructions, (g) keeping choices within a test paper to a minimum, (h) when using less reliable methods, increasing the number of questions, observations or examination time, (i) conducting tests under identical and ideal examination conditions.

## Usability

In selecting tests and other evaluation instruments, practical considerations cannot be neglected. Tests are usually administered and interpreted by teachers with only a minimum amount of training in measurement. Factors that contribute to the usability or practicability are ease of administration, moderate time required for administration, ease of scoring, ease of interpretation and application and affordable cost of testing.

# CONSTRUCTION AND ADMINISTRATION OF ACHIEVEMENT TEST

Construction and administration of achievement test involves the following steps:

## Planning an Achievement Test

This step is concerned with determining the maximum time, marks and nature of the test. These should be decided in terms of the nature and scope of the unit or units involved in the testing. A test for a single unit may be generally of 40 to 45 minutes duration, with a maximum of 20 to 25 marks. But in the case of test conducted at the end of a term, a semester or a session, the duration may be about 2 to 3 hours and the maximum marks may be 50, 80 or 100.

## Developing Test Design

The objective, content, form of question and the weightage of difficulty level are the most important factors to be considered while designing the test. What is required is to analyze the syllabus in terms of the objectives and the content area and determine the relative weightage to each of the predetermined objectives as well as the subunits into which the contents have been divided. In the same way, the weightage for the different forms of the questions to be included and for the difficult levels to be maintained also are considered while finalizing the design. This will be followed by the scheme of option (choice of questions), if any and scheme of sections into which the test has to be divided in case it is required.

A sample design for a unit test with a maximum of 50 marks and duration of one and a half hours is given below. This is designed to measure behaviors in the cognitive domain only.

## Design for a Unit Test

### a. Weightage to Instructional Objectives

| Sl. No. | Objective | Marks | Percentage |
|---|---|---|---|
| 1. | Knowledge (information) | 10 | 20 |
| 2. | Understanding | 20 | 40 |
| 3. | Application | 8 | 16 |
| 4. | Analysis | 5 | 10 |
| 5. | Synthesis | 5 | 10 |
| 6. | Evaluation | 2 | 4 |
|  | Total | 50 | 100 |

### b. Weightage to Content Areas

| Sl. No. | Sub unit | Marks | Percentage |
|---|---|---|---|
| 1. | I | 15 | 30 |
| 2. | II | 10 | 20 |
| 3. | III | 10 | 20 |
| 4. | IV | 5 | 10 |
| 5. | V | 10 | 20 |
|  | Total | 50 | 100 |

### c. Weightage to Form of Questions

| Sl. No. | Form of questions | No. of questions | Marks | Percentage |
|---|---|---|---|---|
| 1. | Objective-type | 25 | 25 | 50 |
| 2. | Short answer-type | 5 | 15 | 30 |
| 3. | Long essay-type | 1 | 10 | 20 |
| | Total | 31 | 50 | 100 |

### d. Weightage to Difficulty Level

| Sl. No. | Level of difficulty | Marks | Percentage |
|---|---|---|---|
| 1. | Easy | 10 | 20 |
| 2. | Average | 30 | 60 |
| 3. | Difficult | 10 | 20 |
| | Total | 50 | 100 |

### e. Scheme of Option

There will be no option for any type of questions.

### f. Scheme of Sections

The test will be in two sections. A and B. A will contain all the objective type items and section B is meant for short answer and essay-type questions.

**Guidelines for preparing test designs are:** (a) The design should reflect the predetermined objectives envisaged at the time of instruction. The example mentioned above is not an acceptable pattern for all tests since it is not considering the affective and psychomotor domains. (b) As in the case of the weightage for content, there is no final ruling regarding the number of subunits into which the content has to be divided. It depends on the total content area as well as its nature. In all these, it is the discretion of the teacher who conducts the test is important. One suggestion for fixing the weightage is the scope of each subunit in the curriculum, as indicated by the time allotted for its instruction. (c) Regarding the number of questions under each form also there cannot be any uniformly acceptable design. Whether more weightage has to be given to a particular form of question depends on factors like the nature of the content, the possibility for coverage, etc. Time is another factor determining the nature of questions. (d) Regarding the weightage to difficult level what is suggested in the sample is an acceptable pattern. About 60% of items of average difficulty with 20% on either side is a distribution that will suit to students of all levels. (e) Modern trend is to avoid option.

### Preparation of Blueprint for Test

The next important step in the construction of an achievement test is preparing a blueprint according to the design. Normally a blueprint for a test is prepared as a three dimensional chart, indicating the distribution of questions, objective-wise, content-wise and form-wise.

For example a test blueprint for unit on oxygenation can be prepared as shown in **Table 10.2**.

### Construction of Items

The blueprint gives very definite idea, regarding the number of questions to be set from each subunit, their forms and scope. While setting the questions and making the final selection,

**TABLE 10.2:** Test blueprint for unit on oxygenation.

| Content | Knowledge/ comprehension | Level of knowledge application | Analysis synthesis | Evaluation | Total items |
|---|---|---|---|---|---|
| Principles | 2 | 2 | 2 | | 6 |
| Factors affecting | 3 | 3 | 4 | | 10 |
| Pathophysiology | 3 | 3 | 4 | | 10 |
| Assessment | 1 | 3 | 4 | 2 | 10 |
| Nursing measures | | 3 | 3 | 4 | 10 |
| Evaluation of care | | 1 | 1 | 2 | 4 |
| Total items | 9 | 15 | 18 | 8 | 50 |

*Source*: Sandra Deyoung

care has to be taken to maintain the weightage of difficulty level suggested by the design. It should also be checked where there is sufficient time to answer all the questions included.

## Organization of the Test

After finalizing the items, these have to be arranged according to the scheme of section as suggested in the design. Before that, the preliminary details such as name of the examination, maximum marks and time, instruction for answering each part, etc., have to be written at the appropriate places.

*Next concern is the arrangement of questions.* Psychologically, it will be advisable to arrange the items in the order of difficulty level. Normally, the hierarchical order of the objectives as given in the taxonomy of objectives is an indication of the difficulty level also. That is, an 'information item' will normally be easier than an 'understanding item', which in turn may be easier than an 'application item'. This need not be always true, but may be taken as a clue for arranging items in a test.

## Preparation of the Scheme for Evaluation

One of the steps suggested for maintaining objectivity is to make the scoring strictly in accordance with a predesigned scheme of evaluation. In the case of the objective-type items, a scoring key showing the number of the question and its correct answer is to be prepared. Point method is used to evaluate short answer type questions. Point method or rating method is used to evaluate essay questions.

## TEST ADMINISTRATION

The steps to be followed in the administration of group tests are: (a) motivate the students to do their best, (b) follow the directions closely, (c) keep time accurately, (d) record any significant events that might influence test scores, (e) collect the test materials promptly.

The guiding principle in administering an achievement test is that all students must be given a fair chance to demonstrate their achievement of the learning outcomes being measured. This means a physical and psychological environment conducive to their best efforts and the control of factors that might interfere with valid measurement. Students will not perform at their best if they are tense and anxious during testing. The antidote to anxiety is to convey to the students, by word and deed that the test results are to be used to help them improve their learning. They should also be reassured that the time limits are adequate to allow them to complete the test. This, of course, assumes that the test will be used to improve learning and that the time limits are adequate. The things to avoid while administering a test are: (a) do not talk unnecessarily before the test, (b) keep interruptions to a minimum during the test, (c) avoid giving hints to pupils who ask about individual items, (d) discourage cheating.

## CLINICAL EVALUATION

Clinical evaluation enjoys a dominant position in nursing education so as the clinical teaching. Clinical evaluation is essential to ascertain the attainment of the objectives of clinical posting. Providing fair and reasonable clinical evaluation is one of the most important and most challenging faculty roles. Assessment of clinical performance provides data from which to judge the extent to which students have acquired specified learning outcomes.

According to Caldwell, when clinical performance is evaluated, students' skills are judged as they relate to implementation of an established standard of patient care. Acceptable clinical performance involves behavior, knowledge and attitudes that students gradually develop in a variety of clinical settings. The ultimate outcome of clinical performance evaluation is safe and quality patient care. Clinical performance evaluation gives feedback to the students about performance and provides data that may be used for individual development, assigning grades and making decisions about the curriculum. According to Redman, students have the right to a reliable and valid evaluation that assesses achievement of competencies required to take on the role of the novice nurse when they successfully complete nursing educational program. Good clinical evaluation includes multidimensional evaluation with diverse evaluation methods completed over time, seeking student growth and progress. All evaluation should respect students' dignity and self-esteem.

According to Wanda Bonnel, the faculty have primary responsibility for the student clinical evaluation. Faculty are knowledgeable about the purpose of the evaluation and the objectives that will be used to judge the students' performance. Clarity of purpose provides direction for selection of evaluation tools and process.

Faculty need to be aware of differences between their own value systems and those of their students because this can bias the evaluation process. Additionally, when faculty are supervising a group of students in the clinical area, they can only sample student behaviors. Limited sampling of behaviors or individual biases may result in an unfair or inaccurate clinical evaluation. Because of these limitations, faculty should use a variety of evaluation methods. Additionally, faculty can consider evaluation input from other sources. Potential adjuvant evaluators include students, nursing staff, peer evaluators and patients.

### Purposes of Clinical Evaluation

The purposes of clinical evaluation are: (a) to evaluate the competency, especially the speed and accuracy in providing nursing care, (b) to provide feedback and reinforce positive behavior, (c) to assist students in refining their clinical skills, (d) to diagnose deficiencies and to undertake appropriate remedial measures, (e) to provide information essential for conducting guidance and counseling, (f) to judge the adequacy of the objectives of clinical posting.

### Clinical Evaluation Methods and Tools

According to Gaberson, a variety of approaches should be incorporated in clinical evaluation including cognitive, psychomotor and affective considerations as well as cultural competence and ethical decision making.

Fair and reasonable evaluation of students in clinical settings requires use of appropriate evaluation tools that are effective and ideally efficient for faculty to use. Any evaluation instrument used to measure clinical learning and performance should have criteria that are consistent with course objectives. Instrument content can vary according to the academic level of a student and can also relate to the teaching institution's purpose and philosophy. A faculty group decision about the tools to be used for data collection is essential for fair evaluation. Many clinical evaluation tools have been developed and implemented within clinical settings.

Usually clinical evaluation proforma for each clinical subject is prepared and students are continuously assessed in the clinical area. Class coordinator submits the filled clinical evaluation proforma to the principal or head of the department on a monthly basis.

In Halstead's opinion, strategies for evaluation of clinical experience include: (a) observation, (b) written communication, (c) oral communication and (d) simulation. Because clinical experience is complex in nature, a combination of methods is recommended for conducting evaluation in a fair and reasonable manner **(Table 10.3)**.

Anecdotal records, checklists and rating scales are discussed elsewhere in this chapter.

## Charting and Patient Progress Notes

In Higuchi's opinion, writing cogent nursing and progress notes is an important clinical skill. Evaluating the charting done by the student provide faculty with an opportunity to assess the student's ability to process and record relevant data. Students' skill in using healthcare terminology and documentation practices can be examined and critical thinking process can be demonstrated in these notes.

## Nursing Care Plans

Nursing care plans allow faculty to evaluate students' ability to determine and prioritize care needs according to the understanding and interpretation of individual patient's health problems. Because of the availability of numerous standardized care plans, students rarely use their critical thinking ability to prepare care plan. Hence care plan is not a reliable tool to assess critical thinking ability of students.

## Standardized Patient Examination

According to Borbasi and Koop standardized patient examination, sometimes referred to as **objective structured clinical examinations (OSCEs)** can be described as "pretend patients" in an artificial environment designed to simulate actual clinical conditions. A simulation

**TABLE 10.3:** Commonly used sample evaluation strategies and tools by category.

| | |
|---|---|
| Observation | • Anecdotal notes<br>• Checklists<br>• Rating scales |
| Written | • Charting/progress notes<br>• Care plans<br>• Process recordings (especially in psychiatric nursing)<br>• Paper and pencil tests |
| Oral | • Student interviews and case presentation<br>• Clinical conferences |
| Simulations | • Standardized patient examination<br>• Role play |

center, modeled as an authentic clinical environment with standardized patients, can provide a safe setting in which to observe and document student competencies. Standardized patients can provide feedback to students and help ensure competence before students begin practice in the "real" world. Multiple evaluators can observe and test students in the performance of numerous skills during brief examination periods. Many faculty members consider OSCE process as an acceptable and powerful instrument in clinical performance evaluation. OSCE is a quick and efficient evaluation method, allowing for rapid feedback to students about identified clinical deficits.

## CLINICAL EVALUATION PROCESS

According to Halstead and Billings, before the evaluation process begins faculty and students need a clear understanding of the outcomes to be attained from the clinical experience. Clinical evaluation is a systematic process with three consecutive phases: (1) preparation, (2) clinical activity phase, and (3) final data interpretation and feedback. A listing of sample tasks within each phase are provided in **Box 10.2**.

## INTERNAL ASSESSMENT

In nursing education, internal assessment is equally important as university examinations. Results of the internal assessment are considered along with the university examination scoring while grading the students. Moreover, a minimum prescribed internal assessment score is essential for writing the university examinations. Internal assessment should be incorporated wisely into the total nursing educational program and should supplement the university examinations.

Internal evaluation enables the teacher to diagnose the students' difficulties in the clinical area and the classroom so that she can take timely remedial measures. Since internal evaluation

---

**Box 10.2:** Role of faculty evaluator during the clinical evaluation process.

**Phase I: Preparation**
- Determine objectives and competencies
- Identify evaluation methods and tools
- Choose clinical site
- Orient students to the evaluation plan
- Focus on objectivity in evaluation

**Phase II: Clinical Activity**
- Orient students and staff to the student role
- Provide students clinical opportunities
- Ensure patient safety
- Observe and collect evaluation data
- Provide student feedback to enhance learning
- Document findings, maintain privacy of records

**Phase III: Final Data Interpretation and Presentation**
- Interpret data in a fair, reasonable and consistent manner
- Assign grade
- Provide summative evaluation conference (ensure privacy and respect confidentiality)
- Evaluate experience

*Source*: Halstead and Billings
*Courtesy*: Evolve Publications

is continuous, it builds regular study habit among students. This will in turn help students to prepare well for the university examinations. Properly conducted internal evaluation provides feedback and thereby motivate the students. Misuse of internal assessment by the teachers can be minimized by setting guidelines intended to safeguard the rights of students and through increasing the validity and reliability of test items.

## SELF-ASSESSMENT AND SELF-REPORTING TECHNIQUES

There are some areas of student development, however, in which the teacher's evaluation of behavior is apt to be inadequate unless observations are supplemented and complemented by the students' self-assessment through employing self reporting techniques. By self-assessment, we mean an assessment system which involves the students in establishing the criteria and standards they will apply to their work and then making judgments about the degree to which they have been met. Anecdotal records, rating scales, interview, questionnaire, sociometric techniques and personality inventories can be used for self-reporting.

## SUMMARY

Evaluation is the process of judging the value or worth of an individual's achievements or characteristics. Educational evaluation is concerned with judging the value or worth of the goals attained by the education system. Evaluation, measurement, assessment and testing are interrelated but have unique features. Evaluation is based on sound principles. Evaluation is closely linked to instructional objectives and instructional process. Functions of evaluation can be divided into functions related to instructional process and functions related to education system as a whole. Based on the frequency of conducting, evaluation can be classified into summative evaluation and formative evaluation. According to the nature of measurement, evaluation can be classified into maximum performance evaluation and typical performance evaluation. Based on the method of interpreting results, evaluation can be classified into criterion-referenced evaluation and norm-referenced evaluation.

Techniques of evaluation are written examination, oral examination, practical examination, interviews, observation, projective techniques and sociometric techniques. Tools of evaluation include tests, anecdotal records, checklists, cumulative records, interview schedules, inventories, questionnaires and rating scales. Achievement test is a systematic procedure for determining the amount a student has learned through instruction. Achievement tests employed in nursing can be classified into oral test, written and performance test. Written test include essay tests and objective tests. Essay test is classified into extended response type and restricted response type. Objective test offers a variety of test items like true-false item, multiple choice item, matching type, extended matching type, multiple-response item, assertion-reason item, and interpretive item, short answer type and completion type. Each test item has its own advantages and disadvantages.

Validity, reliability and usability are the three main characteristics of an achievement test. Steps involved in the construction and administration of an achievement test are planning, developing test design, preparation of blueprint, construction of items, organization of the test, preparation of a scheme for evaluation and test administration. The guiding principle in administering any achievement test is that all students must be given a fair chance to demonstrate their achievement of learning outcomes being measured. Clinical evaluation is concerned with the judging of the quality of the student's performance in the clinical area. Most frequently used tools for clinical evaluation are checklists, rating scales and anecdotal records. Internal assessment should be incorporated wisely into the total nursing educational program and should supplement the university examinations. It is better to enrich teacher's evaluation with students' self-assessment. Anecdotal records, rating scales, interviews, questionnaire, sociometric techniques and personality inventories can be used for self-reporting.

## MULTIPLE CHOICE QUESTIONS

1. Judging the worth or value of a situation is called:
   a. Measurement
   b. Evaluation
   c. Test
   d. Assessment
2. Systematic procedure for measuring a sample of behavior is called:
   a. Measurement
   b. Evaluation
   c. Test
   d. Assessment
3. Assessment for learning is:
   a. Formative evaluation
   b. Summative evaluation
   c. All of the above
   d. None of the above
4. Assessment for learning is:
   a. Formative evaluation
   b. Summative evaluation
   c. All of the above
   d. None of the above
5. Which is an example of a tool of evaluation?
   a. Checklist
   b. Oral examination
   c. Interview
   d. Observation
6. Which is an example of a technique of evaluation?
   a. Interview
   b. Checklist
   c. Intelligence test
   d. Performance test
7. Anecdotal record is used mainly for:
   a. Observation
   b. Interview
   c. Tests
   d. Practical examination
8. Short essay is an example of which achievement test:
   a. Selection type
   b. Supply type
   c. Restricted response type
   d. None of the above
9. Multiple choice is an example of which achievement test:
   a. Selection type
   b. Supply type
   c. Restricted response type
   d. None of the above
10. OSCE is an example of:
    a. Clinical evaluation method
    b. Written test
    c. All of the above
    d. None of the above

### ANSWER KEY

| 1. b | 2. a | 3. a | 4. b | 5. a | 6. a |
| 7. a | 8. c | 9. a | 10. a | | |

# CHAPTER 11

# Guidance and Counseling

## LEARNING OBJECTIVES

**After completing this chapter, reader will be able to:**

- Define guidance.
- Define counseling.
- Explain the characteristics of guidance.
- Explain the characteristics of counseling.
- Describe the bases of guidance and counseling.
- Identify the aims of guidance.
- Describe the principles of guidance.
- Explain the functions of guidance and counseling.
- Identify the need for guidance and counseling in nursing education.
- Recognize the guidance areas.
- Explain the guidance and counseling services.
- Classify counseling.
- Describe the levels of counseling.
- Explain the approaches to counseling.
- Describe the phases of counseling.
- Identify the qualities of a counselor.
- Recognize the do's and don'ts in counseling.
- Explain the role of class teacher as counselor.
- Identify the problems of student counseling.
- Explain the organization of guidance and counseling services in nursing institutes.

## GUIDANCE

One of the most important areas in education which has acquired considerable importance and received much attention in recent years is guidance and counseling. Present day teachers have to acquire some specialized knowledge regarding guidance and counseling in order to guide the students tactfully in this highly competitive world. As students are living in a materialistic and consumer-driven society under the influence of media, the possibility of deviating from the healthy lifestyle is more than ever before, making guidance and counseling an integral part of the modern education system. Guidance and counseling ensures a healthy climate in the institution, which is essential for the harmonious and integrated personality development of students. Let us see in detail regarding guidance and counseling with special reference to nursing education.

### Concept of Guidance

According to NCERT, guidance can be explained as assistance made available by a competent person to an individual to help him direct life course, develop a point of view, make decisions and be better adjusted with situations. Guidance does not mean giving directions, nor is it an imposition of one's point of view on another person. The person who is giving guidance does not take the responsibility of making decisions on behalf of the client. We can see that guidance is more about assisting people to find their way rather than giving instructions or readymade solutions.

## Definition of Guidance

Hamrin and Erikson define guidance as "that aspect of educational program which is concerned especially with helping the pupil to become adjusted to his present situation and to plan his future in line with his interests, abilities and social needs".

According to Crow and Crow, "Guidance is not direction. It is not making decisions for an individual which he should make for himself. It is not carrying the burden of another's life. Rather, guidance is assistance made available by competent counselor to an individual of any age to help him direct his own life, develop his own points of view, make his own decisions and carry his own burdens."

In the educational context, guidance means assisting students to select courses of study appropriate to their needs and interests, achieve academic excellence to the best possible extent, derive maximum benefit of the institutional resources and facilities, inculcate proper study habits and satisfactorily participate in curricular and extracurricular activities or in other words, guidance is a process of assisting or helping the students in developing their potentialities, in solving their immediate or future problems and in planning their own future wisely thereby enabling them to lead a successful personal and social life.

## Characteristics of Guidance

Guidance offers all-round assistance to individual in all aspects of his/her development whenever required. Thus, guidance connotes the function of giving the needed enlightenment–particularly in unknown areas. Guidance makes use of the science of psychology to determine the aptitudes, interests, intelligence, personality, attitudes, etc. and the discipline of education for providing the right and suitable assistance. Guidance has the following characteristics:

1. **It is a process:** As a process, it helps every individual to help himself, to recognize and use his inner resources to set goals, to make plans and to work out his own problems of development.
2. **It is a continuous process:** It is needed right from early childhood, adolescence, adulthood and even in the old age.
3. **Choice and problem points are the distinctive concerns of guidance:** Guidance operates in the zones in which the individuals own unique world of perceptions interacts with the external order of events in his life context.
4. **It is the assistance to the individual in the process of development rather than a direction of that development:** The aim of guidance is to develop the capacity for self-direction, self-guidance and self-improvement through an increased understanding of one's problems, resources available to solve the problems and limitations to solve the problem.
5. **Guidance is a service meant for all:** It is a regular service, which is required at every stage for every student, not only for awkward situations and abnormal students. It is a positive program geared to meet the needs of all students.
6. **Guidance is both generalized and a specialized service:** It is a generalized service because everyone—teachers, parents, advisors—play a part in the program. It is a specialized service because especially qualified personnel, such as counselor, psychiatrists and psychologists render their services needed to help the individual to get out of his problem.
7. **Guidance is an organized service and not an incidental activity of the school:** It is broad based and has a definite purpose. It makes use of the entire facilities available in the school to achieve its objectives and if needed brings about changes in the guidance program in order to meet new demands or challenges.

8. **Guidance is not a branch of any discipline:** Even though it draws insights and methods from psychology, sociology, anthropology, philosophy, economics, etc. It is not a branch of any of these disciplines.
9. **Guidance has limits:** It has limits to what it can accomplish.
10. **Guidance is more an art than science:** While guidance should always utilize the tested results, guidance practice most often makes decisions on the basis of best judgment in the absence of complete scientific verification.
11. **Guidance has its roots in the education system:** Guidance program followed in a particular country must be based on the broad educational objectives of that country.
12. Above all, guidance is centered around the needs and aspirations of students.

# COUNSELING

## Concept of Counseling

Counseling is a scientific process of helping an individual by an expert to manage a difficult situation. Counseling involves relationship between two persons in which one of them (counselor) attempts to help the other (counselee or client) to adjust with a life situation or attain self-actualization. It is a relationship of natural respect between counselor and counselee. By the process of counseling counselee acquire independence and develop sense of responsibility. Counseling process is carried out around the felt needs of the counselee.

The main objective of counseling is to bring about a voluntary change in client. For this purpose, the counselor provides help to achieve the desired change or make a suitable choice. The client alone is responsible for the decisions or choices he makes, though the counselor may assist in this process by his warmth and understanding relationship. Thus, counselor helps counselee to discover and solve his problems independently.

## Meaning

Counseling is a process of enabling the individual to know himself and his present and possible future situations in order that he may make substantial contributions to the society and to solve his own problems through a face-to-face personal relationship with the counselor. Thus, *counseling is an enabling process.* Counseling is also a learning-oriented process carried on in a social environment in which the professionally competent counselor attempts to assist the counselee using appropriate procedure to become a happy and productive member of the society by formulating realistic and purposeful goals for attaining total growth.

In the educational context, counseling is a method of intervention when the teacher observes that a student under her care or supervision exhibits a problem that may be affecting his role performance. Ideally, counseling is a therapeutic process, wherein a student seeks the teacher's help is assisted to clearly identify his problem and to find methods of resolving his problem by utilizing all the resources available to him.

## Definition

❖ Stone and Shertzer define student counseling as 'an interaction process that facilitates meaningful understanding of self and environment and result in the establishment and/or clarification of goals and values for future behavior'.
❖ Roges writes of effective counseling as 'a definitely structured permissive relationship which allows the client to gain an understanding of himself to a degree which enables him to take new positive steps in the light of his new orientation'.

- According to counseling consortium, "counseling is a professional relationship that empowers diverse individuals, families and groups to accomplish mental health, wellness, educational and career goals".
- This definition highlights the following aspects of counseling:
  - Counseling deals with wellness, personal growth, career, education and empowerment concerns.
  - Counseling is conducted with persons individually, in groups and in families.
  - Counseling is diverse and multicultural and
  - Counseling is a dynamic process.

## Characteristics of Counseling

Analysis of the above definitions reveal the following characteristics of counseling.
- Counseling involves two individuals—one seeking help and the other a professionally trained person who can help the first. The one who seeks the help is known as the counselee and the one who provide the help is the counselor.
- There should be a relationship of mutual respect between the two individuals. The counselor should be friendly and cooperative and the counselee should have trust and confidence in the counselor.
- Counseling is aimed at bringing about desired changes in the individual for self-realization and providing assistance to solve problems through an intimate personal relationship.
- The counselor discovers the problems of the counselee and helps him to set up realistic goals and guide him through difficulties and problems.
- If the counselee is a student, counseling helps him to take a decision, make a choice or find a direction in matters related to an educational program or career.
- It helps the counselee acquire independence and develop a sense of responsibility. It also helps him explore and fully utilize his potentials and actualize himself.
- It is more than advice giving. Solution emerges through the thinking that a person does for himself rather than through solutions suggested by the counselor.
- It involves something more than offering an assistance to find a solution to an immediate problem. Its function is to produce changes in the individual thereby enabling him to deal with the difficulties in a more productive and independent manner.
- Counseling is democratic. Counseling takes place in a non-threatening and democratic atmosphere, which allows the counselee to think independently with the counselor and not under the counselor.
- Counseling concerns itself with attitudes as well as actions.
- Emotional rather than purely intellectual attitudes are the raw materials of the counseling process. Information and intellectual understanding have their place in the counseling, but it is the emotionalized feelings which are most important.
- Counseling is a body of techniques that helps individuals to grow up normally through guided learning. It helps an individual to know himself better, gives him confidence, encourages his self-directiveness and provides him with new vision to grow and flourish.
- In the educational context, counseling is centered around the needs and aspirations of students.

## DIFFERENTIATION OF GUIDANCE AND COUNSELING

Very few terms have been more freely or interchangeably used than the terms 'guidance' and 'counseling'. Guidance is mainly preventive and developmental, whereas counseling is remedial as well as preventive and developmental. Intellectual attitudes are the raw materials of the guidance process but emotional rather than purely intellectual attitudes are the raw materials of the counseling process. Thus, in guidance, decision making operates at intellectual level, whereas in counseling it operates at emotional level.

As far as education is concerned, the counseling service is one among various services offered by the guidance program. *Thus, in education, our goal is guidance and our technique among others is counseling.* Counseling is called the crux, heart, essence or pivot of the guidance program. The success or failure of the guidance program is determined by counseling service. This importance has helped the counseling to outgrow all other services of the guidance program and to achieve a status more or less equal to the guidance. *Thus, in strict sense, mentioning guidance and counseling instead of guidance in the educational context is just like mentioning central nervous system and brain.*

Guidance focuses on helping individuals choose what they value the most, whereas counseling helps them to make change. In other words, guidance helps an individual in choosing the best alternative. Counseling helps to change the perspective for helping individual to find the solution of the problem by himself or herself.

Guidance is mainly preventive in nature. Counseling is mainly remedial and curative in nature. Guidance usually focuses on education and career related matters. Counseling focuses on personal and socio-psychological aspects. Guidance can be given by a superior or an expert. Counseling is given by a person who possess high level of skill and professional training.

Counseling and guidance are not synonymous terms. Guidance is a relatively more comprehensive process which includes counseling as one of its functions. Counseling is a part of guidance, not all of it. Counseling is a specialized and important part of total guidance process. Thus, all counseling is guidance but all guidance is not counseling.

## BASES OF GUIDANCE AND COUNSELING

A program of guidance and counseling is based on sound philosophical, psychological, sociological and pedagogical grounds.

### Philosophical

A guidance and counseling program enables the student to adjust himself to the ethics of life by assisting him to develop a sound philosophy of life in accordance with the realities of day to day living. Students need to be helped to keep themselves balanced and adjusted so that they may be receptive to the great values which their student years offers them.

### Psychological

Guidance and counseling program has to consider the individual differences among students and should provide each student with the greatest opportunity to know himself. This will help the student to manage the problems of maladjustment. Above all, self-awareness will enable the student to utilize the opportunities waiting for him in life. In short, psychological basis of guidance and counseling advocates for the personal as well as social development of the student.

### Sociological

This deals with the proper utilization of human resources, good citizenship, vocational awareness and building better relationship between students and their family members. Through the creation of vocational awareness among the students, guidance and counseling program can assist students to formulate sound educational and vocational plans based on realistic self-appraisal. Sociological basis is also concerned with integrating education system with the needs of the society, developing a positive attitude towards change, finding solutions to problems arising out of coeducation and controlling indiscipline.

## Pedagogical

As the word meaning indicates, this basis correlates with the ultimate aim of education, i.e., the all-round development of the student. According to the pedagogical basis, as a counselor or guidance worker, teacher has to understand the needs, abilities and interests of the students in order to promote their all-round development. Teachers have to ensure optimum achievement or academic growth by assisting students in the choice of curricular and cocurricular activities, increasing the holding power of schools and helping students to solve the pedagogical problems.

## FUNCTIONS OF GUIDANCE AND COUNSELING

Guidance and counseling have three-fold functions, namely—adjustmental, orientational and developmental. They also assist the teachers in understanding their students, especially in identifying the gifted and backward children. This will help the teachers to recognize the individual difference among students.

## Adjustmental

Guidance and counseling are adjustmental in the sense that they help the students in making the best possible adjustment to the current situations in the educational institution, in the home and the community. Professional and individual aid is given in making immediate and suitable adjustment at problem points. At the same time, the adjustive attitude as per the below mentioned words of Reinold Neibuhr is to be developed in individuals.

"God grant me the serenity,
To accept the things, I cannot change,
The courage to change the things I can,
And the wisdom to know the difference".

In accordance with the words of Reniold, guidance and counseling should enable the students to accept the things which they cannot change in life, to modify or change the things which they can in order to achieve success in life and to differentiate between what they can change and cannot change in life. For instance, a student cannot change his short stature but he can change, i.e., get rid of the inferiority complex that has arisen out of the short stature by giving more importance to his good character and academic achievements. *In fact, the ability to differentiate between the things which we can change and cannot will help us a lot in leading a happy life.*

## Orientational

Guidance and counseling have orientational function also. They orient the students in the problems of career planning, educational programming and direction towards long-term personal aims and values. This orientation will serve as a foundation for formulating realistic plans regarding future education and after education career.

## Developmental

Guidance is developmental in that it is concerned with helping the pupils to achieve self-development and self-realization. Through assisting in the achievement of self-development and self-realization, they can prevent problems and maladjustments rather than curing the damage occurred as a result of problems.

## PURPOSES OF GUIDANCE AND COUNSELING

The guidance and counseling purposes include assisting students, teachers and school administrators to:

- Promote readiness to learn. "Readiness to learn" involves the attainment of skills, knowledge and attitudes. Readiness to learn prepare students to achieve learning objectives of the curriculum.
- Make students aware of their abilities, assets, liabilities and potentials.
- Assist students in making appropriate and satisfying personal, vocational and educational choices.
- Assist students to develop a positive image of self through understanding their needs and abilities.
- Assist teachers in understanding the needs and problems of each student.
- Assist school administrators in educational planning.
- Mobilize all the available resources of the school or home for attaining the learning aims of students.
- Help students to develop proper attitude, values, morals, beliefs and discipline.
- Help students to optimize and utilize their skills and correct their shortcomings.
- Assist students to live within the framework of an institution.
- Help students to develop a good sense of self-awareness, ability to acquire good knowledge and ability to make good decisions or choices.
- Help students to attain positive mental health and value human endurance or human effectiveness.

## NEED OF GUIDANCE AND COUNSELING

The problems of students must be properly tackled with an intention to solve them. Unresolved problems may affect not only the academic performance of students but also their personality development. Guidance and counseling help teachers to solve the student's problems with their active involvement. They also assist the teacher in creating a healthy climate in the institution by ensuring harmonious and integrated personality development of students.

The need for counseling and guidance can be summarized as follows: (a) to help in the total development of students, (b) to assist students in leading a healthy life by abstaining from whatever is deleterious to health, (c) to help in the proper selection of educational programs, (d) to help in the selection of careers according to their interests and abilities, (e) to help the students in vocational development, (f) to develop readiness for changes and to face challenges, (g) to minimize the mismatching between education and employment and help in the efficient use of manpower, (h) to help freshers establish proper identity, (i) to identify and motivate the students from weaker sections of society, (j) to help students overcome the period of turmoil and confusion, (k) to identify and render help for students who are in need of special help, (l) to ensure proper utilization of time spent outside the classrooms, (m) to help in tackling problems arising out of student explosion and coeducation, (n) to make up the deficiencies at home. (o) To minimize the incidence of indiscipline, (p) to motivate the youth for self-employment, (q) to assist the needy students in availing financial assistance from appropriate organizations.

In a survey conducted by all India educational and vocational guidance associations for assessing college students' needs, major problems reported by 50% of the respondents highlights the need of guidance and counseling in educational institutions. The major problems are:
- Gap between expectations and performance
- Lack of knowledge regarding careers and professions
- Anxiety regarding the future
- Lack of concentration in studies
- Inability to make friends or deal with members of the opposite sex
- Lack of knowledge regarding sexual matters
- Lack of awareness regarding one's strengths and weaknesses
- Lack of awareness regarding one's aptitude and abilities
- Lack of awareness regarding resources
- Lack of knowledge regarding effective learning strategies
- Inability to live in the present moment by forgiving oneself for past mistakes.

**Developmental needs of adolescents** also underlines the need of a robust guidance and counseling program. According to Okon, a need is a condition within an individual that motivates him to adopt certain kind of behavior. Durojaiye stated that developmental needs of adolescents include:
- Attaining individuality
- Making progress towards an organized personality pattern
- Developing philosophy of life
- Developing concepts of values and desirable behavior
- Achieving a place in the society
- Understanding of personal assets and liabilities
- Preparing plans for future living
- Establish healthy personal relationships with individuals of both sexes
- Learning to live independently
- Learning to adjust to changes resulting from physical and social relationships
- Learning to attain adult status by vocational plans, family and social relationships and citizenship plans.

All these needs of adolescents underlines the need of guidance and counseling program.

## NEED FOR GUIDANCE AND COUNSELING IN NURSING EDUCATION

The need for guidance and counseling in nursing education is very obvious. Different from their past learning experiences, nursing students are exposed to a situation where errors are detrimental and commitment is the way of life. Many students who have joined for nursing are unaware about the realities waiting for them as nursing students. They opted nursing just because of a promising future ensured by the nursing career. Guidance and counseling will assist them in developing proper attitude, commitment, dedication and other qualities required for a successful nursing practice. Moreover, emerging and re-emerging diseases, technological advancements in the patient care, evolving of new specialities, especially in the clinical areas, changing role of nurses in the healthcare sector, impact of consumer protection act, etc., underlines the need of a viable guidance and counseling service in all nursing institutes. The need for guidance and counseling in nursing education can be summarized as follows:
- To help students adjusting with the new environment of the nursing institute

- To help in developing qualities required for a successful nursing practice.
- To help students in getting adjusted with the clinical environment.
- To help students keeping in touch with the latest trends in nursing and to reap benefits from the trends.
- To help students in developing positive learning habits, especially in skill learning so that they can retain and transfer the learned lessons in a better way.
- To help in the development of appropriate coping strategies in order to deal with stress in a productive manner.
- To help nursing students in establishing proper identity.
- To help them develop a positive attitude towards life.
- To help them to overcome periods of turmoil and confusion.
- To help students in developing their leadership qualities.
- To motivate them for taking membership in professional organizations after completing their studies.
- Help them to make advantages of the technological advancements in the patient care.
- Help them develop readiness for changes and to face challenges both in the personal as well as professional life.
- Help them to carry out the responsibilities as a worthwhile health team member.
- Help them in the proper selection of careers both in India and abroad.
- Motivate them to do higher studies according to their abilities and interest.
- To assist the needy students in availing financial assistants from appropriate organizations.

## AIMS OF GUIDANCE

According to National Guidance Association of America, the aims of guidance can be stated as follows: (a) to help the schools adapt the needs of the pupils and the community and to make sure that each child obtains the equality of opportunity which is the duty of the schools to provide, (b) to assist individuals in choosing, preparing for, entering upon and making progress in occupation, (c) to provide knowledge regarding the characteristics of the common occupations and problems of the occupational world, (d) to secure help for the worker to understand his relationship to workers in his own and other occupational settings and to society as a whole, (e) to secure better cooperation between schools on the one hand and the various commercial, industrial and professional pursuits on the other hand, (f) to encourage the establishment of courses of study in all institutions of learning that will harmoniously combine the cultural and practical studies.

Humphrey and Traxler state that the aims of guidance are to help the individual: (a) to understand himself, (b) to make the most of his capacities, interests and other qualities, (c) to adjust himself satisfactorily to the varied situations within his total environment, (d) to develop the ability to make his own decisions, (e) to make his own unique contributions to society to the finest possible extent.

## PRINCIPLES OF GUIDANCE

According to Hollis and Hollis, there are eight principles on which any guidance program should be based. They can be modified in order to meet the requirements of the local context where guidance is carried out. The principles are: (a) the dignity of the individual is supreme, (b) each individual is different from every other individual, (c) the primary concern of guidance is the individual in his social setting, (d) the attitudes and personal perceptions of the individual are the basis on which he acts, (e) the individual generally acts to enhance his perceived self, (f) the individual has the innate ability to learn and can be helped to make choices that will lead to self-direction consistent with social improvement, (g) the individual needs a continuous guidance process from early childhood through adulthood, (h) each individual may at times need the information and personalized assistance best given by competent professional personnel.

According to Crow and Crow there are fourteen significant guidance principles. They are:

1. Every aspect of a person's complex personality pattern constitutes a significant factor of his total displayed attitudes and forms of behavior. Guidance services which are aimed at bringing about desirable adjustment in any particular area of experience must take into account the all-round development of the individual.
2. Although all human beings are similar in many respects, individual differences must be recognized and considered in any efforts aimed at providing help or guidance to a particular child, adolescent or adult.
3. The functions of guidance is to help a person:
   - Formulate and accept, stimulating, worthwhile and attainable goals of behavior,
   - Apply these objectives in the conduct of his affairs.
4. Existing social, economic and political unrest is giving rise to many maladjustive factors that require the cooperation of experienced and thoroughly trained guidance workers, counselors and the individual with a problem.
5. Guidance should be regarded as a continuing process of service to an individual from young childhood through adulthood.
6. Guidance service should not be limited to the few who give observable evidence of its need, but should be extended to all persons of all ages who can benefit there from either directly or indirectly.
7. Curriculum materials and teaching procedures should evidence a guidance point of view.
8. Although guidance touches every phase of an individual's life pattern, the generally accepted areas of guidance include—concern with the extent to which an individual's physical and mental health interfere with his adjustment to home, school and vocational and social demands and relationships or the extent to which his physical and mental health are affected by the conditions to which he is subjected in these areas of experience.
9. Parents and teachers have guidance appointed responsibilities.
10. Specific guidance problems of any age level should be referred to persons who are trained to deal with particular areas of adjustment.
11. To administer guidance intelligently and with as thorough knowledge of the individual as is possible, programs of individual evaluation and research should be conducted and accurate cumulative records of progress and achievement should be made accessible to guidance workers. Through the administration of well selected standardized tests and other instruments of evaluation, specific data concerning degree of mental capacity, success of achievement, demonstrated interests and other personality characteristics should be accumulated, recorded and utilized for guidance purposes.
12. An organized guidance program should be flexible according to the individual and community needs.
13. The responsibility for the administration of guidance program should be centered in a personally qualified and adequately trained chairman or head of guidance, working cooperatively with his assistants and other community welfare and guidance agencies.
14. Periodic appraisals should be made for existing school guidance programs. The success of its functioning should rest on outcomes that are reflected in the attitudes towards the program of all who are associated with it—guider, guide, etc., and in the displayed behavior of those who have been served through its functioning.

# GUIDANCE AREAS

Guidance help students to make proper adjustments with the environment which they are living and also make the best possible contributions commensurate with one's strengths and limitations. Every individual, at sometime or other needs help to become happier, more creative and better adjusted in his family and society. There are several areas where student require assistance. These areas can be classified into education, vocation, personal, social, avocation, health, moral, religion and financial. Let us see each area in detail with special emphasis to nursing education.

# EDUCATIONAL GUIDANCE

Educational guidance help the students to get maximum benefit out of education and to solve their problems related to education. The emphasis is on providing assistance to students to perform satisfactorily in their academic work, choose the appropriate course of study, overcome learning difficulties, foster creativity, improve levels of motivation, utilize institutional resources optimally, such as library, laboratory, etc. The function of guidance in this area are: (a) to help the students make educational plans consistent with their abilities, interests and goals and to select appropriate courses and cocurricular activities which will enable them to join careers of their choice. They also need to be guided for developing good study habits, prepare for examinations properly and face examinations with confidence, (b) help the students to explore educational possibilities beyond their present educational level. They need to be guided in selecting subjects for specialization and additional courses of studies. They also need to be made familiar with the various fellowships, scholarships, competitive examinations, etc., so that their journey ahead becomes smooth and profitable, (c) provide help at crisis points of students in their academic and personal life, (d) monitor academic progress of students and help the students who are not studying as expected, (e) identify special learners, such as academically backward, gifted and creative and provide help in meeting their educational needs, (f) diagnose the learning difficulties of students in different subjects and assist them to overcome the difficulties, (g) help students in their adjustment to curricular and cocurricular demands of the educational programs.

## Principles of Educational Guidance

The strategies that teachers adopt to plan and implement educational guidance must be appropriate to the problems for which they are needed. The following are some of the principles on which educational guidance must be based: (a) they should be based on clear cut objectives, (b) every student is capable of achieving the best of his ability, (c) individual differences in academic achievement of students must be recognized, (d) the strategies adopted must be student oriented, (e) the strategies must take into consideration the resources and facilities available to the students, (f) educational guidance is not meant for a few students only; they need to be provided to all.

## Educational Guidance in Nursing Education

In nursing education, guidance must perform the following functions in the educational area: (a) provide an orientation regarding the aim and philosophy of nursing education, (b) help them to differentiate between previous learning experiences and the learning experiences they are going to receive in the nursing institute, (c) help them to develop an awareness regarding the qualities required for a successful nursing practice, (d) help students to develop a realistic educational planning, (e) help them to make an objective analysis regarding their own abilities and interests, (f) help students in developing positive learning habits, especially in skill learning so that they can retain and transfer the learned lessons in a better way, (g) provide an orientation regarding the clinical area and the methods of teaching employed there with special reference to the student's role in terms of active participation, (h) help them to utilize institutional resources, such as clinics, library, various labs, etc. to the maximum extent possible, (i) provide knowledge regarding the latest trends in nursing education and nursing service. This will help them to plan their career and higher education, (j) motivate them to do higher studies and help in choosing specialization according to their needs and interests. This can be done by providing information regarding higher education, such as qualifying examinations, fellowships, etc. (k) assist them in preparing for the internal assessments and university examination.

## VOCATIONAL GUIDANCE

Vocational guidance is the assistance provided for selection of a vocation and preparation for the same. It is concerned with enabling students to acquire information about career opportunities, career growth and training facilities. For organizing an effective vocational guidance program, the teacher has to consider the student's goals, needs, interests and emotional characteristics.

The functions of vocational guidance are: (a) enabling the students to discover information about themselves–their abilities interests, needs, ambitions and above all what is expecting from them, (b) providing them information regarding the dynamic nature of the modern world, the advantages and disadvantages of different occupations and educational courses, the qualifications necessary for entry into them and the range of opportunities available to them, (c) provide them with a frame of reference in which to see themselves in relation to these educational and vocational opportunities; to orient them to the helping agencies available to them and to alert them to future decision making points in their career, (d) promote self-understanding and to develop educational and occupational plans, (e) providing placement services to help them implement those plans, (f) providing follow-up service to help them; if necessary, when faced with future decision making situations, (g) train students for entrepreneurship. This function is very important in the light of the new world order where money is not a problem for starting a new venture. Individuals with adequate knowledge and commitment can easily convert their knowledge into money by starting new ventures with the help of financial institutions.

### Vocational Guidance in Nursing Education

The functions of vocational guidance in nursing education are: (a) provide a clear picture regarding the latest trends in nursing service and nursing education, such as changing roles of nurses, emerging new specialties, especially in the clinical areas, etc. (b) help the nursing students to find a suitable career either in the nursing education or service according to their skills, abilities and interests, (c) orient them to the abroad opportunities and assist them in preparing for the qualifying examinations, such as CGFNS, NHS examination, etc. (d) *since good English is the key to success around the world,* provide them an idea regarding the English language tests conducted in various countries, such as TOFEL, IELTS, OET, etc. (e) guide students in preparing curriculum vitae or biodata and conduct mock interviews to prepare them for the upcoming interviews, (f) conduct placement services in association with reputed man power consultants and do the follow-up services. This function can be carried out easily due to the advancements in the communication and information technology. Many nursing institutes have tie-ups with well-known manpower consultants, which will help them in ensuring promising careers to the students either in India or abroad, (g) another important function is to collect opinions and suggestions from the passed out students regarding the various aspects of the educational program. Guidance service should also try to get a feedback from the institutions regarding the performance of the passed out students placed through it. Valuable suggestions from the passed out students and employers should be handed over to the curriculum committee for further actions. This will also help in the curriculum revision.

An increasing global demand for qualified nurses and the emergence of various specialties in nursing in order to meet the challenges of the modern healthcare system has given a face-lift to this area of guidance in nursing education. More than ever before nursing institutions are giving much consideration to vocational guidance. Some institutes even renamed their guidance and counseling services into guidance, counseling and placement services to show their commitment towards vocational guidance. Even though placement service is a part and parcel of vocational guidance, the word placement is separately mentioned with an intention to highlight the help rendered to the students by the institute in the matter of finding a promising career. Of course, this renaming does not carry any sense except some cosmetic advantages, but it is a clear indication of the elite status grabbed by this area of guidance.

## PERSONAL GUIDANCE

Personal guidance refers to the guidance offered to students for enabling them to adjust themselves to their environment so that they become efficient citizens. Adolescent behavior, to a great extent, depends upon the moods and attitudes of the adolescent. Emotional instability is a characteristic of adolescents and this is often the cause of many of their personal problems. Personal guidance will help them to solve these problems. Severe competition and irrational expectations of the parents also lead to personal problems.

Students may find it difficult to follow the lectures, especially when exposed to a new medium of instruction. Difficulty in understanding in turn leads to disliking of teachers and ultimately results in poor achievement. Guidance needs to be provided to such students to enable them to adjust to the situation which they cannot change.

The functions of personal guidance can be summarized as follows: (a) help students improve mental health, (b) assist students in becoming progressively responsible for their own development, (c) assist students to understand and resolve their emotional problems, (d) assist students in exploring various mechanisms of adjustment, (e) assist students to get control over emotions, (f) assist students to deal with the difficulties of personal as well as academic life, (g) help students to develop interpersonal skills, (h) help students to accept themselves and others, (i) help students to solve the problems of coeducation, (j) help students to maintain healthy heterosexual relationships, (k) assist students to deal with the stress in a productive manner, (l) assist students to overcome the times of turmoil and confusion, (m) help students to find suitable accommodation if needed and to adjust with the hostel life.

### Personal Guidance in Nursing Education

Since a large number of students opt nursing without prior knowledge regarding nursing education, personal guidance has to play a vital role in nursing education. In addition to the above listed functions, personal guidance has the following functions in the nursing education: (a) assist students to deal with homesickness: Many nursing students are staying in the hostel for the first time in their life and this creates a lot of homesickness. A well-planned interaction with the parents by the teachers in presence of students, assigning *a teacher guardian* for every group of ten students, arrangements for a comfortable hostel stay and a well-organized orientation program in an informal atmosphere will reduce their homesickness within a short period of time, (b) protect students from the ragging: Now-a-days, ragging is not a problem in a civilized campus, even then precautions should be taken to avoid any incident of ragging. Even though prevention of ragging is an administrative aspect, many institutes seek the help of guidance and counseling service to prevent it. Ragging can be prevented by constituting an antiragging committee with the active participation of senior students, motivating first year students to report any incidents of ragging, educating all students regarding the consequence of ragging and conducting surprise visits to the hostel where first year students are staying, (c) assist students to develop proper attitude required for a successful nursing practice: In addition to the routine teaching sessions, personal guidance also contributes to the proper development of attitudes among students. Personal guidance helps the students differentiate between empathy and sympathy and contributes to the nurturing of the former. In the presence of empathy, compassion and commitment will naturally develop to the needed extent, (d) assist students to adjust with the new learning experiences and to overcome learning difficulties: Personal guidance help students to adjust with the new learning experiences, especially those provided in the clinical areas, special help should be rendered to students in the matter of developing mastery in English. Maintaining a wall magazine for displaying literary works in English, insisting to speak in English rather than the local language, encouraging to read English periodicals and newspapers and placing a vocabulary board outside the library to display meaning of five words per day will help them in developing fluency in English. This will also help them in scoring high grades in the future qualifying examinations like TOFEL, IELTS, etc., (e) help students develop emotional maturity: In the clinical area, nurses have to face many situations which may cause an emotional breakdown in the case of freshers. Helping students to develop empathy rather than sympathy, teaching them to analyze events in the clinical area with a rational basis, teaching them the healthy ways to ventilate emotions and above all, educating them regarding the role of a nurse in the critical situations will help develop emotional maturity, (f) assist Students to cope with the Stress: In fact, nursing students are the only student group who are forced to bear the responsibility of staff before completing their studies. In many hospitals, nursing students are posted in the place of staff nurses to look after the patients. This immature shouldering of responsibility creates enormous stress among nursing students. Unfortunately, in many of the cases, nursing faculty are helpless and only thing they can do is to equip the student to convert this stress laden situation into an opportunity oriented one. Teaching relaxation techniques, ensuring the availability of teachers round the clock to help students in the crisis situation, constituting peer groups and assigning senior students to look after juniors are some of the ways to deal with the stress among nursing students, (g) help students achieve balance between personal and professional life: From the very beginning itself students should be taught how to achieve balance between personal and professional life and the danger of giving more importance to professional life at the cost of personal life and vice versa. Equal importance should be given to both and there should be a clear cut demarcation between the two for a successful life. Students should be instructed to concentrate on other responsibilities after returning from the clinics instead of being preoccupied with the matters related to patient care, (h) help students develop a healthy interpersonal relationship with other health team members, patients and others related to patient care.

## SOCIAL GUIDANCE

Social guidance enables the student to make substantial contributions to the society, assume leadership, confirm to the social norms, work as team members, develop healthy and positive attitudes, appreciate the problems of society, respect the opinions and sentiments of fellow human beings, acquire traits of patience, perseverance and friendship. Its main purpose is to enable the student to become an efficient citizen.

## Social Guidance in Nursing Education

In nursing education, social guidance has to perform the following functions: (a) train students for leadership and followership qualities—since nursing is experiencing a shortage of capable leaders, this function of guidance deserves special attention. Various leadership development programs should be conducted under the guidance service in cooperation with the student nurses association to promote leadership qualities among nursing students, (b) help students to carry out their responsibilities as a responsible health team member—nurses constitute 50% of the total healthcare workers and to a certain extent success of any health team is determined by how well the nurses render their service. So special care should be taken to inculcate a sense of accountability and responsibility among nursing students, (c) assist them in acquiring desirable set of values and developing a positive life philosophy, (d) motivate students to become a responsible member of professional organizations, (e) social guidance also help students develop a healthy interpersonal relationship with other health team members, patients and others related to patient care, (f) motivate students to contribute towards bridging the gap between nursing education and nursing service.

# AVOCATIONAL GUIDANCE

Avocational guidance is the assistance to be provided to students to spend their available leisure time profitably. Activities and programs outside the formal classrooms provide many opportunities for the blossoming of talents of students.

## Avocational Guidance in Nursing Education

Functions of avocational guidance in nursing education are: (a) help students prepare for the monthly educational and cultural programs conducted by SNA, (b) assist students to conduct programs related to World Health Day, Nurses Day, etc. (c) assist students to participate in the activities of National Service Scheme, Drug Bank, Blood Donors Forum, etc. (d) help students to use their leisure time to increase their vocabulary by reading English periodicals, newspapers and hearing English news, (e) help students who are spiritually inclined to meet their spiritual needs, (f) help students to develop hobbies related to nursing care, such as collecting drug literature.

# HEALTH GUIDANCE

Health guidance implies the assistance rendered to students for maintaining sound health. Sound health is a prerequisite for participating in curricular and cocurricular activities. This type of guidance focuses on enabling students to appreciate conditions for good health and take steps necessary for ensuring good health, maintaining sound physical and mental health.

## Health Guidance in Nursing Education

The functions of health guidance in nursing education are: (a) conduct periodic health check-up of students and maintain the health records, (b) insist students to take universal precautions strictly, especially when posted in infectious departments, (c) alert students to take vaccines correctly, (d) motivate students to take food regularly, especially breakfast for maintaining good health, (e) motivate students to seek help of the faculty members when they are under stress, (f) ensure the availability of faculty members round the clock to help students in matters related to health, (g) motivate students to seek medical help in the initial stage of disease itself, (h) supervision of college facilities, such as hostels and canteen to see that healthful condition are maintained.

## FINANCIAL GUIDANCE

The function of financial guidance is to help the needy students in determining the financial assistance they need in the light of the expected expenses and to get it from financial organizations after completing the formalities. Earlier financial guidance was included along with the personal guidance. Nowadays, a new guidance area, namely—finance and welfare is also mentioned along with other areas of guidance. Some students are hard-pressed for finances. They need to be guided regarding fee concessions, scholarships, stipends, etc., available in the institution or offered by other welfare agencies and how and when to apply. The provision of financial assistance has to be ensured so that no meritorious student is denied education for lack of financial assistance. In this era of liberalization, securing an educational loan is not a big task. Any talented student can pursue education by seeking hassle free, easily repayable educational loans. Nursing students also require financial guidance just like other students.

## GUIDANCE AND COUNSELING SERVICES

According to Kochar, in order to meet the diversified needs of the students, an effective guidance program will have to offer the following services: (a) the preadmission service, (b) the admission service, (c) the orientation service, (d) the student information service, (d) the information service, (e) the counseling service, (f) the placement service, (g) the remedial service, (h) the follow-up service, (i) the research service, (j) the evaluation service.

It needs to be pointed out that different labels have been given to the different services for practical considerations only. A good guidance program, in fact, is a unified program—all the specific services woven into it. The various services have to be supportive of one another for best results. We will discuss the services which are related to the nursing education. The pre-admission service helps the high school students get admission into the right course once they complete their schooling.

## ADMISSION SERVICE

Admission service is concerned with:
- Admitting the right candidates for the right course for the maximum advantage both to the individual and the society.
- Selecting those candidates most likely to succeed and to keep wastage figures and dropout rate at the minimum level. Admission service, to be effective, will comprise a carefully framed criterion of admission, some entrance test and interview. For admission to reputed nursing institutes this triple measure is adopted. Admission service in nursing institutes should be centered around the attitude of the candidates. As far as nursing education is concerned, it is easy to train a student with right attitude compared to a student with undesirable attitude and high intelligence.

## ORIENTATION SERVICE

Orientation service is essentially a "welcome service" as it is concerned with welcoming freshers to the world of nursing. Orientation program is organized by the guidance and counseling department in association with other faculty and staff. Usually a two day orientation program is arranged. First day sessions are mainly interactive sessions with the freshers and their parents or guardians with an intention to convince them about the facilities available for students. Principal, faculty members and other staff introduce themselves to the students, and students also introduce themselves through a brief introduction. On the first day, parents are allowed to see the nursing institute, hostels and parent hospital where students are posted for clinical experience so that they can compare the facilities with the brochure. Principal gives a brief note regarding the philosophy, vision, mission, rules and regulations of the institute and request the cooperation of parents towards the smooth functioning of the institute. She also explains the measures taken to prevent ragging of any form in the campus. The counselor speaks about the student welfare programs and highlights the role of parents in transforming the freshers to well qualified professional nurses. Head of the office department explains about the expected mess bill per month, formalities to be completed for opening a bank account, etc. Wardens of the boys and girls hostel also clarifies their roles and request cooperation for the smooth running of the hostels. First day sessions mainly aims to reduce the severity of the impending homesickness among freshers and to minimize the anxiety of parents. Second day sessions are meant only for freshers and deals with confidence building measures and matters related to nursing education, such as role of the student, role of the faculty, utilization of resources, etc.

## STUDENT INFORMATION SERVICE

The student information service is concerned with:
- Assist the student to obtain a realistic picture of his abilities, interests, personality characteristics, achievements, levels of aspirations, state of health, etc.
- Enable the student to know himself on a socio-comparative basis.
- Provide a record of students' progress.
- Help the guidance workers and others to understand him more adequately. This service involves collecting essential data about the students and orderly maintenance of records to assist the students as well as their advisers in making important decisions.

## INFORMATION SERVICE

Information is an essential part of every guidance program, whether we want to assist the student to make better choices, help him in better adjustment or optimum development. Information provided under this service can be categorized under three headings, namely: (a) educational information, (b) occupational information, and (c) personal-social information.

### Educational Information

Educational information usually provide the following information to the students:
- Information regarding higher studies, such as post-certificate BSc nursing, postgraduate programs, MPhil and PhD. Regarding postgraduate educational programs, the information should include the merits, limitations and scope of each speciality. Information regarding entry criteria and institutions offering these programs should also be made available to students.
- Detail information pertaining to clinically oriented higher studies, such as trauma nursing, dialysis nursing will help them select the appropriate one according to their interests and abilities. Current trend in nursing favors clinically oriented higher studies than others.
- Information regarding the trends in nursing education and nursing service and ways to make advantage from the prevailing trends.

- Information related to the sources of knowledge, such as textbooks, journals, internet and the ways and means to utilize these sources effectively.
- Information regarding ways to develop positive learning habits, especially skill learning and positive transfer of learning.

### Occupational Information

Occupational information serves the following purposes: (a) provide a clear picture regarding the scope of nursing in terms of career opportunities so that they can prepare in advance for selecting a good career, (b) give information regarding the ways of selecting a good career in nursing and achieving career growth, (c) give information regarding the skills, abilities and other attributes required for a particular career in nursing, (d) furnish detailed information related to internationally reputed qualifying examinations, such as CGFNS, NHS examinations, etc. and English language tests, such as TOFEL, IELTS, etc. (e) give information regarding the ways to acquire mastery in English, (f) provide details regarding the sources of information related to job vacancies, such as advertisement columns of nursing journals and publications like employment news, assignments abroad, etc.

### Personal-Social Information

Personal-social information provides the following information to students: (a) information regarding the ways to lead a well-rounded life, (b) information pertaining to the ways to inculcate essential qualities of a nurse, such as empathy, compassion, commitment, perseverance, etc. (c) information regarding the ways to deal with stress, (d) information related to the development of a philosophy of life, (e) information regarding the ways and means to achieve success in professional life without undermining the personal life.

A variety of activities, such as educational and career conferences, work experience seminars, discussion groups and individual interviews constitute the main media for implementing the information service.

## COUNSELING SERVICE

The counseling service involves helping the student to: (a) Understand what he can do and what he should do, (b) understand the choices he faces—the opportunities open to him and the qualifications he possesses for the goal he has chosen, (c) handle his difficulties in a rational way and strengthen his best qualities, (d) make his own decisions and plans on the basis of self-understanding, accept responsibility for the decisions and actions.

Counseling is helpful in crystallizing the problem and reaching a reasonably good solution. That way counseling is one of the most distinctive of all the guidance services.

## PLACEMENT SERVICE

An increasing global demand for qualified nurses has considerably improved the status of placement service in the nursing institutes. Thus, this service is considered as an important service in the guidance program. Realizing the need of an efficient placement service many nursing institutes have already renamed their guidance and counseling service into guidance, counseling and placement service. The functions of placement service in nursing institutions are: (a) help students to be in proper scholastic track so that placement service can easily place them in good careers when they pass out with flying colors, (b) help students realize their career expectations by assisting them in finding a suitable job according to their attributes, (c) organizing campus selection interviews in association with man power consultants and reputed hospitals and teaching institutions, (d) provide information regarding the current trends in nursing and motivate students to reap benefits out of the trends, (e) conduct career conferences with an intention to provide information regarding the qualifying exams, such as CGFNS, NHS examination, etc., and the English language tests, such as TOFEL, IELTS, etc. This will also help the students develop their competitive abilities and to boost their morale, (f) conduct periodic talks of the passed out students who are working in reputed positions both in India and abroad, (g) conduct mock interviews and other tests for the outgoing students in order to equip them for the upcoming interviews and tests, (h) conduct workshops to improve the English handling skill of students. This will help them to become global nurses with adequate communication skills.

## REMEDIAL SERVICE

In nursing education, remedial service is mainly oriented towards helping the students to improve their study habits, improve their adjustment in the clinical areas, reducing the stress and to guide properly in matters related to the relationship between other health team members. Major defects noted are handled by the counseling service with the help of professionals.

## FOLLOW-UP SERVICE

Follow-up is that review or systematic evaluation which is carried out to find out whether guidance service in particular and educational program in general satisfies the needs of the students. It has to be seen to what extent have the students been able to achieve according to their abilities and aptitudes, to what extent curricular and cocurricular choices have been wise and how are the passed out students adjusting with their jobs. The typical follow-up techniques employ one or more of the following techniques-interview, post-card survey or questionnaire.

The follow-up service can be maintained through follow-up interviews with the passed out students or sending follow-up questionnaires to them. Follow-up services also concerned with seeking the opinion of employers regarding the performance of passed out students.

Information obtained through follow-up techniques can be used for improving the curriculum, stimulating better teaching, increasing the value of the guidance services and establishing better college and community relationship. In nursing education, it is not uncommon that the clinical posting schedules and durations are changed on the basis of the follow-up services without changing the minimum requirement prescribed by the curriculum.

## RESEARCH SERVICE

Research service is intended to examine both the personnel in the college guidance program and the techniques of guidance used by them so as to discover their strong and weak points and ultimately strengthen the whole program. Research can give the guidance staff greater psychological security because of a knowledge of the effectiveness of their efforts. It can also provide a basis for guidance development program. Research has to be a continuous process, it cannot be "done" and "forgotten".

## EVALUATION SERVICE

The evaluation service completes the entire process of guidance. Evaluation service determines the effectiveness and efficiency of the guidance program. Less number of dropouts, harmonious relationship between teachers and students, good results, well placed passed out students, long standing relationship with man power consultants and reputed organizations or institutions, sense of security feeling expressed by the students, appreciation of students' performance in the clinical area, less number of problematic students and above all, a satisfied student body are the indicators of a well-functioning guidance and counseling department.

Guidance and counseling program in a college can work effectively if all these services are organized in an efficient manner. If organized well and implemented effectively, these services will facilitate good teaching and efficient learning and thus prove as necessary supplements to academic achievement, which is the primary responsibility of educational institutions.

## GUIDANCE AND COUNSELING PERSONNEL

According to Kochar, guidance is an all inclusive program intend to help the students achieve their optimum potential. It is both a generalized and a specialized service. Naturally, therefore, in such a program the total needs of the students need to be met by the total staff. One cannot assign the teaching-learning relationship to the teacher, the counseling relationship to the counseling officer and the smooth functioning relationship to the administrator. Infact, everybody who comes into contact with the student, contributes in one way or the other in his growth and development. Hence, guidance is a cooperative responsibility of all the members of staff-professionally and technically qualified counseling officers and deans and not well qualified—in terms of counseling—but very important are the: administrators, teachers, advisors, wardens, physical education instructors, doctors, librarians, parents—in fact all those who come into contact with the student in some form or the other. Each one can contribute his share according to his capabilities and training.

## GUIDANCE FUNCTIONS OF TEACHERS

According to Zeran and Riccion, the following are the guidance functions of teachers.
- Know and use basic principles of human behavior
- Develop skills in observing and analyzing student behavior in order to identifying problems at the earliest.
- Provide information to student about his abilities so that he can set realistic goals in accordance with the abilities.
- Place emphasis on self-understanding, self-direction, utilization of potentials and acceptance of responsibilities for actions by the student.
- Assist principal in establishing an organized program of guidance services
- Recognize the need of specialized guidance personnel and refer needy students to them.
- Assist in providing data for the student's cumulative record and utilize these data in a professional manner.
- Review constantly course content and curriculum to meet student needs.
- Give attention to all phases of the student's developmental patterns rather than just with his intellectual achievements.
- Assist students whenever possible and refer to specialized personnel if needed.
- Attend in-service programs for acquiring new competencies in performing the guidance activities.

## WHAT GUIDANCE IS NOT?

Guidance is not compulsion, prescription, domination, cut and dried planning regimentation. It is not making decisions for the one guided. It is not an advice. Guidance does not mean cuddling or pampering the student; but it provides more suitable programs for him.

## PURPOSES OF STUDENT COUNSELING

Dunsmoor and Miller are of the view that the core of student counseling is to help the student help himself. From this point of view, they describe the following purposes of student counseling: (a) to give the student information on matters important to success, (b) to get information about student which will be of help in solving his problems, (c) to establish a feeling of mutual understanding between student and teacher, (d) to help the student work out a plan for solving his difficulties, (e) to help the student know himself better—his interests, abilities, aptitudes and opportunities, (f) to encourage and develop special abilities and right attitudes, (g) to inspire successful endeavor toward attainment, (h) to assist the student in planning for educational and vocational choices.

It is obvious that goal of counselling is problem clarification and self-directed needs. The counselor helps the student to understand the problems and helps the student to help himself. In this process, the role of the student is objective self-assessment of the situation and the role of counselor is to formulate the decision making process and to act as a stimulator of insights and sensitivities of the student.

Counseling does not solve the problems but helps in solving and if solution is not possible, to help face challenges and to live with them. In short, counseling aims at developing students' self-understanding, self-acceptance and self-confidence.

## WHEN COUNSELING IS REQUIRED?

The following are some of the situations in which counseling is needed: (a) when the student needs not only reliable information but an interested interpretation of such information in order to meet his own personal difficulties, (b) when the student needs a wise, sympathetic listener with broad experience than his own, to whom he can reveal his difficulties and from whom he may gain suggestions regarding his own proposed plan of action, (c) when the counselor has access to facilities for helping in the solution of a student's problem to which the student does not have easy access, (d) when the student is unaware that he has a certain problem but for his best development to make him aware about the problem, (e) when the student is aware of a problem and of the strain and difficulty it is causing, but is unable to define and understand it and is unable to cope with it independently.

## WHO SHOULD BE COUNSELED?

The following types of students are in urgent need of counseling: (a) students who have a consistent record of under achievement, (b) students whose scholastic achievement drops suddenly, (c) students who find it difficult to participate in class and extra-class activities, (d) students who use exhibitionism for gaining recognition or attention in class, (e) students who find it difficult to adjust to the college or clinical areas, (f) students who suddenly decide to dropout of college, (g) students who display unusual ability in any direction—intellectual, artistic, musical, etc., (h) students who have behavioral problems, such as drug addiction, aggressiveness, bullying, stealing, shyness, timidity, etc.

## CLASS TEACHERS AS COUNSELORS

Given the desirability of student counseling, who is to act as a counselor? The student's teacher? An outside expert? The continuing controversy on this question has been reviewed by and on the one side are those who maintain that all counselors must be classroom teachers: They best understand the problems of behavior in the classroom; they have experience of aberrant behavior; they can meet their students as partners in search for an answer to behavioral problems. On the other side are those, such as and who states categorically that 'the nature of the relationship to the student-client must be necessarily be different from that of the teacher to the pupil'. Students, it is claimed, feel 'safer' in discussing their problems with someone who does not represent 'authority' and who seems to be neutral in matters concerning the college. Because effective counselors need to be well grounded in psychology and its applications, it is not possible for the practising teacher to move easily—even should he possess appropriate expertise-from one role to another. According to SK Mangal are 'while some teachers might become good counselors, all counselors need not be classroom teachers, nor need not necessarily have ever been classroom teachers'. A rational division of labor would involve the training of the classroom teacher in the recognition of stress signs, for example, severe learning difficulties and behavioral problems and knowledge of when to hand over consideration of the problem to a trained counselor.

## LEVELS OF COUNSELING

There are three levels of counseling namely, informal counseling, nonspecialist counseling by professionals and professional counseling. *Informal counseling* is any helping relationship by a responsible person who may have little or no training for the work. *Nonspecialist counseling by professionals* is the help provided by physicians, nurses, lawyers, teachers and others who do a great deal of face-to-face work with psychological problems in the course of their other work. Sometimes, special titles are used, such as "religious counseling", "financial counseling", etc., to denote this level of counseling. *Professional counseling* is helping another person with decision and life plans, whether personal, educational or vocational, by a person especially trained for this work. Professional counselors are usually psychologists or educational psychologists.

## CLASSIFICATION OF COUNSELING

Counseling can be classified according to the nature of the problem, the complexity of treatment and the competence of the counselor. In one way, we can classify counseling into surface level counseling, next level counseling and therapeutic counseling.

*Surface level counseling* is offered when the student wishes only some item of information. The counseling given may be casual; it is brief, and it may be superficial in that it is not extensive or intensive. *Counseling at the next level* requires a more prolonged contact because the counselee needs more and complicated information. When the student is seriously disturbed, *therapeutic counseling* may be needed.

In another way, we can classify counseling into: (a) developmental, (b) preventive, (c) facilitative, and (d) crisis counseling.

Developmental counseling aims the all-round development of the individual by helping him to: (a) achieve personal growth by making him aware about himself and his opportunity-aden environment, (b) Formulate goals commensurate to his abilities and attaining them, (c) Develop right attitudes, values, etc. Preventive counseling helps the individual face the untoward incidents, such as failure in the examinations, not getting the desired job, etc., in the future life. In education, preventive counseling mainly focus on the prevention of drug abuse, suicides, etc., among students. Facilitative counseling is intended to correct an undesirable behavior. It is also known as remedial or adjustive counseling. Crisis counseling helps the individual overcome the crisis situations with minimum damage. Counselor helps the individual to get a realistic view regarding the crisis situation and to develop appropriate pattern of behavior so that he can deal effectively with the feelings associated with the crisis situation, such as anxiety, guilt, etc.

## DIFFERENT COUNSELING TECHNIQUES/APPROACHES TO COUNSELING

Based on the nature of the counseling process and the role of the counselor, there are three approaches to counseling, namely—directive, nondirective and eclectic counseling.

### Directive or Prescriptive or Counselor-centered Counseling

Directive counseling is an approach in which the counselor uses a variety of techniques to suggest appropriate solutions to the problem of counselee. In this approach, the counselor plays a leading role. The basis of directive counseling advocated by EG Williamson is that counseling is possible only when an individual is able to accumulate adequate data to form the basis for an analytic diagnosis of the problem. The counselor's role in this type of counseling is to assist his student in getting such data and to suggest suitable solutions. He tries to direct the thinking of the counselee by informing, explaining, interpreting and advising. However, the decision has to be taken by the counselee.

### Nondirective or Permissive or Client-centered Counseling

Nondirective counseling is a counselee-centered approach in which he is guided to use his own inner resources to solve the problem. In this approach, the counselee plays a predominant role. Carl R Rogers is the exponent of the nondirective technique of counseling.

### Eclectic Counseling

In eclectic counseling, the strategy arises out of the appropriate knowledge of student behavior and a combination of directive, nondirective and other approaches. Irrespective of the differences, all approaches should have developmental, preventive, and remedial values.

## PHASES OF COUNSELING

Phases of counseling are described in a variety of ways. Generally phases of counseling include:
1. Appointment and establishing relationship
2. Assessment
3. Diagnosis
4. Setting goals
5. Interventions
6. Termination and follow-up.

The phases may overlap each other and each phase enriches the other phase.

### Appointment and Establishing Relationship

Since counseling is essentially a face-to-face relationship between the counselee and counselor, this phase is the most important one in the process of counseling. Appointment with the counselee is fixed according to the convenience of both the counselor and counselee. The principle governing the counseling relationship are uniqueness of student, his capacity to choose and decide what is good for him, belief in his ability to make changes, teacher communicating respect, maintaining confidentiality, being non-judgmental and a trusting relationship. It may take several sessions to establish a trusting relationship with the counselee.

### Assessment

This phase is concerned with data collection, analyzing the data and clarification of expectations. The counselee is encouraged to talk about his problems, ventilate his feelings, whereas the counselor asks questions, collects information, observes and possibly helps the counselee clearly state his problem. Counselee also talks about his expectations.

### Diagnosis

In this phase, the counselor diagnosis the problem of the student and decides the areas of intervention.

### Setting Goals

In this phase, the counselor explains to the student what is possible, i.e., setting goals which will in turn provide direction to the counselee and counselor. Goals may be of two types—immediate or short-term goals and long-term goals. Short term goals ultimately lead to the attainment of long-term goals. Goals can be changed according to the new information or new insight.

### Intervention

Interventions are needed to achieve the goals. In this phase, counselor explains to the student how the goals can be achieved. The intervention employed will depend upon the technique used by the counselor, the problem and the students. Intervention is a process of adaptation and the counselor should be prepared to change the intervention when the selected intervention is not yielding results.

### Termination and Follow-up

Successful termination is an important aspect in counseling. It must be done without destroying the accomplishment gained and should be done in a phased manner covering few sessions. This will prevent the development of a feeling of sense loss in the counselee. Follow-up appointments, i.e., planning for the next sessions, if needed should also be carried out.

## COUNSELING INTERVIEW

While undertaking the formal functions of a counselor, the class teacher has to follow the below mentioned generally accepted guidelines without forgetting the importance of an individual approach to a particular, often unique, situation.

As far as possible an attempt should be made to alter the physical environment, i.e., the room in which the interview will be held so as to avoid any suggestion of an authoritative relationship between counselor and student. One of the objectives of the interview must be to put the student at ease so as to establish a friendly atmosphere in which conversation will flow naturally; this requires an absence of any trappings suggesting an impassable gulf between the parties. Wide tables separating the parties, furniture which stresses hierarchical status, will not be conducive to the creation of a relaxed atmosphere in which confidence is to be established. A couple of easy chairs, not separated by table or desk, is often found suitable.

The interview which is designed to build a foundation of trust and confidence requires openness from both parties; this will require patient work on the part of the counselor. He must use a style of language appropriate to the occasion and must remember the significance of body language and its interpretation by the student. Gestures which might be interpreted as indicating impatience, hostility, incredulity, disapproval are out of keeping with the nature and purpose of this type of interview, in which existing anxieties may be fed by perceptions of hostility in the counselor.

Careful questioning, based on the use of open-ended questions and designed to give no suggestion of a forensic cross examination, is essential. The purposes of questioning in this situation are to elicit information and to present the student with an opportunity of explaining the basis of behavior and perhaps, anxieties. Hence, questions must not embarrass; where they do, silence or obfuscation and evasion will be the response. A teacher placed in the position of counselor must be prepared to hear unstructured, incomplete, contradictory sets of responses to his simple questions; it is for him to listen, to ask for elucidation, but not to criticize the form or content of those responses. Probing will be resented and may be perceived as an attack on the student's self-esteem.

Hambling advocates utilization of the technique of 'funneling'. This involves the counselor approaching the particular problem at its 'broad end', with appropriately wide, open questions and then narrowing the questions until the kernel of the problem is reached. The process requires an atmosphere of confidence and an absence of any mutual suspicions as to integrity. Understanding, on the part of the counselor, will emerge, Hamblin suggests, only if he is able to put himself in the 'student's shoes' and is prepared to await results. The diagnosis which may follow the first interview and the creation of confidence are to be seen as the most important objectives of that occasion.

## QUALITIES OF A GOOD COUNSELOR

The counselor should possesses certain qualities in order to conduct counseling in a successful manner. These qualities are depicted in the **Table 11.1**. Do's and Don'ts are depicted in **Table 11.2**.

## PROBLEMS IN STUDENT COUNSELING

The major problems inherent in the counseling process derive from its very nature. It demands certain personal qualities, such as spontaneity, genuineness, nonpossessive warmth and sensitivity to low-level signals coming from the student; the counselor must not only possess these qualities, he must convince the student that he does possess them. Counseling also requires skills of a high order—an ability to establish a confidential relationship with students of all types, a knowledge of the techniques of eliciting and analyzing information, an understanding of the prevalent, so called, 'youth culture' and acquaintance with a variety of social environments. Its success involves patience and persistence. In Roger's words, it requires the creation of a nonthreatening, nonjudgmental environment, characterized by an attitude of empathy and respect for the student. Above all, perhaps, it requires more than a superficial acquaintance with the principles of psychotherapy. The formidable list of desirable qualities in the student counselor is a pointer to and a warning against, the morass in which the well-intentioned, but ill-equipped, amateur may find himself.

Further problems may arise from the possible clash of goals and beliefs in the interviewing process which is inseparable from counseling. How is the strong-minded counselor, possessed of a morality founded on deeply-held ethical principles, to react when faced with 'values of nihilism'? How does the professional teacher respond to the expressions of an 'anticulture' which denies the validity of that in which he believes? In short, how does the counselor achieve the 'understanding neutrality' said to be required in the counseling process?

The complexities of the counseling relationship are outlined by Munro in the enumeration of essential conditions of such a relationship. These conditions are described as 'of an ethical

**TABLE 11.1:** Qualities of a good counselor.

| | |
|---|---|
| Good listener | Has resources, or knows where resources are available |
| Nonjudgmental warm | Will refer if and when appropriate |
| Approachable | Has a comfortable office and privacy |
| Genuine | No telephone or other interruptions |
| Mature | Looks after plants properly (so may hopefully be nourishing and supportive objective to clients) |
| Confidential sense of humor | Long experience as a good counselor |
| Has/makes time | Dresses appropriately |
| Common sense | Not easily embarrassed |
| Creative | Free or fees not too expensive |
| Imaginative | Cares about clients |
| Perceptive | Has 'good vibes' |
| Notices nonverbals | Looks healthy |
| Notices what is felt out | Does not use jargon, or at least |
| Notices where pain is | Translates jargon |
| Focuses | Looks interested, alive and friendly |
| Good pacing/timing | Strong minded and able to speak about |
| Confronts appropriately | Upsetting things |
| Calm | Does not want to take over or make you like himself |
| Keeps fairly still | |
| Empathic | Encourages independence of himself and others |
| Knowledgeable | |
| Supportive | Can deal with panic, knows about physiology of anxiety, tension, stress, headaches, breathing, etc. |
| Does not advise | |
| Does not preach | |
| Makes good, pleasing eye contact | Can recognize and deal with neurotic and psychotic behavior |

nature' and include: a higher degree of confidentiality than is normally expected from a teacher, an insistence on the essentially voluntary nature of the relationship; insistence on the client's responsibility for his/her own behavior.

Some teachers who have practised as counselors have reported their feelings of inadequacy when the complex reality of problems of a classroom deviance is uncovered. Family backgrounds, financial difficulties, health concerns and emotional entanglements may have woven a web from which the student cannot be extricated, save by a long term process of adjustment, requiring assistance which is totally beyond the counselor's power and resources. Frustration on both sides is deepened when the counselor's diagnosis reveals a situation from which escape seems quite impossible.

The problem of confidentiality often emerges at an early stage in student counseling, sometimes in the first meeting where the interviews produce criticisms of a counselor's

**TABLE 11.2:** Do's and don'ts in counseling.

| Do's | Don'ts |
|---|---|
| • Do have a liking for people, especially young people<br>• Do have a caring attitude<br>• Do know that you are 'learning'<br>• Do listen well<br>• Do know that you are not a 'knowall"<br>• Do remember each of the principles of counseling<br>• Do maintain a record<br>• Do work on assessment, diagnosis and prognosis<br>• Do discuss with experienced professionals<br>• Do maintain confidentiality<br>• Do be punctual for appointments<br>• Do prepare in advance for the next appointment<br>• Do be aware of 'transference' | • Do not label the student<br>• Do not get too close to the student emotionally or physically<br>• Do not take sides<br>• Do not share secrets with your student<br>• Do not abuse or manipulate the student<br>• Do not talk loosely about the student<br>• Do not use their lingo<br>• Do not jump to conclusions<br>• Do not accept gifts or favors<br>• Do not protect the student<br>• Do not be manipulated by the students |

teaching colleagues, is it to be conveyed to them? Where an interview reveals activities of a criminal nature, are the police to be informed? What is the legal situation of a counselor who, aware of such activities fails to inform the authorities? Is it possible to create the conditions necessary for a successful counseling interview if the student is aware that the principle of confidentiality may be breached?

## ORGANIZATION OF GUIDANCE AND COUNSELING SERVICES

School level, size of the school, student needs, community interests, faculty attitudes and budgetary provisions are some of the factors that determines the nature of guidance and counseling service in any institution.

## FORMS OF ORGANIZATION

### Centralized Services

In a centralized guidance and counseling service, entire responsibility of the guidance service is vested upon a group of trained personnel or department of guidance and counseling service.

Counseling activities are done by the selected members of the teaching staff under the direction and supervision of the guidance staff.

### Decentralized Services

In decentralized services, the responsibility of rendering guidance service is vested upon the teachers. Guidance minded teachers may give excellent and timely assistance to their students. Absence of a specially trained person to give professional assistance to students is the drawback of this type of service.

### Combination of Centralized and Decentralized Services

Adopting the midway between centralization and decentralization is the best way to organize an effective guidance and counseling service. The counseling department headed by the counselor and the faculty will cooperate with each other for the welfare of the students. Counselor provides the specialized service in a professional manner with the help of faculty members and the faculty members provide nonspecialized services and refer students who need special service to the counselor.

## BASIC CONCEPTS RELATED TO GUIDANCE AND COUNSELING SERVICES

### Purposes to be Achieved

The purposes of the guidance and counseling service should be formulated on the basis of needs and should be communicated to all who are concerned. The purposes are usually stated in the form of objectives of the guidance program.

### Functions to be Served

After finalizing the purposes or objectives, the next step is to determine the specific functions to be performed in order to achieve the guidance goals.

### Allocation of Responsibility and Authority

The guidance abilities and interests of the individual members of the staff have to be assessed so that specific functions can be assigned according the personal capacity. Establishing clear cut line of authority will help everyone distinguish his duties from those of others. This will prevent any occurrence of misguidance at the cost of students.

### Appraisal of the Program

Appraisal of the guidance program is essential to maintain its relevance. The efficiency of the program should be tested against the changing needs of the students and the society. Appropriate measures should be taken to rectify any noted defects in order to keep the program more students friendly.

## REQUIREMENTS FOR ORGANIZING GUIDANCE AND COUNSELING SERVICES

Requirements for organizing guidance and counseling services are: (a) trained counselors and guidance workers, (b) planned programs to meet objectives, (c) consultation services, (d) evaluation instruments, such as psychological tests, inventories, etc. (e) student data bank, (f) educational and vocational information service, (g) programs for cooperation between home and school, (h) programs for integrating community services with guidance services, (i) in-service educational programs for teachers, counselors and other personnel to provide knowledge regarding the current trends in guidance, (j) physical facilities, (k) budgetary provisions.

Physical facility include rooms, furnitures and other equipment needed for guidance and counseling department. In order to have privacy for personal advises, the space can be divided in such a way that there will be several private offices as well as general offices.

## GUIDANCE COMMITTEE

The main purpose of guidance committee is to "carry forward the total guidance program through the united efforts of management, principal, guidance personnel, teachers, parents and students." To this end, the committee should be a representative of all these groups, with the possible exception of the parents and students. However, in some circumstances, it might be advisable to obtain the views of both parents and students as well. The guidance committee serves the following additional purposes: (a) it establishes and maintains policy, (b) it articulates the program between the school and the community, (c) it acts in a planning capacity to ensure that the various functions of guidance are properly coordinated, (d) it helps clarify particular roles, offers support when these roles are challenged, (e) it prepares the way for guidance personal to function in cooperation with community agencies, such as business organizations, employer groups, voluntary agencies, etc. (f) it serves a source of ideas and recommendations to be submitted to appropriate bodies, such as curriculum committees, professional associations of teachers and department of education.

## PRINCIPLES OF ORGANIZATION OF GUIDANCE SERVICES

- **Child centeredness:** Guidance services should be organized while keeping in view of the needs and interest of students.
- **Continuity:** Guidance services should be continuous because development and learning is a continuous process.
- **Wholeness:** Guidance services should be concerned with the whole individual in his total environment and with specific needs and principles.
- **Prevention as well as cure:** Guidance should be organized to deal not only with problems after they arise but also with the prevention of problems.
- **Specialization:** Guidance is a specialized service. It should be provided by competent individuals.
- **Self-knowledge and self-directive:** Guidance should be directed towards improvement of self-knowledge and self-direction among students.
- **Securing and recording adequate information:** Guidance service should provide for securing and recording adequate information regarding educational and occupational requirements and opportunities.
- **Leadership and coordination:** Guidance service should provide for leadership and coordination of all the agencies of school and community for long term guidance of youth.
- **Cooperation:** Guidance service should ensure active cooperation of parents for achieving the aims of guidance.
- **Simplicity:** Guidance service should be as simple as possible.
- **Collection and analysis of data:** Up-to-date data related to guidance service should be maintained.
- **Latest ways and means:** Latest trends in educational guidance should be incorporated in the guidance service.
- **Budgetary provisions:** There should be enough budgetary provision for guidance service.

## ORGANIZATION OF GUIDANCE AND COUNSELING SERVICES IN NURSING INSTITUTIONS

Since many nursing institutes are conducting a bunch of programs, such as diploma in Nursing, BSc Nursing, Post-certificate Nursing and MSc Nursing, the number of nursing students per institute has increased considerably. This ever increasing number of nursing students along with other factors, such as rapid social changes, changing role of nurses, more demanding patients, changes in the healthcare system, complexity of modern life and global demand for qualified nurses resulted in the formation of guidance and counseling services in many nursing institutes.

Regarding the organization, a midway between centralization and decentralization is preferred. Department of guidance and counseling is headed by a qualified counselor and she is assisted by one or two clerical staff. With the help of the counselor the faculty members are trained to provide nonspecialist guidance and counseling to students. Any student who is in need of specialized service is referred to the counselor and she provides counseling with the help of the faculty members.

As a part of the guidance program many nursing institutions have successfully implemented the *"teacher guardian program"*. In teacher guardian program, each faculty member is given the full responsibility of a group of ten students. The class coordinator also looks after the entire students in her class. Thus, a student is looked after by the teacher guardian at the ground level and the class coordinator at the next level. Teacher guardian has to conduct periodic meeting with her assigned group of students and assess their performance in the class as well as in the clinical area. She has to fill a proforma during the meeting with the student and send the filled proforma to the counseling department for further verification and filing through the principal. During the meeting, she has to fix the date for the next follow-up also. Students can approach the teacher guardian as needed to seek help in the academic and personal matters.

When the teacher guardian feels that a student under her supervision needs more specialized help, she reports the details of the student simultaneously to the student's class coordinator, counselor and principal. The counselor then takes over the student and renders help as needed with the help of the faculty members and other concerned personnel, such as parents and peers. A considerable amount of student problems are solved at the teacher guardian or class coordinator level and students who need specialized service only are referred to the counselor. In this way, the counselor is not overloaded and can concentrate on another areas/services of guidance and counseling also. The proformas send to the counseling department through the principal is verified by the counselor before filing. A monthly meeting under the chairmanship of the principal is held to review the functioning of the guidance and counseling services. In this meeting, teacher guardians, class coordinators and the counselor presents a brief report.

## ISSUES IN GUIDANCE PROGRAM

- Guidance program is not considered as an integral part of the educative process; even though it is recommend so.
- Lack of formal training to teachers in matters related to the implementation of guidance program.
- Guidance program is mainly viewed as a remedial measure to improve academic performance rather than contributing to the whole well-being of students.
- Lack of adequate resources for the successful implementation of the program.
- Lack of cooperation from parents and students in the proper implementation of the program.
- Faculty members overloaded with academic matters fails to appreciate the need of proper guidance program.
- Referring students to professional counseling is misinterpreted as a failure from the side of teachers. This misinterpretation often motivate teachers to ignore guidance program.
- Lack of proper follow up in the case of students seeking guidance result in poor implementation of guidance program.
- Non-cooperation of professional counselors with teachers also is an important issue in the guidance program.
- Inability of teachers to recognise properly when a student needed professional counseling also adversely affect guidance program.

❖ Failure of teachers and professional counselors to address ethical aspects of guidance is also a major problem in implementing guidance program.

## SUMMARY

Guidance and counseling enjoys a dominant role in the present day education system. Guidance and counseling services are aimed at enabling students to acquire ability which promote self-direction and self-realization. In education, our goal is guidance and our technique among others is counseling. Knowledge regarding the characteristics of guidance and counseling is essential to integrate them properly into the education system. Basics of guidance and counseling are philosophical, psychological, sociological and pedagogical. Guidance and counseling have three-fold functions namely adjustmental, orientational and developmental. Guidance and counseling are needed to maintain a healthy climate in the educational sector. In nursing education, guidance and counseling help the teachers and students become more professional so that they can face the challenges boldly.

Guidance program is based on the principles of guidance. Areas of guidance in education can be classified into education, vocation, personal, social, avocation, health, moral, religious and financial. The guidance and counseling services are the preadmission service, admission service, orientation service, student information service, information service, counseling service, placement service, remedial service, follow-up service, research service and evaluation service.

Guidance and counseling is a cooperative responsibility of the members of the staff. Professional services are offered by the qualified counselor, whereas nonspecialized services are rendered by other members of the staff. The main purpose of student counseling is to help the student help himself. The teacher should possess sound knowledge regarding when counseling is required and who should be counseled. There are three levels of counseling, namely, informal counseling, nonspecialist counseling rendered by professionals and professional counseling. In one way, counseling can be classified into surface level counseling, next level counseling and therapeutic counseling. In another way, counseling is classified into developmental, preventive, facilitative and crisis counseling. Different approaches to counseling are directive, nondirective and eclectic counseling. Phases of counseling are appointment and establishing relationship, assessment, diagnosis, setting goals, interventions, termination and follow-up. The counselor should possess certain qualities inorder to conduct counseling in a successful manner. Knowledge regarding do's and don'ts in counseling is essential for effective counseling.

While organizing guidance and counseling service, midway between centralized and decentralized organization structure is preferred. Basic concepts related to organization of guidance and counseling services are the purposes to be achieved, functions to be served, allocation of responsibility and authority and appraisal of the program. Requirements for organizing guidance and counseling services ranges from trained counselors to budgetary provisions. Availability of requirements is a must for conducting guidance and counseling service in an organized manner. The main purpose of guidance committee is to carry forward total guidance program with the support of all concerned.

Nursing institutes also follow the midway organization structure while organizing guidance and counseling services. The counselor will provide the professional service and other faculty members render the nonspecialized services. Teacher guardian program plays a vital role in providing guidance and counseling services. An increased global demand for qualified nurses motivated many nursing institutions to set up well functioning guidance and counseling departments.

## MULTIPLE CHOICE QUESTIONS

1. **Counseling is mainly:**
   a. Remedial
   b. Preventive
   c. Developmental
   d. All of the above
2. **Diagnosis is which phase of counseling:**
   a. First
   b. Second
   c. Third
   d. Fourth
3. **Who is taking care of students at first level in guidance service:**
   a. Teacher guardian
   b. Class coordinator
   c. Class leader
   d. Course director
4. **Philosophical basis of guidance help students to:**
   a. Develop values
   b. Develop knowledge
   c. Develop skills
   d. Develop attitude
5. **Psychological basis of guidance help students to:**
   a. Develop self-awareness
   b. Develop attitude
   c. Develop values
   d. Develop knowledge
6. **Ultimate goal of counseling is helping counselee to attain:**
   a. Self-actualization
   b. Knowledge
   c. Skill
   d. Attitude
7. **Guidance is based on:**
   a. Knowledge of students
   b. Skill of students
   c. Attitude of students
   d. Needs of students
8. **Counseling is basically an:**
   a. Supportive service
   b. Helping service
   c. Enabling service
   d. Facilitating service
9. **Guidance is basically:**
   a. Preventive in nature
   b. Remedial in nature
   c. Curative in nature
   d. None of the above
10. **Sociological basis of guidance focus on:**
    a. Relationship
    b. Learning
    c. Personality
    d. None of the above

## ANSWER KEY

| 1. a | 2. c | 3. a | 4. a | 5. a | 6. a |
| 7. d | 8. c | 9. a | 10. a | | |

# CHAPTER 12

# Discipline

## LEARNING OBJECTIVES

**After completing this chapter, reader will be able to:**

- Define discipline.
- Explain the modern concept of discipline.
- Realize the need for discipline.
- Identify the aims of discipline.
- List down the functions of discipline.
- Explain the principles of discipline.
- Maintain classroom discipline while conducting class.

Discipline is essential for maintaining a conducive environment in educational institutions. Modern education has given due recognition to this vital aspect of educational management. Since discipline comes under the purview of administration, we are limiting our discussion to some cardinal features only.

## MEANING AND DEFINITION

The term discipline comes from the Latin word 'disciplina' which means "instruction given to a learner". Thus, discipline should be considered as an integral part of teaching learning process rather than a mean of intimidation or humiliation.

The word discipline is derived from *disciplus* (pupil) and *discipere* (to comprehend). In the context of education, it should refer to group conduct held to be desirable in the teaching situation and in relation to the personal development of individual students who comprise the learning group. Percynunn defined discipline as follows: "Discipline consists in the submission of one's impulses and powers to a regulation which imposes form upon chaos and brings efficiency and economy where there would otherwise be ineffectiveness and waste. Though part of our nature may resist this control, its acceptance must on the whole be willing acceptance, the spontaneous movement of a nature in which there is an inborn impulse towards greater perfection."

An analysis of the above said definition reveals the following facts about discipline: (a) it is a vital component in the process of education, (b) it is the control of behavior to attain a goal and purpose, (c) it implies a good understanding of right conduct, the formation of desirable habits and attitudes and an adherence to such standards as are just and necessary, (d) it implies the subordination of individual interests to group interests in order to bring efficiency and economy, (e) it implies the willing acceptance of the control, i.e., the individual must do either what he is expected to do or must not do what he is forbidden to do.

According to Allen Mendler, "discipline is the process of learning how to get along with others, to solve problems and to make responsible choices"

This definition focuses on responsible behavior of students. By making students more responsible, aims of discipline can be easily achieved. Encouraging responsible behavior among students requires: (a) clear understanding of student expectations, (b) proper explanation of teacher expectations, (c) valuing what students think, (d) seeking more student participation in the teaching–learning process, (e) teaching students how to make good decisions and choices, and (f) maintaining better relationship with students.

## MODERN CONCEPT OF DISCIPLINE

The authoritarian discipline began to lose its significance at the beginning of the eighteenth century. Today, we teach students to obey, but we want this obedience to be a thinking obedience, not merely a reliance upon authority. Students are led gradually to discipline themselves. They are taught that there is a time for leisure and a time for learning, a time to converse and a time to listen and so on. Guarded freedom is granted to students. Many of the superimposed and unnecessary restrictions have been wiped. The teacher instead of working as a hard-task master, is viewed as a friend and a guide. Modern discipline satisfies the needs of self-respect and security. Present day discipline is of positive and creative type. The teacher who is a skilled disciplinarian always tries to inculcate good behavior among students, in this way right attitude and habits are formed in students.

The modern educator believes in self-discipline. In self-discipline, the source of control is largely within the individual and not external to him. It is a combination of self-control and self-direction. In this sense, it is something internal and may be regarded as a response to an inner stimulus. It implies not only bringing under control but also submitting one's behavior to self-imposed regulations. The student who controls his own behavior, willingly and spontaneously identifies himself with what is right. Thus, self-discipline creates an earnest desire in the student to do the right thing and thereby enabling him to become an active member in the educational process. The student makes decisions and assumes responsibility for his actions even in the absence of supervision. In short, modern discipline helps the student become self-propelled, self-controlled and self-guiding person.

## NEED FOR DISCIPLINE

Discipline is the most significant prerequisite for the successful implementation of the educational program. It is essential for helping the child in the growth of individual personality, for giving him the feeling of security, a sense of confidence and the knowledge of boundaries of his freedom.

Discipline is essential for the teacher also. Before he can teach the children, there must be proper conditions to do so. For good teaching, good conditions are as necessary as good ideas and good teachers.

Discipline is a necessary condition for good administration. If the administration is interpreted as all those things administrators do for the purpose of creating a situation favorable to learning, it becomes evident that maintaining discipline is one of his major tasks.

Discipline in an educational institution is also the requirement of the society. Without constructive and proper discipline, aims and aspirations of society cannot be realized.

## FUNCTIONS OF DISCIPLINE

Discipline as a universal cultural phenomenon is considered as serving a number of specific functions in the growth process of young people: It facilitate learning; it assists in learning those standards of conduct acceptable within society; it helps to acquire characteristics of positive nature, such as self-control and persistence; it assists in securing stability of the social order within which the young may achieve security and maturity.

## AIMS OF DISCIPLINE

Heidgerken describes the aims of discipline in nursing education as follows:
- To create and maintain desirable conditions in the teaching–learning situation (classroom or clinical setting). This will in turn assist in the achievement of objectives.
- To create favorable attitudes toward the establishment and the maintenance of conditions essential to effective work, in order to achieve the desired objectives.
- To assist in the development of self-control and cooperation which are regarded as essential traits in the daily living as well as in professional functioning.

## PRINCIPLES OF DISCIPLINE

Below listed principles of discipline will help in maintaining discipline in a student friendly manner:
- Disciplinary procedures should be in harmony with the total goals of education.
- Discipline should be based on and controlled by love and not by fear.
- The discipline should be mainly positive and constructive.
- Discipline should ensure equal justice for all, respect for the rights and dignity of the individual and humanitarian treatment for all.
- Discipline is not an end. It is just a means for the successful implementation of the educational program.
- Disciplinary policies and procedures should be primarily preventive, secondarily corrective and never retributive.
- Discipline should be designed to place upon the student more and more responsibility in respect of his own choices, purposes and behavior as he grows in the ability to shoulder such responsibility.
- Discipline is something which the teacher helps children to attain not something that a teacher maintains.
- Make most disciplinary talks in private.
- Definitely relate the act of misconduct to the act of correction. Be sure that the student understands the correction, otherwise it is not educative. Unless the correction contributes to the development of the student, it is not justified.
- Avoid collective punishments, such as punishing a whole class when only one or two individuals are culpable. Such action will provoke unnecessary resentment from the innocent members.
- As far as possible do not let disciplinary measures interfere with other educative opportunities. Avoid banishing a student from the classroom if possible. Where you feel isolation is needed try to let it be within the classroom.
- Only send a student to the head of the institution as a last resort or when you are confronted with a particularly serious case of misbehavior. However, do not hesitate to seek advice from other faculty members.

## TYPES OF DISCIPLINE

Based on the nature, discipline can be classified into authoritarian discipline, democratic discipline, self-discipline and assertive discipline. Since the authoritarian and democratic discipline is known to all, we will discuss the other two types in detail.

## SELF-DISCIPLINE

The modern educator believes in self-discipline. In self-discipline, the source of control is largely within the individual and not external to him. It is a combination of self-control and self-direction. In this sense, it is something internal and may be regarded as a response to an inner stimulus. It implies not only bringing under control but also submitting one's behavior to self-imposed regulations. The student who controls his own behavior, willingly and spontaneously identifies himself with what is right. Thus, self-discipline creates an earnest desire in the student to do the right thing and thereby enabling him to become an active member in the educational process. The student makes decisions and assumes responsibility for his actions even in the absence of supervision. In short, self-discipline helps the student to become self-propelled, self-controlled and self-guiding person.

Self-discipline is regarded as true discipline. Conditions for self-discipline to grow are: (a) a common purpose sufficiently to control the action of the individual, (b) a compelling desire to achieve that purpose and willingness to take up a common endeavor, (c) a clear understanding of functions to be performed by each member of the group, (d) an agreement on the regulations to be imposed on the group.

## ASSERTIVE DISCIPLINE

According to Louschan, this comparatively recent approach to behavior management is based on five key principles: (a) clear expectations for the required behavior are set out by the teacher, (b) specific, concrete and verbal praise and rewards are given for the behavior, (c) there is a graded sequence of negative consequences of undesirable behavior, (d) the teacher is assertive in insisting on the application of the rewards and sanctions, (e) power resides with the teacher, while informed choice of whether to follow a path that leads to rewards or sanctions resides with the student.

In this approach, a student who is misbehaving is told to stop and told explicitly what will happen, if he/she does not stop. The student can choose to comply with the teacher's orders (i.e., to stop) or not to comply (i.e., to demonstrate the undesirable behavior again and thereby to incur the negative sanctions). If the unacceptable behavior persists, then stronger disciplinary measures are imposed.

## PREVENTIVE DISCIPLINE

Preventive discipline is based on the concept that "most effective discipline is done with students rather than to them". Preventive discipline focuses on measures to avoid disobedience by encouraging responsible behavior among students. Preventive discipline can be achieved by following measures: (a) Making students more responsible for their behaviors, (b) always respect the dignity of students, (c) helping students to manage the feelings of anger, sadness, frustration, etc. (d) seek and value contribution of students in the teaching–learning process, (e) mutual understanding of student expectations and teacher expectations, (f) teaching students how to take good decisions or good choices, (g) build better relationship with students, (h) focus on teaching and learning rather than retribution or punishment, (i) follow good rules to achieve discipline. A good rule is always based on principles, clear and specific, enforceable and aimed on behavioral modification.

## DISCIPLINE WITH DIGNITY

Allen Mendler proposed the concept of discipline with dignity to ensure discipline among students in a desirable manner. Discipline with dignity shares some features of preventive discipline also. Aspects of discipline with dignity are: (a) encourage responsible behavior among students, (b) most effective discipline is done with students rather than to them, (c) students always deserve to be treated with dignity, (d) educational institution is for all students and not just to good ones, (e) effective discipline often demands courage and creativity from teachers, (f) never judge a student with his past experience, and (g) consider individual difference among students.

## ECLECTIC APPROACH TO DISCIPLINE

As discipline is influenced by multiple factors, it is better to follow an eclectic approach to discipline by combining good features of self-disciplines, assertive discipline, preventive discipline and discipline with dignity.

Teachers have to use positive reinforcement and punishments to manage student behavior. Teachers need to give proper assistance to students in developing capacities to regulate their own behavior. Emphasis should also be given to building a trusting and caring relationship with students. An effective students support and guidance program also helps to identify problems of students as early as possible.

In eclectic approach emphasis is on prevention of problem behaviors, early detection and correction of problem behaviors, promotion of behavior and social competencies.

## DISCIPLINE STRATEGIES/APPROACHES

Even though teachers have their own style of discipline for their classrooms, most discipline strategies can be categorized into three main styles or approaches:

### Preventive Discipline

Teachers with effective classroom management strategies establish expectations, guidelines and rules for behavior in classroom. Clearly explaining expectations is an essential component of preventive discipline. The goal of preventive discipline is to provide proactive interventions to potential disruptive behavior by clearly explaining to students what behaviors are appropriate and not.

### Supportive Discipline

When a teacher offers a verbal warning or a suggestion for correcting behavior while a student is disobeying the teacher is using supportive discipline. Supportive discipline is distinct from punishment because it provides opportunity for correcting behavior.

### Corrective Discipline

When a student not complies with supportive discipline, a teacher may opt for a corrective discipline strategy. Corrective discipline refers to the set of consequences faced by student following an information corrective discipline strategies vary from simple verbal warning to suspension.

## SPECIFIC MEASURES TO MAINTAIN CLASSROOM DISCIPLINE

There are no golden rules for the maintenance of discipline in class; each problem requires a separate analysis and set of responses as it occurs. The following measures suggested by Curzon should be found useful, always provided that they are interpreted not in a mechanical way, but in accordance with the exigencies of specific classroom situations. The strategies involved in class control must always match context.

- Ensure, as far as possible, that the classroom conditions appropriate to your lesson requirements have been prepared. Seating arrangements are important—thus, to seat students where they are unable to see or hear important parts of the lesson is to create an atmosphere in which order can breakdown.
- Prepare your lesson thoroughly. Pitch it at a suitable level so that an appropriate climate is established. Make sure that you do not depress class morale by demanding impossible standards. Ensure, similarly, that students do not feel degraded by being asked to participate in trivial activities which obviously require minimum standards only. Students who believe that their time is being wasted—no matter what the pretext—are unlikely to approach their tasks in disciplined fashion. Provide opportunities for success in class.
- Where the objective of a task is not immediately obvious, be prepared to explain its significance. It is difficult to maintain discipline when students are asked to engage in activities for incomprehensible ends.
- Know your class. The teacher who is interested to learn the names of his students and to study their backgrounds is demonstrating an interest in those for whose instruction he is responsible. Teacher-student cooperation can be intensified in this way, with a corresponding, positive effect on problems of behavior in class.
- Adopt an appropriate professional style in the classroom and keep to it. To be either too friendly or too remote is, almost always, to forfeit respect, with marked effects on class discipline.
- Watch very carefully for signs of trouble. Just as a successful navigator learns to recognize and react to storm signals, so the teacher must learn to watch for those events which can lead to loss of class control. The conversations which continue after the teacher has complained of their interference with the lesson, the 'clenche silence' which follows a request for cooperation, the continued failure to complete assignments, a record of unexplained absence or unpunctuality—these are some signals which require swift assessment and action.
- Establish momentum at an early stage. Avoid over-long introductions to lessons and focus attention swiftly. Keep up a reasonable pace of class activity and involvement. Periods of inactivity can produce the boredom which spills over easily into indiscipline. Check performance regularly.
- Do not confuse the trivial and the important. Over-reaction to a minor breach of a rule can be counter-productive. Learn to assess swiftly the real significance of events in the class.
- Be seen as fair-minded and impartial: Favoritism of any kind, conscious or unconscious, bias and prejudice, will be interpreted by a class as an indication that fair consideration from the side of the teacher cannot always be expected. Students have a rudimentary but keen sense of justice which, when outraged, often leads to a withdrawal of cooperation.
- When you have to issue orders, do so firmly and unambiguously. 'Be sparing of commands. Command only when other means are inexplicable or have failed…….. But whenever you do command, command with decision and consistency **(Spencer)**.
- The reprimand is the most common form of primary reaction to misbehavior in the college. The teacher must know when and how to reprimand. Reprimands are based on overt responses to unacceptable behavior; they may be verbal or nonverbal, formal or informal. The precise form will be dictated by the situation, the nature of the behavior and the effect desired by the teacher. The rules are do not over-react; use the reprimand sparingly, avoid expressions of hostility and idle threats, do not injure a students' self-esteem, consider the

effect of the reprimand in the short-term and long-term on the offender and the rest of the class. Learn when to ignore a minor, 'one-off', manifestation of misbehavior, but watch for a build-up of potentially disruptive activities and reprimand firmly any important violation of previously announced rules.
- If you feel that you have to punish, ensure that the situation really demands it and that the consequences seem worthwhile. You must decide what constitutes misbehavior and when it requires punishment; your judgment on the necessity for punishment may vary from group to group or student to student, but it must be based consistently on principle. The decision to punish is in no sense a confession of failure. On the contrary, it may be a perfectly appropriate response to behavior which critically threatens the maintenance of class control. Punishment should be consistent in nature and neither random nor haphazard. The alternative desirable behavior ought to be understood by the person who is being punished and should be reinforced immediately on its occurrence. Let the punishment follow a warning; let it be just and exemplary.
- Without hesitation consider the dismissal of a student who continuously threatens the maintenance of class control. Dismissal ought to be followed by discussions with the student and his family. Note, however, Dewey's warning on the use of the dismissal: 'It may strengthen the very causes which have brought about the undesirable antisocial attitude, such as desire for attention or show off'.
- Follow-up all important disciplinary matters. Analyze what initiated and precipitated the breakdown of discipline. Do not confuse symptom and underling cause. Learn and apply in the future whatever lessons you have learned from your solution of disciplinary problems.

## PRACTICAL GUIDELINES TO DISCIPLINE

Below mentioned practical guidelines help to maintain discipline in classroom and clinical area:
- Abide by rules and be a role model to students. For example, meet deadline and due dates promptly and be in class and clinical area on time.
- Adopt eclectic approach to discipline by following good aspects of various types of discipline.
- Be an active listener, proper listening of students' issues itself avoid many problems.
- Respect dignity of students. Never judge a student with his past behavior.
- While disciplining provide good choices and limits
- All rules should contribute to the success of students.
- Limit assignments according to syllabus rather than curriculum. As far as possible evaluate clinical assignments in the clinical area itself.
- Never compare performance of students and respect individual differences among students.
- Inform students periodically about their academic progress and attendance percentage. This will avoid issues related to attendance and internal marks.
- Ensure active role of students support and guidance program to monitor academic progress and timely implementation of remedial measures.
- Prepare students to become an achiever than winner by fostering collaboration.
- Motivate students to limit use of social media
- Assist students to embrace boredom. Explain students the need to embrace boredom to achieve success.
- If possible convert disciplinary actions to a learning opportunity. For example, if a student uses social media excessively, give him an assignment on evil effects of social media in learning process.

## SUMMARY

Discipline is a vital component in the process of education. It is the control of behavior to attain a goal and purpose. Discipline can be classified into authoritarian discipline, assertive discipline, democratic discipline and self-discipline. Self-discipline is a combination of self-control and self-direction. Discipline is the most significant prerequisite for the successful implementation of the educational program. Discipline is essential for the teacher also. It plays an important role in the growth process of young people. Without constructive and proper discipline, aims and aspirations of the society cannot be realized. In nursing education, discipline helps in the development of proper attitude, self-control and cooperation, which are regarded as essential traits in the daily living as well as in professional functioning. Knowledge about the principles of discipline and specific measures to maintain classroom discipline will help the teacher to create a student-centered classroom atmosphere.

## MULTIPLE CHOICE QUESTIONS

1. **Who proposed discipline with dignity?**
   a. Allen Mendler
   b. Plato
   c. Skinner
   d. Mahatma Gandhi
2. **Modern education mostly believes in:**
   a. Self-discipline
   b. Preventive discipline
   c. Autocratic discipline
   d. Democratic discipline
3. **The term discipline is derived from:**
   a. Discipline
   b. Disciplus
   c. Discipere
   d. Disciples
4. **Providing suggestion for correcting behavior is:**
   a. Supportive discipline
   b. Preventive discipline
   c. Corrective discipline
   d. Assertive discipline
5. **Conveying teacher expectations is a part of:**
   a. Preventive discipline
   b. Supportive discipline
   c. Assertive discipline
   d. Democratic discipline

### ANSWER KEY

| 1. a | 2. a | 3. a | 4. a | 5. a |
| --- | --- | --- | --- | --- |

# CHAPTER 13
# Ethics and Evidence-based Nursing Education

## LEARNING OBJECTIVES

**After completing this chapter, reader will be able to:**

- Define ethics.
- Explain branches of ethics.
- Describe process of ethical decision making.
- Explain ethical standards for students.
- Appreciate value-based education in nursing.
- List down value development strategies.
- Explain evidence-based education in nursing.
- Describe student–faculty relationship.
- Explain role of ICT in education.

As in life ethics is an important aspect in education also. Ethics helps to attain the objectives of nursing education in a right manner. Evidence-based education allow nursing faculty to conduct classes in a learner-friendly manner. In this chapter, we will briefly discuss about ethics, ethical decision making, ethical standards for students, value-based education in nursing, value development strategies, evidence-based education in nursing and student–faculty relationship.

## ETHICS-REVIEW

### Definition

Ethics refers to the concept of right and wrong conduct or behavior. Ethics is basically a branch of Philosophy dealing with the issue of morality. Ethics involves rules of behavior. It certainly defines how a person should behave in specific situations. The term ethics is derived from the Greek word "ethos" which means custom, habit, character or disposition. Ethics are the set of moral principles that guide an individual's behavior. It is concerned with beliefs about what is right, what is wrong, what is unjust, what is good and what is bad in terms of human behavior.

### Branches of Ethics

Ethics is divided into two parts **(Fig. 13.1)**—theoretical ethics and applied ethics. Theoretical ethics include normative ethics, descriptive ethics and meta ethics. Applied ethics refers to professional ethics.

### Normative Ethics

Normative ethics deals with certain norms that explain how an individual should behave or act. Therefore, normative ethics is concerned with the rightness or wrongness of actions or behaviors. In other words normative ethics is the study of ethical behavior. Normative ethics is concerned with criteria of what is morally right and wrong. It includes the formulation of moral rules that guide action of institutions as well as individuals. These moral rules will in turn create moral standards.

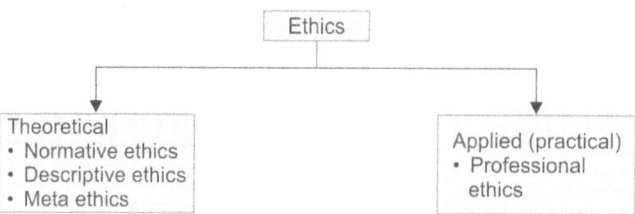

**Fig. 13.1:** Branches of ethics.

Normative ethics involves creating moral standards that regulate right and wrong conduct. The Golden Rule is a classic example of a normative principle. As per Golden Rule, we should do to others what we would want others to do to us. For example, we should behave gently to others if we are expecting gentle behaviors from others. So, based on the Golden Rule, it would be wrong if we harass, victimize, assault or kill others. The key assumption in normative ethics is that there is only one ultimate criterion of moral conduct. Another name of normative ethics is perspective ethics.

### Descriptive Ethics

Descriptive ethics is the study of individuals' beliefs about morality. It is regarding what individuals actually believe to be right or wrong. On the basis of this, the law decides whether certain human actions are acceptable or not. Thus, descriptive ethics describe how individuals should behave or what moral standards they have to follow. Descriptive ethics is also known as comparative ethics. This is because, it compares the ethics of past and present as well as ethics of one society and another.

Descriptive ethics are individuals' judgment about "rightness and wrongness" or moral beliefs. For example, some people support abortion whereas some oppose it in accordance with their moral beliefs.

### Meta Ethics

Meta ethics is also known as analytic ethics. It deals with origin of ethical concepts themselves. Meta ethics is not concerned whether an action is good or bad, rather, meta ethics tries to find out what morality itself is. Thus, it is the study of moral thought and moral language. Meta ethics attempts to explain the underlying assumption behind moral theories, therefore, it is the branch of ethics that tries to understand the nature of ethical properties, statements, attitudes and judgments. Meta ethics questions the very essence of goodness or rightness.

Examples of meta-ethical questions are: (a) What does it mean to say something is good? (b) How, if at all, do we know what is right and wrong? (c) How do moral attitudes motivate actions? (d) Are there objective or absolute values? and (e) What is the source of our values?

## ETHICAL DECISION MAKING

Ethical decision making refers to the process of evaluating and choosing among alternatives in a manner consistent with ethics principles. In making ethical decisions, it is necessary to understand and eliminate unethical options and select the best ethical alternative.

An ethical decision is one that represents responsibility, fairness and trust for an individual. Ethical reasoning is essential for taking good ethical decisions. Ethical reasoning is a way of thinking about issues of right and wrong.

## Factors Influencing Ethical Decision Making

Factors influencing ethical decision making can be classified into: (a) individual, (b) organizational, and (c) opportunity factors.

### Individual Factors

Significant individual factors that affect the ethical decision making process include personal moral philosophy, stage of moral development, motivation, ethical maturity and other personal factors such as gender, age and experience.

Moral philosophies are the principles or rules that individuals apply in deciding what is right or wrong. Moral philosophies can be briefly classified as consequentialism, ethical formalism and justice. Consequentialist philosophies consider a decision to be right or acceptable if it accomplishes a desired result such as knowledge, career growth, the realization of self-interest or utility. Ethical formalism focuses on the rights of individuals and on the intentions associated with a particular behavior rather than on its consequences. Justice theory is related to evaluation of fairness or the ability to deal with justices from others. Kohlberg's theory of moral development includes six stages such as: (a) obedience and punishment, (b) individualism and exchange, (c) maintaining interpersonal relationship, (d) laws and order, (e) social contract, and (f) universal principles.

### Organizational Factors

The culture of organization as well as superiors, peers and subordinates can have a significant impact on the ethical—decision-making process. Organizational culture can be defined as set of values, beliefs, goals, norms and rituals shared by members of the organization. Organizations ethical climate focuses especially on issues of right and wrong. Organizational culture needs to foster a good ethical climate to prevent its member from engaging unethical activities.

### Opportunity Factors

Opportunity is a set of conditions that limit unethical behaviors and provide rewards for ethical behaviors. If an individual takes advantages of an opportunity to act unethically and escapes punishment that person may repeat such acts when circumstances favor them.

## Steps in Ethical Decision Making

The 'PLUS' ethical decision making model suggests 7 steps for ethical decision making. At key steps in the process, one should use ethical filters to ensure adequate ethical reasoning in decision making. Ethical filters are grouped into the mnemonic PLUS. (*Courtesy:* www.ethics.org)

- **P-Policies:** Is it consistent with my organization's policies, procedures and guidelines?
- **L-Legal:** Is it acceptable under the applicable laws and regulations?
- **U-Universal:** Does it confirm to the universal principles/values my organization has adopted?
- **S-Self:** Does it satisfy my personal definition of right, good and fair?

The plus fitters work as an integral parts of steps 1, 4 and 7 of the decision making process. Steps in ethical decision making are:

Step 1: Define problem (consider PLUS filters)
Step 2: Seek out relevant assistance, guidance and support
Step 3: Identify alternatives

Step 4: Evaluate the alternative (consider PLUS filters)
Step 5: Make the decision.
Step 6: Implement the decision
Step 7: Evaluate the decision (consider PLUS filters)

## ETHICAL STANDARDS FOR STUDENTS

In student life, ethics can be interpreted as the discipline of dealing with good and bad with commitment and moral duty. Following ethical standards enable students to make right choices and this will in turn lead to building a better life. It is the duty of teachers to make students aware about ethical standards. Awareness regarding ethical standards help students to achieve academic responsibility, integrity and practice self-discipline.

The components of ethical standards for students are: (a) awareness regarding rights as a student, (b) awareness regarding responsibilities as a student, (c) honesty, (d) integrity, (e) truthfulness, (f) trust worthiness (g) loyalty, (h) respect for others, especially teachers, (i) concern for others, especially towards classmates, (j) obedience to law, (k) commitment to excellence, and (l) focus on collaboration than competition.

## VALUE-BASED EDUCATION IN NURSING

Value education is the process of enabling students to develop values essential for leading a successful life by way of educative process. Values are essential for the proper development of personal, social, moral and spiritual behaviors along with academic excellence.

Considering the major role of technology in education and influence of social media among youngsters special attention is needed to inculcate value among students.

Value-based education in nursing is essential to develop proper attitude and behavior needed to practice as a successful professional nurse. Values help students to distinguish between good and bad. Thus, values are essential for making good choices in life. Good choices in turn create success in life.

Value education in nursing helps students to identify their rights and responsibilities as students. It motivates students to become more proactive in learning. This is evident by spending more time on learning, increase in attendance and reduction in the unhealthy use of mobile phones and social media.

For providing value-based education in nursing, faculty need to focuses on personal, social, moral and spiritual development of students along with other aims of nursing education. Nursing curriculum should include provision for developing values, such as responsible behaviors, loyalty, empathy, passion, honesty, reliability, dependability, optimism and commitment along with subject matter. A sound system of values helps nursing students to grow and live as good human beings as well as a successful nursing professional. Quality of nursing education can be improved by making it more value oriented one.

## VALUE DEVELOPMENT STRATEGIES

Nurse educators can assist nursing students to develop proper values through below mentioned strategies.
- Incorporating values through existing curriculum.
- Value—inculcation through co-curricular activities.
- Development of value—consciousness through role play.
- Development of values through classroom discussion.
- Development of values through assisting students in proper journaling.

- Value inculcation through appropriate feedback during clinical supervision.
- Development of value—consciousness through narrating good stories.
- Assisting students to enhance emotional intelligence.

# EVIDENCE-BASED EDUCATION

The concept of evidence-based practice has its origins in medical science. Evidence-based education is the educative process-based on empirical evidence to make informed decisions about educational interventions. Education interventions can be classified into educational policies, practices and educational programs. Evidence-based education is supported by high-quality evidence that ensure better learning outcomes. It provide specific approaches and programs that improve student performance.

Evidence-based education recommends use of scientific principles and rigorous research methods in the educative process instead of depending on old traditions. It is a set of principles and practices for enhancing educational policy and practice.

Key components of evidence-based education have four key components:
1. Promoting best-practices research and development
2. Facilitating review and evaluation of scientific research
3. Disseminating scientific research
4. Developing and supporting "evidence-based culture"

## Evidence-based Educative Process

According to Philip Davis evidence-based education operates at two levels. The first is to utilize existing evidence from worldwide research and literature on education and associated subjects. Educationists at all levels need to be able to:
- Pose an answerable question about education
- Know where and how to find evidence systematically and comprehensively using electronic (computer-based) and non-electronic (print) media.
- Retrieve and read such evidence competently and undertake critical appraisal and analysis of that evidence according to agreed professional and scientific standards.
- Organize and grade the power of this evidence
- Determine its relevance to their educational needs and environments.

The second level is to establish sound evidence, where existing evidence is lacking or of a questionable, uncertain or weak nature. Teacher following evidence-based education working at this level need be able to plan, carry out and publish studies with highest standards of scientific research and evaluation. The objective of evidence-based education at this level is to ensure that future research on education meets the criteria of scientific validity, high quality and practical relevance that is sometimes lacking in existing evidence on educational activities, processes and outcomes.

## Advantages of Evidence-based Education

According to Larry Wexler the advantages of evidence-based education for teachers and students are:
- An increased likeliness of positive student outcomes.
- Increased accountability because there are data to back up the selection of a practice or program, which in turn facilitates support from administrators, parents and others.
- Less wasted time and fewer wasted resources because educators adopt an effective practice or program and are not forced to find a method that works through trails and error.
- An increased chance for responding to learner's needs in a positive manner.

## Application of Evidence-based Education in Nursing Education

Evidence-based nursing education is the process of attaining objective of nursing education by combining the nurse educator's reliable and valuable evidence-based knowledge regarding subject matter from personal experience with evidence from systematic research.

Evidence-based nursing education involves use of evidence as suggests by Geofmaster.

According to Geoffmaster, evidence-based teaching involves the use of evidence to:
- Establish where students are in the learning or their previous knowledge.
- Decide on appropriate teaching strategies and interventions.
- Monitor student progress and evaluate teaching effectiveness

## Evidence to Identify Starting Points for Teaching and Learning

At first, essential form of evidence for teaching is information about level of attainment by learners or their previous knowledge. Their previous knowledge is the starting point for teaching and to ensure that learners are provided with well-targeted learning opportunities and appropriately challenging learning goals. Understanding where learners are in their learning is important to clinical teaching as understanding a patient's symptoms and health is important for providing effective nursing care.

In evidence-based teaching, assessments are undertaken to gather evidence and draw conclusions about where students are in their learning. The objective is to use observations of students' performance and work to draw inferences about their current level of attainment. A thorough understanding of where a student is in their learning may require a detailed analysis of errors they are making or the misunderstandings they have develop. This understanding serve as essential evidence for removing obstacles for further progress and a key element in providing effective clinical teaching. Instead of grading, this evidence is used to identify what students know, understand and can do.

## Evidence to Decide on Appropriate Teaching Strategies and Interventions

From the teaching experience of the teacher and systematic research teacher can collect evidence to find answers to the following questions for deciding on appropriate teaching strategies and intervention.
- Which interventions are likely to improve students' level of understanding and skills?
- What teaching strategies help in attain clinical teaching objectives?
- For which learners?
- Under what conditions?

In general, evidence provides best ways to implement effective teaching strategies and interventions in subject-specific contexts.

## Evidence to Evaluate Student Progress and Teaching Effectiveness

A third form of evidence for teaching is information about the progress students make in their learning over time. This is important information for evaluating learning success and for making judgments about the effectiveness of teaching strategies and interventions.

Evidence about the progress students make is crucial information for teaching. It provides a basis for establishing whether and how effectively students are learning. Low levels of progress may indicate lack of student effort and /or ineffective teaching and demands remedial action. Information about progress provides the most direct indicator of teaching effectiveness as well as necessary for the evaluation of educational policies, progress and teaching methods.

# STUDENT–FACULTY RELATIONSHIP

An effective student–faculty relationship is essential to attain aims of nursing education. It is also essential to create a positive learning climate both in classroom and clinical area. The educator must have qualities, such as love and care, respect, responsibility, morality, patience, good listening capacity, being open to new ideas, motivation, willingness to spend more time, and punctuality to build a trusting relationship with students. Such as any relationship, those between faculty members and students require nurturing. A sense of connection with teachers helps students feel like they belong to the institution.

Regardless of the environment (online or offline) in which learning takes place, students feel more satisfied when faculty members function as an active part of their lives. Through positive relationship, faculty can motivate students to excel academically and help students to realize their potential. Students also feel faculty members are approachable and often are willing mentors in the learning process.

The most important aspect of student–faculty relationship is that it helps faculty members understand the learning needs and interests of their students. This will in turn help faculty members in the instructional process.

## Elements of Student–faculty Relationship

According to Kimlee, one of the most pure and deeply inspirational relationships is that of a devoted teacher and a willing student. He suggests following four elements of student-teacher relationship:
1. Consistent communication
2. A positive learning environment
3. Mutual respect, trust and feedback
4. True equity (all students have equal access to learning recourses without disparity)

# INFORMATION AND COMMUNICATION TECHNOLOGIES IN EDUCATION

Information and communication technologies (ICT) are influencing education in many ways. In this digital era, ICT use in the classroom is important for giving students opportunities to learn and apply the required 21st century skills. ICT improves teaching and learning by helping teachers in performing their role in a better manner. Integrating ICT in formal teaching and learning is essential to achieve the aims of education in a better manner.

## Meaning

Information and communication technology in education is the mode of education that use information and communications technology to support, enhance and optimize the teaching-learning process. Information and communication technology includes computers, mobile phones, the internet apps and electronic delivery systems, such as radios, televisions and projectors among others and is widely used in today's education system. As ICT is being applied successfully in teaching, learning and assessment, it is considered as a powerful tool for educational change and reform.

Through ICT, learning can occur anytime and anywhere. Online course materials, for example, can be accessible anytime of the day. Based on ICT, learning and teaching need not depend on print materials only. Various resources are available on the internet and knowledge can be acquired through video clips, audio sounds, visual presentation, etc. In short, ICT assists in transforming a teaching environment into a learner-centered one.

## Benefits of Using ICT in Education

Jo Shanfu explains the benefits of ICT in the following manner:

- **Assist students in accessing digital information efficiently and effectively:** ICT helps students to access relevant content, solve problems and provide solutions to the problems in the learning process. ICT makes knowledge acquisition more accessible and concepts are easily understood through application of ICT.
- **Support student-centered and self-directed learning:** ICT help students to build knowledge through accessing, selecting, organizing and interpreting information and data. Based on learning through ICT, students are more capable of using information and data from various sources and critically assessing the quality of the learning materials.
- **Provide a creative learning environment:** ICT helps students to develop new understanding in their areas of learning. ICT provides more creative solutions to different types of learning inquiries. For example, learners can access all types of texts from beginning to advance levels with ease through computers, laptops, personal digital assistants or I pads. Thus, ICT involves purpose-designed applications that provide innovative ways to meet a variety of learning needs.
- **Promote collaborative learning in a distance-learning environment:** Using ICT enables students to communicate, share and work collaboratively anywhere, anytime. For example, a zoom-based videoconferencing helps all students in a class to attend class simultaneously. In such a class, students not only acquire knowledge together but also share diverse learning outcomes.
- **Offer more opportunities to develop critical (higher-order) thinking skills:** Based on a constructive learning approach, ICT helps students focus on higher level concepts rather than less meaningful tasks. A longer exposure to the ICT learning environment can foster students' critical thinking skills.
- **Improve teaching and learning quality:** According to Lowther, there are three important characteristics are needed to develop good quality teaching and learning with ICT— **autonomy, capability and creativity**. Autonomy means that students take control of their learning through use of ICT. In this way, they become more capable of working by themselves and with others. ICT also foster autonomy by allowing teachers to create their own teaching material, thus providing more control over course content than possible in a traditional classroom setting. With regard to capability once students are more confident in the learning process, they can develop the capability to apply and transfer knowledge while using new technology with efficiency and effectiveness. By using ICT, students' creativity can be optimized. They may discover new multimedia tools and create materials essential for learning with a combination of students' autonomy capability and creativity the use of ICT can improve the quality of both teaching and learning.
- **Support teaching by creating quality course content:** Through ICT teachers can integrate technology with education. Through ICT teachers get more opportunity to access quality teaching materials and this will enhance the confidence of teachers.

## SUMMARY

Ethics refers to the concept of right and wrong conduct or behavior. Ethics is basically a branch of philosophy dealing with the issue of morality. Ethics involves rules of behavior. It defines how a person should behave in specific situations. Branches of ethics include normative ethics, descriptive ethics, meta ethics and professional ethics. Ethical decision making refers to the process of evaluating and choosing among alternative in a manner consistent with ethical principles. Factor influencing ethical decision making are: (a) individual, (b) organizational and (c) opportunity factors.

Ethical standards for students can be interpreted as the discipline of dealing with good and bad with commitment and moral duty. Value-based education is the process of enabling students to develop values essential for leading a successful life by way of educative process. Nurse educators need to support students in developing appropriate values. Evidence-based on empirical evidence to make informed decisions about educational interventions An effective student faculty relationship is essential to attain aims of nursing education.

## MULTIPLE CHOICE QUESTIONS

1. **Applied ethics refers to:**
   a. Normative ethics
   b. Professional ethics
   c. Descriptive ethics
   d. Meta ethics

2. **Normative ethics is otherwise known as:**
   a. Perspective ethics
   b. Comparative ethics
   c. Analytic ethics
   d. None of the above

3. **Descriptive ethics is otherwise known as:**
   a. Perspective ethics
   b. Comparative ethics
   c. Analytic ethics
   d. None of the above

4. **Meta ethics is otherwise known as:**
   a. Perspective ethics
   b. Comparative ethics
   c. Analytic ethics
   d. None of the above

5. **Moral philosophy is related to which factor of ethical decision making:**
   a. Individual
   b. Organizational
   c. Opportunity
   d. Social

6. **Value-based education mostly influence:**
   a. Attitude
   b. Skill
   c. Knowledge
   d. Patience

7. **Evidence-based education recommends:**
   a. Use of scientific principles
   b. Use of research
   c. Both of the above
   d. None of the above

8. Golden rule is an example of:
   a. Normative ethics
   b. Descriptive ethics
   c. Meta ethics
   d. Professional ethics
9. Which branch of ethics tries to find underlying assumption behind moral theories?
   a. Normative ethics
   b. Descriptive ethics
   c. Meta ethics
   d. Professional ethics
10. The way of thinking about issues of right and wrong is known as:
    a. Moral reasoning
    b. Ethical conduct
    c. Attitude
    d. None of the above

## ANSWER KEY

| 1. b | 2. a | 3. b | 4. c | 5. a | 6. a |
|------|------|------|------|------|------|
| 7. c | 8. a | 9. c | 10. a | | |

# CHAPTER 14

# Communication and Human Relations

## LEARNING OBJECTIVES

**After completing this chapter, reader will be able to:**

- Describe the communication process.
- Identify the techniques of effective communication.
- Establish effective interpersonal relations with patients, families and coworkers.
- Develop effective human relations in the context of nursing.
- Teach individuals, group, and communities about health with their active participation.

Nursing is regarded as the most caring one among healthcare professions. This image is mainly due to the high proportion of human element involved in the practice of nursing. Effective communication skills, ability to maintain healthy interpersonal relationships, awareness regarding the complexity of human relations and ability to communicate health messages in a down-to-earth manner will enable you to uphold the humanitarian nature of our profession. Through different sections of this chapter we will discuss communication process, interpersonal relations, human relations and information, education and communication for health.

## COMMUNICATION PROCESS

### Definition

- In Heinz's opinion, "Communication is the transfer of information from a sender to a receiver, with the information being understood by the receiver." This definition focuses on the sender of the communication, the transmission of the message and the receiver of the message.
- In Shirley Taylor's words, "Communication is the giving, receiving or exchanging information, opinions or ideas by writing, speech or visual means, so that the message communicated is completely understood by the recipients." This definition is highly comprehensive in nature and focuses on effective communication.
- According to Stephen R Robbins, "Communication is the transfer and understanding of meaning." This simple definition emphasis the "transfer" of meaning. As per this definition, if no information or ideas have been conveyed, communication has not taken place. Communication also involves the "understanding of" the meaning. For communication to be successful, the meaning must be imparted and understood.
- In simple terms, Brooks and Heath defined interpersonal communication as "The process by which information, meanings and feelings are shared by individuals through the exchange of verbal and nonverbal messages".

## Significance of Communication in Nursing

The significance of communication in nursing is evident from one specific reason: Everything a nurse does for patients involve communication. Ineffective communication can give rise to problems, sometimes may even results in the loss of precious human life. Manreen N believes that communication is significant in nursing practice due to following reasons:

- Good communication is essential for providing competent nursing care. If nurses are not communicating properly, patient's safety is at risk for several reasons such as lack of important information, misinterpretation of information and unclear orders over telephone. Thus, good communication is essential for providing meticulous nursing care.
- Communication is a vital element in all areas of nursing interventions such as prevention, treatment, rehabilitation, education and health promotion.
- Comprehensive nursing care based on nursing process approach involves group activity with specific skills of verbal communication.
- Coordination with other healthcare professionals is essential for better treatment outcomes. As advocate of patients, nurses need excellent communication skills to coordinate patient care.
- Good communication of nurses with patients reduce their anxiety, thus good communication enhances the health of patients.
- Good communication makes patient feel valued. When nurses listen to patients and try to understand their problems, patients develop a feeling as a valuable person.
- Communication is a core component of sound relationship, collaboration, and cooperation, which in turn are essential aspects of professional practice.
- The quality of communication between nurse and patients influence outcome of nursing care. Good communication reduces medical errors and results in positive outcomes.
- Communication is the means by which behavior is modified, change is affected, information is made productive and goals are achieved. Since education aims behavior modification of learner, communication is important in nursing education also.
- Communication is the means by which people are linked together in an organization to achieve a common purpose. Thus, nurses working in managerial positions need effective communication skills to organize the activities of nursing department in an effective manner.

## Principles of Communication

To make communication effective we have to follow certain principles. They are:

- **Principle of readiness and motivation:** Both sender and receiver of communication should be ready and remain motivated throughout the process of communication. Then only communication can be effective.
- **Principle of competence and worth:** The sender and receiver should be competent and efficient in terms of communicating and receiving the desired message. Communication skills of the sender and receiver is essential for the effective transmission and receiving of message.
- **Principle of sharing and interaction:** Communication is a two-way process maximum sharing of information and interaction between sender and receiver is needed for effective communication. More the interaction, more will be benefits of communication.
- **Principle of suitability of the message:** The message to be communicated in the communication process should be appropriate for sender and receiver. The sender must be able to transfer the message properly to the receiver. The receiver grasp the message and respond properly.

- **Principle of appropriate channel:** The effectiveness of communication depends the selection of appropriate channel or media. The channel should be appropriate for the message, situation and receiver.
- **Principle of appropriate feedback:** Desired feedback from both the receiver and sender is essential for effective communication. Feedback helps the sender to modify the aspects of communication in favor of the receiver.
- **Principle of facilitators and barriers of communication:** Communication process is influenced by many variables lying between the sender and receiver of communication. Proper understanding of facilitators and barriers will help to communicate effectively.
- **Principle of communication situations:** Depending on the individuals involved and environment, communication situations can be one to one communication, small group communication, large group or public communication, mass communication and organizational or institutional communication. Selection of channel of communication should be appropriate to the situation of communication.

## Communication Process and Elements

**Figure 14.1** illustrates the seven elements of the communication process: the source of the message or sender, the message, encoding, the channel, decoding the receiver and feedback. Communication process can be defined as transferring of meaning from one person to another through the seven elements involved in communication.

In addition, the entire process is susceptible to noise disturbances that interfere with the transmission, receipt or feedback of a message. In other words, anything that interferes with understanding can be noise, and noise can create distortion at any point of communication process. Typical examples of noise, include illegible print, phone static, inattention by the receiver or background sound of equipment or colleagues. Let us discuss the elements in brief.

The sender or source of a message initiates the communication. The sender will be a person with information, needs or desires and a purpose for communicating them to one or more other people.

Before communication can take place, a purpose, expressed as message to be conveyed, must exist. It passes between the sender and receiver. Thus, message can be defined as a purpose to be conveyed. The message must be formulated with the receiver's background in mind. If the message does not reach the receiver, communication has not taken place.

The receiver is the individual to whom the message is directed. In broad sense, receiver is the person whose senses perceive the sender's message.

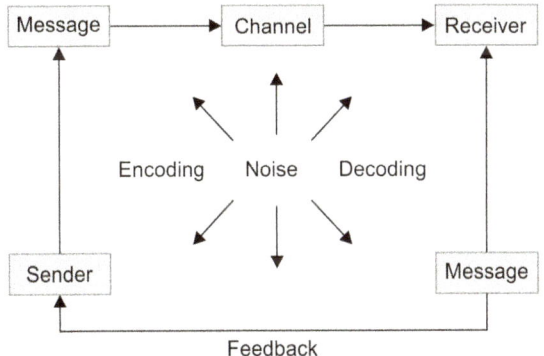

**Fig. 14.1:** The communication process.

A sender initiates a message by encoding a thought. Encoding takes place when the sender translates the information to be transmitted into a series of symbols. Encoding is necessary because information can be transferred from one person to another only through representations or symbols—gestures, sounds, letters, number, and words. Four conditions influence the effectiveness of the encoded message: the skills, attitudes and knowledge of the sender, and sociocultural system.

Decoding is the process by which the receiver interprets the message and translate it into meaningful information. It is a two-step process. The receiver must perceive the massage then interpret it. Decoding is influenced by the receiver's past experience, personal assessment of the symbols used, expectations, and mutuality of meaning with the sender.

Channel is the formal medium of communication between a sender and a receiver. Common channels in organizations include meetings, memos, letters, reports e-mail and telephone calls. The channel chosen to communicate the message influence the communication process. Appropriate selection of the channel will help minimize the effect of noise. In healthcare organizations, certain channels are more appropriate for certain messages. For example, during an emergency we cannot wait for a written order from a physician to safeguard the life of a critically ill patient. Instead, we follow the verbal order and later obtain the written order. After decoding the message, the receiver has the option of responding through feedback. Feedback enables the sender to evaluate the effectiveness of the message. Feedback often initiates another cycle through the communication process, which can continue until both parties are satisfied with the result. Thus, there exists considerable value for feedback in the communication process.

### Types of Communication

Communication can be divided into verbal and nonverbal communication (**Fig. 14.2**). Verbal communication is the expression of ideas with the help of speech sounds or written symbols combined into words and words into sentences that could effectively convey meaning.

Nonverbal communication is done with the support of physical expression. The study of how one's head, arm, hand and facial expression get into act when one speaks is called kinesics. Mehrabian has stated that communication takes place 45% verbally and 55% nonverbally. The elements of nonverbal communication are personal appearance, posture, gestures, facial expression, eye contact and space distancing. Space distancing is the personal territory maintained around each communication. Space distancing is found to differ among different cultures.

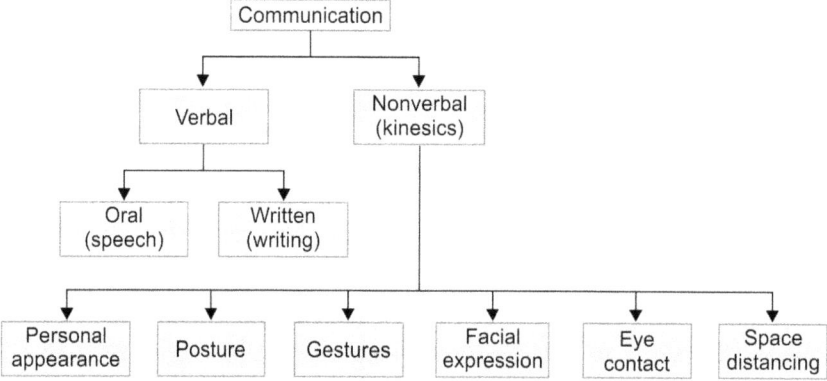

**Fig. 14.2:** Types of communication.

## Different Media or Channel of Communication

Various types of media used in communication processes are the following:
1. **Audio media:** While using audio media, the sender and receiver depend only on audio media. The receiver receives the communication only through hearing. The communications through radio, tape recorder, etc., also are examples of audio media.
2. **Visual media:** The communication may involve only visual media for transmitting and receiving message. The receiver may receive information or message by reading out a written or printed statement or through the visual interpretation of the graphic material (chart, diagrams, graphs, etc.).
3. **Audio-video media:** It is the combination of audio and visual media. When a teacher writes on the blackboard, draws a diagram, display a model or graph, he also makes use of his skill of narration explanation and lecturing along with visual display.
4. **Multisensory media:** Depending on the involvement of each of five senses (sight, hearing, smell, taste and touch) effectiveness of communication can be enhanced. Involving as many as senses possible is the best way of effective communication.
5. **Mass media:** Mass media is useful in carrying out communication with the masses. Radio, television, video, cinema, printed media, like books, newspapers and magazines are example of mass media. Internet communication in the form of e-mail, WhatsApp, Facebook also is an example of mass media. Teleconferencing and satellite communication also comes under the classification of mass media.
6. **Multimedia:** A communication is based on multimedia approach when it employees a number of media in a planned and organized combination for deriving maximum result in a particular communication situation. On-line education courses follow multimedia approach to enhance learning.

Fiske described three types of media in the following manner:
1. **Presentational:** For example, voice, face, body, etc.
2. **Representational:** For example, good picture, photograph, etc.
3. **Technological/mechanical:** For example, internet, phone, television, radio, CD, MP3, etc.

## Benefits of Effective Communication in Nursing

Effective communication provides numerous benefits as shown in **Figure 14.3.**

## Effective Communication Techniques

Effective communication is the process of sending a message in such a way that the message received is as close in meaning as possible to the message intended. Following are some of the effective communication techniques:

* **Organize information coherently and completely:** Organizing information in a clear and intelligible manner is essential for effective communication.
* **Express and present information coherently and persuasively:** Presenting information in a way to convince the audience by influencing their thoughts or actions is regarded as an effective communication technique. Maintaining eye contact is important while employing this technique.
* **Listening to others effectively:** Effective listening requires conscious effort. Good listening skill is essential to communicate effectively with patients.
* **Consider the background and experience of the audience:** Since decoding is influenced by the receiver's background, past experience and expectations, it is essential to have a knowledge regarding the background of the audience.

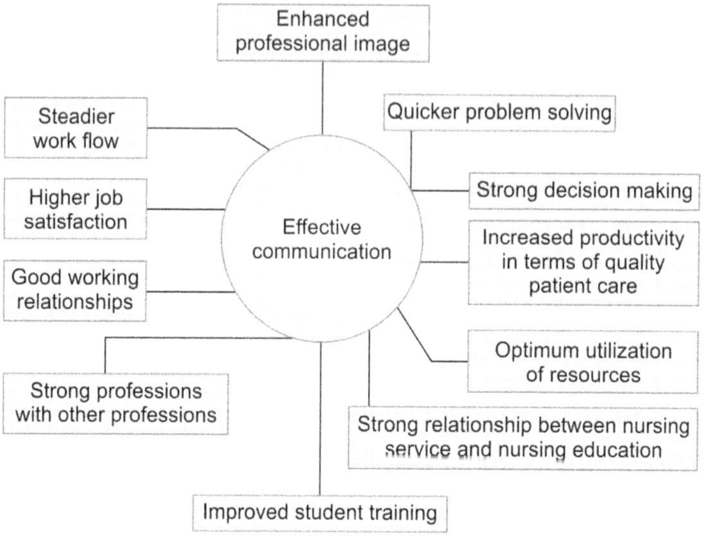

## Fig. 14.3: Benefits of effective communication in nursing.

Effective communication leads to:
- Enhanced professional image
- Steadier work flow
- Higher job satisfaction
- Good working relationships
- Strong professions with other professions
- Improved student training
- Strong relationship between nursing service and nursing education
- Optimum utilization of resources
- Increased productivity in terms of quality patient care
- Strong decision making
- Quicker problem solving

- ❖ **Use communication technologies effectively and efficiently:** Effective use of technological tools like E-mail, electronic presentations, web conferencing, etc., will enhance effectiveness of communication.
- ❖ **Communicate in a civilized manner that reflects contemporary expectations of nursing etiquette:** Even in a stressful situation, we are expected to communicate with courtesy and respect in a manner that is appropriate to the situation. This technique holds true especially in the clinical area.
- ❖ **Utilize the magical effect of touch:** When appropriately used, touch is a powerful form of communication. According to Battorff, support, encouragement, and tenderness are conveyed through touch. Janes believe that comfort touch is important for vulnerable patients experiencing severe illness with its accompanying physical and emotional losses. Hence appropriate use of touch is regarded as an effective communication technique.
- ❖ **Communicate ethically:** While communicating, it is essential to uphold ethical considerations for transmitting message in a pleasing manner.
- ❖ **Provide practical information:** Give recipients useful information, whether it is to help them perform a desired action or understand a new disease. For example, while giving health education on essential nutrients, it is better to advice on foods that are locally available rather than ready to eat commercially available ones.
- ❖ **Give facts rather than impressions:** Use concrete language, specific detail and information that is clear, convincing, accurate, complete and relevant. This technique is important when you explain a disease condition to a patient. This technique also assists you in giving health education pertaining to subjects, which contain specific details like developmental milestones.
- ❖ **Clarify and condense information:** Highlight the most important information rather than overloading the recipient with a flood of data and information. For example, while giving health education on myocardial infarction, you have to give emphasis on predisposing factors, preventive measures and warning symptoms rather than explaining the physiology and anatomy of the cardiovascular system in detail.

- **State precise responsibility:** Communicate messages to generate a specific response from a specific audience. Clearly state what you expect from audience or what you can do for them. For example, while you conduct a class on developmental milestones and weaning to postnatal mothers, you have to explain very clearly about what they are expected to do after discharge, and what help you can offer them through nearest health care providers.
- **Elicit feedback:** Explain to the audience precisely how they will benefit if they respond to your message in the desired manner. Eliciting feedback is essential when you convey health messages.

## Facilitators of Communication

Since communication is a dynamic process, many factors influence it in many ways. According to Potter and Perry, following are the facilitators of communication: (a) the message, (b) level of development, (c) individual background, especially culture and attitudes, (d) emotions, (e) past experiences, (f) relationships and roles, (g) the grapevine, (h) space and territory, and (i) environmental factors. As we have already discussed about message along with the elements of communication process, let us discuss the other facilitators.

- **Level of development:** Language skills of children develop as they grow. By adulthood, one is usually quite fluent in a language. During old age or suffering from health problems, language skills may be affected. When communicating, we have to consider the individual's level of development.
- **Individual background:** The background of the individual includes one's culture, language, attitudes and values. Culture influences the message of communication, its style, the gestures used and the value placed on the messages. Nurses need to be aware about their personal values and not allow them to interfere while communicating. Attitude strongly influences communication. Individuals with negative attitudes are less likely to receive complete message. Knowledge regarding the background of the receiver will help you send messages in a more comprehensible manner. Communication and
- **Past experiences:** Past experiences can have an impact on communication. For example, communicating effectively with a patient who had a bitter experience during previous hospital stay is difficult.
- **Emotions:** Emotions are feelings and how one feels about the subject strongly influences the sending and receiving of messages. Since emotions can be easily misunderstood, it is important be aware about your emotions as well as receiver's emotions. Developing an awareness of your own emotions and keeping an open mind will help you communicate in a clear manner.
- **Relationship and roles:** Communications are affected by roles people assume. Based on relationships and roles, communication can be classified as downward communication, upward communication, lateral communication, and diagonal communication.
- **The grapevine:** The grapevine is the most important informal communication system within any organization. Communications within the grapevine are usually based on relationships rather than roles. Grapevine flourishes when people do not receive information they want or need. The grapevine satisfies the need for people to communicate. The grapevine carries information that is of interest. Naturally, that information can become distorted or incomplete. People will fill the missing pieces; thus, further distorting the communication. Since grapevine can have a negative impact, nurses working in managerial positions need to be more aware about it.
- **Space and territory:** When people interact they keep a certain amount of space or distance between themselves. Territoriality is an important consideration when communicating

and nurses involved with direct patient care frequently work at the intimae distance levels of 18 inches or less. Hein recommends following interactive distances for different communications: (a) Intimate distance (18 inches or less). (b) Personal distance (18 inches to 4 feet). This is the space at which most managerial communications take place. They are usually one-on-one interaction, but they can involve small group. (c) Social distance (4 feet to 12 feet). It is commonly used when working in groups. (d) Public distance (more than 12 feet). This is used when addressing a large group. The speakers usually use a microphone and little group interaction occurs.

- **Environmental factors:** The sending and receiving of message is much more effective when people are free of physical and emotional discomfort. The best physical environment for communicating is one that is private, warm and free of noise or distractions. The effectiveness of communication is also decreased when one is emotionally disturbed. Person who is hungry or worried is much less likely to send or receive messages effectively.

## Barriers to Communication

Barriers to communication can be classified as information-related barriers, physical barriers, language barriers, psychological barriers, and background barriers.

- **Information-related barriers:** Information-related barriers include filtering and information overload. Filtering is the deliberate manipulation of information to make it appear more favorable to the receiver. Information overload occurs when the information we have to work with exceeds our assimilating capacity. Information overload may result in ignore, pass over, or forget information.
- **Physical barriers:** Physical barriers include noise, invisibility, environmental and physical discomfort, distraction, and ill health. Physical distractions range from bad connections and poor acoustics to illegible printing and uncomfortable meeting rooms.
- **Language barriers:** Language barriers include verbosity, unclear graphics, and symbols. Sometimes, Jargon may also serve as language barrier. A jargon is a specialized terminology or technical language that members of a group use to communicate among themselves. For example, nurses say "mc" instead of mouth care. As far as possible, use the correct term instead of jargon to minimize communication errors.
- **Psychological barriers:** Extreme emotions, prejudice, disinterest, inattention, redundancy, unpleasant experience and defensiveness are some of the psychological barriers. Psychological barriers may cause selective perception. Selective perception occurs when people selectively interpret what they see or hear on the basis of their interests, experience and attitudes.
- **Background barriers:** Background barriers include previous learning, cultural differences, etc.

## Methods to Overcome Barriers to Communication

- **Methods to overcome information related barriers:** Organization of information and objective analysis of the situation will help prevent filtering of information. Written mode of communication reduces filtration because communication is more directing in manner. By the judicious selection of relevant information and organizing information according to relevance and priority, we can prevent information overload.
- **Methods to overcome physical barriers:** Measures like (a) proper seating arrangement, (b) ensuring adequate audibility and visibility, (c) reduction of visual and aural distractions, and (d) provision of conducive environment will help overcome physical barriers.

- ❖ **Methods to overcome language barriers:** Words mean different things to different people. Age, education, and cultural background are the main factors that influence the language a person uses, and the definitions he or she gives to words. Using simple language, proper explanation with adequate examples, appropriate use of audiovisual aids, adopting different methods of communication and above all obtaining frequent feedbacks are some of the measures that will help overcome language barriers.
- ❖ **Methods to overcome psychological barriers:** Initiating a healthy interpersonal relationship with the receiver, creation of a nonthreatening atmosphere, encouraging feedback, calling by name and motivating the receiver, showing empathy, judicious use of audiovisual aids, and appropriate use of touch are some of the methods suggested to overcome psychological barriers.
- ❖ **Methods to overcome background barriers:** Clear understanding of the receiver's background, explaining the receiver about the significance of message and explanation about the merits of the proper comprehension of the message are some of the techniques to overcome background barriers.

## Communication Theory

Communication takes place intrapersonal (within the self) or interpersonally (with others).

Intrapersonal communication occurs in the form of person's inner thoughts that influence behavior. Intrapersonal communication is defined as a reciprocal, interactive and dynamic process involving transmission and reception of information. According to Elizabeth Arnold, interpersonal communication theories are concerned with the transmission of information and how people create meaning from this information. Through speech, touch, listening and responding people construct personal meanings and share them with others. Relational communication is an important way of personal expression and influence communication takes place by means of language, gesture, body movements, eye contact and personal cultural symbols.

Bateson put forward below mentioned basic assumptions of communication theory
- ❖ All behavior is communication and it is impossible to not communicate.
- ❖ Every communication has a content and a relationship aspect.
- ❖ We only know about ourselves and others through communication.
- ❖ Wrong communication results in wrong feelings and actions.
- ❖ Feedback is the only way to know about how the message is perceived by others.
- ❖ Silence is a form of communication.
- ❖ All elements of a communication system are interrelated and influence one another.
- ❖ People communicate through nonverbal behaviors; both forms are needed to interpret a message appropriately.

## Communication Theories in Nursing

Multiple communication theories are used in nursing to guide interactions between nurses and patients, as well as nurse and other healthcare professionals. Among communication theories, Peplau's interpersonal relations theory is most widely accepted by the nursing community.

### *Peplau's Interpersonal Relations Theory*

This theory focuses on the nurse-patient relationship and the therapeutic process that takes place. Communications involves many factors such as environment in addition to attitudes, practices and beliefs determined by the culture. Peplau's interpersonal relations theory defines four stages of the relationship that achieve a common goal.

The four stages are:
1. **Orientation phase:** Nurse explains her role in treatment and the patient is motivated to ask questions and receive explanations and information. This stage helps the patient develops trust and get an idea about health care.
2. **Identification phase/working phase:** The patient and nurse begin to work together. Due to interactions between nurse and patients, patient becomes more active participant in treatment.
3. **Exploitation phase:** The patient takes advantage of all services offered, exploiting the nurse-patient relationship to attain treatment goals.
4. **Resolution phase:** As a result of effective communication, the patient's needs are met and now patient moves toward full independence. The patient no longer needs help and the relationship ends.

## Principles of Effective Communication in Nursing Practice

In Lambrini Kourkouta's opinion, communication is a key part of all nursing practices including treatment, prevention, rehabilitation, education and health promotion. She proposes following principles for effective communication in nursing practice.

- **Effective communication is bilateral:** Effective communication is bilateral. The person sending the message also becomes the receiver of messages. Nurses should be aware of this while communicating with patients. Listening and speaking are equally important in communication.
- **Effective communication is possible only by deeply understanding all parts of a message:** Effective communication goes beyond merely understanding the message. Effective communication requires an understanding of the intention of the message, the sender's purpose and sender's expectation about what the receiver will do with the received message.
- **Effective communication requires active listening:** Active listening is the key of successful communication. Active listening requires attending the content, intent and feeling of the sender. Active listeners asks questions and give nonverbal and visual cues to indicate that they are interested in the words of speaker. In nursing, listening skill is very important for collecting relevant data about illness of patients.
- **Effective communication is both verbal and nonverbal:** Communication theory focuses on verbal communication. However, effective communication also requires consideration of nonverbal cues. Nurses need to be aware about patients' nonverbal cues to learn about what patients are trying to express or communicate. To make the communication effective the nurse's verbal and nonverbal communication should be compatible. If the nonverbal cues doesn't match the verbal communication, it is difficult to understand the message properly.
- **Effective communication in nursing requires good relationships:** Therapeutic relationship is an important prerequisite to effective communication between nurses and patients. Relationship encourages patients to share information with nurses and other healthcare professionals.
- **Effective communication involves conflict resolution:** If managed properly, conflict can encourage communication with others. Maintain respect during conflict is essential to achieve objectives of communication. An open mindset of nurses and patients helps to resolve conflict through communication.
- **Effective communication requires accuracy:** Accuracy should be a guiding principle while sending or receiving information. A message can easily become distorted when it

passes from one person to another. Hence, as far as possible, nurses should speak directly to people to communicate message. This results in correct person receiving the most accurate information.

❖ **Effective communication requires an understanding of the patient and the experiences they express:** Nurses need to understand the concerns of the patients in a sincere manner. Nurses should also convey the message that she is understandable and acceptable.

## Effective Communication in Clinical Area

If healthcare professionals, especially nurses are not communicating properly, patient safety is at risk for several reasons. These include lack of important information or data for patient care, misinterpretation of information and unclear orders over telephone. Lack of effective communication in clinical area leads to medical errors also.

Effective communication in clinical area is defined as the two way exchange of information between patients or patient's relatives and healthcare professionals for ensuring safe and effective patient care. It is an active process for all involved in patient care. Two way communication provides feedback, which enables understanding by both patient and caregivers. Timely, accurate and effective messages that are understood clearly by all concerned help in providing meticulous patient care. In short, effective communication is accurate, clear, concise, concrete complete and courteous.

## Communication Problems in Clinical Area

According to Elizabeth K, communication problems occur when there are failures in one or more categories as discussed below.

❖ System failures occur when the necessary channels of communication are absent or not functioning.
❖ Transmission failures occur when the channels exist but the message is never send or it is not clearly sent.
❖ Reception failures occur when channels exists and necessary information is sent, but the receiver misinterpret the message.

## Standardized Communication Tools

Standardized communication tools help to communicate effectively by ensuring clarity in communication. This is essential to provide meticulous patient care. With the easy access to technology and availability of suitable software, nowadays, most health care facilities develop their own standardized communication tools. Since every member of health team follow the same standard format for communication there is less chance for communication errors.

On example of standardized communication tool is the situation, background, assessment, recommendation **(SBAR)** format.
❖ Situation (what is going on with the patient)
❖ Background (what is the key information/content)
❖ Assessment (what to I think the problem is)
❖ Recommendation (what do I want to be done)

## Assertive Communication

The skill of assertiveness is important to nurses. Nurses are expected to be patient's advocates, so they need to have the assertive communication skills to perform this role effectively. Assertiveness enables a person to be honest with him/herself and in relationship with others.

Assertiveness helps to maintain relationships, avoid misunderstanding and results in clear outcomes.

Being assertive means being able to stand for our own or others legitimate rights in a calm and positive manner, without being either aggressive or passively accepting 'wrong'. Hargis identities four elements of assertive communication as follows:

### Content

Ensure the rights of the individuals involved are stated appropriately in the statement. This could be done by using an explanation, empathy for the listeners or a compromise that is favorable to both individuals.

### Covert Statements

The speaker needs to recognize his rights and the rights of the listener in the communication process. These include respect, expressing feelings, having our own priorities and being able to say no.

### Process

Process is concerned with how people express themselves assertively. Body language, intonation and choice of language need to be reflective of a confident assertive person. The process also involves managing the environment so that people are not embarrassed or the noise levels are kept to a minimum. Providing a feedback that appreciates the role of listener is also important.

### Nonverbal Cues

Gesture, touch, proxemics and posture-also need to reflect confidence, regard and respect for self and others.

## INTERPERSONAL RELATIONSHIP

### Meaning

An interpersonal relationship is an association or connection between two or more individuals. This association may be long-term or short-term depending upon the circumstances and the nature of individuals involved. Interpersonal relationships take place in all walks of life. Generally, interpersonal relationships are based on needs. When two individuals have strong needs and each fills the other's needs, there is powerful interpersonal relationship. When two individuals have weak needs and each fills the other's needs, there is mild relationship. When both personnel has strong needs and those needs are not being filled, there is poor relationship.

### Definition

Haugie defined interpersonal relationship skill as a "process in which the individual implements a set of goal-directed, inter-related, situationally appropriate social behaviours which are learned and controlled". This definition emphasis following aspects:

- ❖ Interpersonal relationship skill is a combination of identifiable units of behavior (In simple terms, verbal and nonverbal).
- ❖ Identifiable units of behaviors are interrelated (verbal and nonverbal messages should be compatible)
- ❖ Goal directed.
- ❖ It can be learned.

* It is under the cognitive control of the individual (cognitive control is how to do certain things and why those things are done the way they are).
* It should be appropriate to the situations.

The acronym CLIPS is useful for remembering the key factors of interpersonal relationship skill:
* **C**ontrolled by the individual.
* **L**earned behavior that improves with practice and feedback.
* **I**ntegrated and interrelated verbal and nonverbal response.
* **P**urposeful.
* **S**mooth manner in which the performance is executed.

## Relationship Quotient

Relationship quotient (RQ) comprises an ability, capacity or skill to perceive, assess and manage one's relationships. According to Dr Yusuf, relationship quotient or relationship intelligence involves gaining an understanding of oneself and others and applying that understanding to build more meaningful and effective relationships. Relationship quotient is closely linked to emotional intelligence. As discussed elsewhere in this book, researchers have identified five components of emotional intelligence, namely knowing our emotions (self-awareness), managing them, motivating ourselves, recognizing emotions in others (empathy), and handling relationships. If one is emotionally stable, understanding, tolerant, and compassionate and has at least an average intelligence, he or she will definitely be able to enjoy good interpersonal relationships. In any relationship, aim is not to avoiding conflicts but managing them constructively. Thus, one of the dimension of relationship intelligence is related to effective problem solving. A good RQ facilitates stable and cohesive relationship in one's life. According to Kripalini, "every relationship has its ups and downs. A person with good RQ is able to focus on the positives and work on the negatives, while maintaining a holistic perspective."

## Purposes of Interpersonal Relations

Since interpersonal relationship is widely discussed under psychology, sociology, social psychology, nursing, and anthropology, it is difficult to list precisely the purposes of interpersonal relationship across various settings and circumstances. Authors believe that the following purposes can be achieved through good interpersonal relationship.
* **Promotion of community living:** Interpersonal relationships involve some level of interdependence. People in a relationship tend to influence each other, share their thoughts and feelings and engage in activities together. Due to this interdependence, any problem faced by one member of the relationship will be solved with the help of other members. Thus, good interpersonal relationship promotes better community living.
* **Promotion of positive thinking:** Positive thinking is essential to lead a healthy and successful life. Good interpersonal relationships always foster positive thinking. Positive thinking also hastens the healing process. By maintaining good interpersonal relationship with patients, we can foster positive thinking among patients. Positive thinking also helps in the reduction of stress.
* **To build a healthy society:** Good interpersonal relationships among individuals in the community will help in the adoption of healthy behaviors. Health programs can be implemented successfully if there exists a good interpersonal relationship between healthcare professionals and the public. Thus, good interpersonal relationships assist in building a healthy society.

- **To promote social harmony:** Good interpersonal relationship among members of a society will help eliminate antisocial elements in a more effective manner. Homicides and suicides are less in a closely held community. Social harmony in turn motivate people to respect and obey the laws existing in the society.
- **To achieve the aims of an organization:** Today, a lot of research works are going on regarding the influence of interpersonal relations among employees in the overall performance of the organization. Good interpersonal relationship among employee is essential for achieving the aims of an organization.
- **To fulfill the responsibilities of a profession:** Good interpersonal relationship among members of a profession is essential to uphold the dignity of the profession. Moreover, social image of a profession is determined by the ability of its members in establishing good interpersonal relationship with the public. Thus, it is very important for us to maintain good interpersonal relationship with the patients and their loved ones to uphold the social image of our profession.

## Purposes of Interpersonal Relationship in Nursing

The ultimate purpose of interpersonal relationship in nursing is to provide the best and safest possible nursing care through achieving below mentioned purposes.
- Building a positive functional multidisciplinary team.
- Improving intra and or inter team communication, coordination and cooperation.
- Helps to understand every nurse about her competencies as an individual and as a professional nurse by proper interaction with team members.
- Improved decision making and problem solving.
- Enhanced collaboration with other healthcare professionals by understanding each member's role in the healthcare team.

## Importance of Interpersonal Relationship in Nursing

Interpersonal relationship is important in nursing because of the following reasons:
- There is a strong relationship between therapeutic interpersonal skill of nurse and patient well-being in nursing care.
- Therapeutic nurse patient relationship is the basis of nursing practice.
- Good interpersonal relationship between nurses and patients is essential for the active participation of patients in health care.
- Good interpersonal relationship helps nurses and patients to share their experience about patient care. This will help in improving nursing care by rectifying deficiencies.

## Types of Interpersonal Relationship

Psychologists believe that all humans have a motivational drive to form and maintain caring interpersonal relationships. According to this view, people need both stable relationships, and satisfying interactions with the people in those relationships. Interpersonal relationship can be classified as friendships, family, romantic relationships, and professional relationships. Friendships consist of mutual liking, trust, respect, and often even love along with unconditional acceptance. They usually imply the discovery or establishment of similarities or common ground between the individuals. Professional relationships are more precise in nature and are governed by predetermined objectives and rules. As a rule, professional relationship follows a predictable path. Nurse-patient relationship is an example of professional relationship. In nursing practice, interpersonal relationship is synonymous with nurse-patient relationship.

## Phases of Interpersonal Relationship

Interpersonal relationships are dynamic systems that change continuously. Like living organisms, relationships have a beginning, a life span and an end. George Levinger argues that natural development of a relationship follows five stages, namely: (a) acquaintance, (b) build up, (c) continuation, (d) deterioration, and (e) termination.

In nursing, interpersonal relationship is synonymous with nurse-patient relationship. According to Barbara Kozier, "Nurse-patient relationship are referred to some as interpersonal relationships, by others as therapeutic relationships and by still others as helping relationships." She believes that process of establishing a nurse-patient relationship involves four sequential phases, each characterized by identifiable tasks and skills. The four phases are preinteraction phase, introductory phase, working phase, and termination phase.

## Barriers to Interpersonal Relationship and Measures to Overcome

Since interpersonal relationship is widely discussed under psychology, sociology nursing, sociopsychology, and anthropology, it is difficult to list down precisely the barriers to interpersonal relationship across various setting and circumstances. Authors believe that following factors can serve as barriers in establishing interpersonal relationship: (a) mistrust, (b) lack of awareness regarding needs, (c) lack of mutual respect, (d) ineffective communication, (e) absence of conducive environment, (f) cultural intolerance, (g) lack of common goal or purpose, (h) professional incompetence, and (i) low relationship quotient. As many of these barriers are self-explanatory, a few only require detailed discussion.

- **Mistrust:** Mistrust is regarded as the major obstacle in maintaining good interpersonal relationship. Integrity, honesty, open communication, mutual respect, and awareness regarding other's needs will help build good interpersonal relationship by avoiding mistrust.
- **Lack of awareness regarding needs:** As discussed earlier, interpersonal relationships are generally based on needs. Finding out what the other person needs and then filling that need is essential to enhance any relationship. Many people fail to discover and recognize other's needs. The way to recognize needs of other people is by their response to you. It is sometimes easier to recognize another person's needs, but we fail to express our own needs due to fear or guilt.
- **Lack of mutual respect:** Mutual respect is an integral requirement of all relationship whether between married couples, parent and child, friends, nurse and patient, peers, or bosses and communication and respectful relationship involves mutually, tolerance, extension of the self, and nonjudgmental attitude. A conscious approach in building a respectful relationship will help in the development of mutual respect.
- **Ineffective communication:** After mistrust, ineffective communication is regarded as the main obstacle in building a good relationship. Sometimes, ineffective communication itself lead to mistrust. Avoiding grapevine by employing effective communication techniques is essential to maintain good interpersonal relationships.
- **Professional incompetence:** This is mainly applicable to professional relationships. For example, when a nurse fails to initiate and maintain interpersonal relationship with a deserving patient, we can say she is professionally incompetent to provide comprehensive nursing care.

## HUMAN RELATIONS

### Definition

Human relationship is the study of how individuals' beliefs, attitudes and behaviors influences in building and maintaining interpersonal relationships. It covers all types of interactions among individuals, their conflicts, cooperative effort and group relationships. Knowledge on human relationships helps to find out and solve issues related to interpersonal relationships in personal as well as professional life. In simple words, human relations refers to the interpersonal and group interactions of individuals.

In nursing perspective, human relations refers to the ability of a nurse to interact appropriately with patients and other health team members to build effective interpersonal relations essential for providing meticulous nursing care.

## Human Relations Skill in Nursing

Most important skills that help nurses to build good human relations are:

- **Communication:** Communication is the most important factor that influence in building relations. The ability to clearly convey messages to others as well as listening sincerely promote relationships. Assertive communication is the most recommended type of communication.
- **Empathy:** How empathetically a nurse interacts with patients definitely influence relationships. Empathy is essential to understand the feelings and needs of patients as well as health team members. Empathy is also essential for providing compassionate nursing care. It will in turn foster good relations.
- **Managing stress:** Stress negatively impacts personal as well as professional life. Good coping mechanisms that helps maintain calmness during stressful situations foster relations.
- **Conflict resolution:** The ability to work well through conflict and reaching conflict resolutions is essential for building good relations. Approaching conflicts with aggressiveness leads to disintegration of relations. Listening others opinions, choosing the right setting and time to solve disagreements is essential for conflict resolution. Being assertive during conflict resolution helps us to safeguard our rights as a nurse.
- **Professionalism:** Highly professional behavior is essential for maintaining good relations in nursing professionalism is essential to provide meticulous nursing care. This will in turn foster good relations with patients and other health team members.

## Understanding Self

### Definition

Understanding self or self-awareness is the process of objective examination of oneself. According to Daniel Goldman, "understanding self is the understanding of one's internal states, preference, resources and intuitions". This definition focuses on awareness about our inner thoughts and feelings. The nonjudgmental aspect is an important element of self-awareness. As we are aware about our inner thoughts, we accept ourselves as being human without regrets. Above all, understanding self helps us to respond appropriately to situations. This will in turn help us to manage our immediate environment in a successful manner.

### Types of Self-awareness

According to Anais Salibain, there are two types of self-awareness. One is conceptual self-awareness and other is embodied self-awareness, of these two, embodied self-awareness is more important. Conceptual self-awareness is what we think about ourselves, which may include judgment, evaluations, logical and things that are easy to express.

Embodied self-awareness is awareness about various types of our inner states. Embodied self-awareness lets us know if we are tired or hungry, excited or in pain, etc. Most importantly, embodied self-awareness lets us know our responses and reactions to internal and external events, our emotions, our impulses, our needs and wants. Embodied self-awareness is as fundamental to health and must be maintained, cultivated, taught and renewed to sustain well-being.

## Importance of Understanding Self

According to Daneil Holeman, understanding self is important for the following reasons:
- Self-awareness is essential for developing emotional intelligence. Good emotional intelligence is needed for achieving success in life by controlling emotions, thoughts and actions.
- Self-awareness individuals possess optimal psychological health and maintain positive attitude in life. Additionally, self-aware individuals are more empathetic to others as well as themselves.
- Self-awareness is essential for developing leadership qualities. Good leaders have a substantial self-awareness.
- Steven covey believes that self-awareness involves deep personal honesty. It is easier for honest people to lead a successful and peaceful life.
- Self-awareness promotes attention of doing tasks by concentrating on the task and living in the present moment. In other words "Mindfulness" is the advantage of good self-awareness".
- Self-awareness is essential to identify our strengths and weaknesses and giving more attention to our strengths.
- Self-awareness allows us to recognize what things we can do best in life. This helps us to attain success in life.
- Above all, understanding ourselves helps us to live fully in any situation or condition by utilizing capabilities as a human being.

## Understanding Self and Nursing Practice

From the above discussions, it is clear that adequate self-awareness contribute to successful nursing practice in the following manner.
- Self-awareness, especially embodied self-awareness is essential for professional nursing practice. Embodied self-awareness helps in finding out the what, how, why and when components of professional practice.
- Since self-awareness is a process of objective examination of oneself it is an important component in building therapeutic nurse–patient relationship.
- Knowing oneself help nurses to understand patients and other health team members in a better manner.
- Good leaders have substantial self-awareness. Hence, good self-awareness help nurses to become good leaders.
- Since self-awareness helps to identify strengths and weaknesses, nurses with good self-awareness can easily attain competency in nursing practice by overcoming weaknesses and focusing on strengths.
- Adequate emotional intelligence associated with self-awareness help nurses to achieve success in professional as well as personal life.
- Self-awareness helps nurses to clearly identify their role in healthcare team and this helps to function as effective health team member.
- Self-awareness helps to develop empathy which is an important quality of a professional nurse.

## Social Behavior and Nursing Practice

In nursing, social behavior is viewed as the patterns of behavior existing between individuals who constitute society. More precisely, in nursing, social behavior deals with the relationships existing between people. The human being as a person is linked by a complex network of social relationships. These social relationships in turn determines the role of a person in the society, for example, the role of a nurse as health team member in the hospital may change to that of a wife or daughter when she reaches home. Understanding social behavior helps the nurse in the following ways: (a) to analyze the relationship of the patient with his loved ones, (b) to establish interpersonal relationship with patients, (c) to analyze the coping strength of patient, (d) to identify the resources available for treating the patient, (e) to clarify her role in various situations, and (f) to achieve a work life balance by fulfilling her roles related to personal and professional life.

## Individual and Groups

Brown argues that every human being living in society is of two things: (a) he is an individual and also (b) a person. Human beings as individuals are subjects of psychologists. The human being as a person is a complex of social relationships. According to CN Shankar Rao, character of social relationships underlie different forms of social groups, such as primary and secondary groups, in groups and out groups, organized and unorganized groups, formal and informal groups or organizations. No man normally lives alone. Men everywhere live in groups. Daily life is possible only through participating in groups activities. Society is made up of groups. A social group exists when two or more people are in direct or indirect contact and communication. Various factors such as psychological factors, biological factors, kinship bond (blood relationship), geographic factor, cultural factor, economic factor, religious factor, and political factor which motivate human beings to lead a social life are known as social bonds. Individuals are motivated to lead a group life because of the following reasons: (a) survival becomes difficult without groups, (b) only a human environment makes a man, (c) group activity is essential for socialization, and (d) groups contribute to the development of personality. As far as health care is concerned, many groups like alcoholic anonymous provide individuals with an opportunity to engage in activities that promote health.

## Groups and Individuals

From the above discussion, it is evident that individuals become individuals only in groups. Group can influence the individual in many ways. Individual may change his opinion, attitude, etc., due to the influence of group. In health care, influence of the group in the behavior of individual is utilized to bring about desired behavioral change in individual.

## Group Dynamics

The communication and behavioral patterns established by the group members is referred to as group dynamics. Each group has its own dynamics because each group is composed of unique individuals. Persons involved in the group should share some characteristics and interact. It is because of this that the group acquires its own characteristics. The effectiveness of group dynamics is influenced by the factors, such as: (a) goals or purpose of the group, (b) commitment of the group members, (c) decision making abilities of group members, (d) leadership style of the group leader, (e) communication among members, and (f) group cohesiveness.

## Teamwork

A team is a group of individuals who functions as a unit for attaining a common goal. In an organization, a team is a group of workers that functions as a unit, often with little or no supervision for carry out organizational functions. In Bragg's opinion, members of the effective teams usually (a) share leadership responsibilities, (b) cooperate each other, (c) share ideas freely, (d) listen affectively and accepts the concerns of others, (e) seek creative solutions when viewpoints differ, (f) for ego personal recognition for the sake of team, and (g) recognize and support the contributions of other members. Needless to say, effective management of conflict is essential for good teamwork.

Tuckman and Jensen have described the phases of team development as forming, storming, and norming, performing and adjourning. In the forming phase, leader provides structure, clarifies goals, communication and refocus as necessary. In the storming phase, differences among group members may arise and often begin to challenge the leader. At this point, it is important for the team leader to allow differences to focus on the problem and not the person. As the group progresses to the norming phase, members solve the differences and start working. At this time, leader needs to clarify roles and responsibilities once again. The performance phase is the most productive. Group members trust each other and work together to achieve the common goal. In the adjourning phase, leader should summarize what the team has accomplished, acknowledge the team effort, and celebrate the team's success.

## Human Relations in the Context of Nursing

A WHO expert committee defined nursing as "the conscious practice of human relationships." This definition itself signifies the importance of human relations in the nursing practice. All nursing actions are based on human interactions. Different roles assumed by a nurse like caregiver, patient advocate, etc., are derived from human relations in the context of nursing. The advent of "high-tech high-touch" approach in nursing practice to preserve the human element in nursing without undermining the technological advancements in patient care underlines the importance of human relations in nursing. The relationships like nurse–patient relationship, nurse–family relationship, nurse–community relationship and nurse–health team member relationship are based on human relations. Nursing is regarded as the most caring one among healthcare professions. This caring image is mainly due to the high proportion of human element involved in the practice of nursing. To a great extent this human element is manifested in the form of human relations.

## ■ INFORMATION, EDUCATION AND COMMUNICATION FOR HEALTH

### Meaning

Information, education and communication (IEC) for health is being widely used as a general term for communication activities in health promotion. Various aspects coming under IEC are health behavior, health education, planning for health education, health education with individuals, groups and communities, communicating health messages, and methods and media for communicating health messages. The relationship between IEC for health and health promotion is evident from **Figure 14.4**.

### Health Education

As per WHO guidelines, health promotion is one of the most important components of health care and consider health education as the core of such promotional activities. According to National Conference on Preventive Medicine in USA, "Health education is a process that informs, motivates, and helps people adopt and maintain healthy practices and lifestyles and advocates environmental changes as needed to facilitate this goal and conducts professional training and research to the same end."

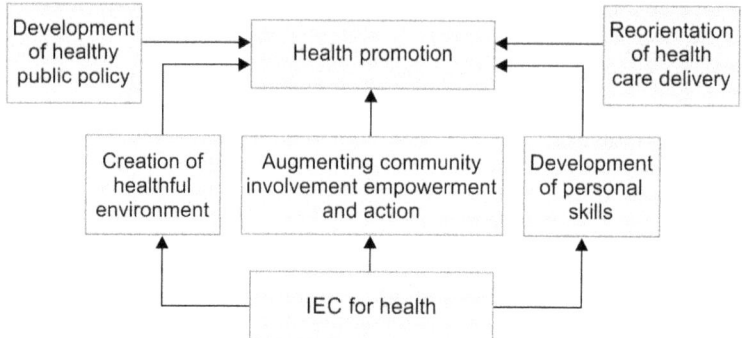

**Fig. 14.4:** Relationship between IEC for health and health promotion.

Almost all healthcare activities provide an opportunity to practice health education, and almost all healthcare providers have an opportunity to serve as a health educator. The interest and needs of the target group and the resources available will decide the content and course of health education. Proper health education is essential for the optimum utilization of health services. In short, the aims of health education can be summarized as follows: (a) to ensure that health is valued as an asset by the community, (b) to equip the people with knowledge, attitudes, and skills essential for leading a healthy life, and (c) to promote the development and proper utilization of health services.

Health education is not a substitute to health service. Presence of accessible and affordable health service is essential for achieving optimum public health. When the behavior of the individual, group or a community is the main reason for a health problem, health education is highly effective in solving that particular health problem.

### Health Behavior and Health Education

The relationship between health behavior and health education is evident from the medical model of health education (**Fig. 14.5**).

Modern concept of health education is based on health behavior and related actions of people. Health education aims to change attitude by providing knowledge which in turn results in the adoption of desired behavior patterns or health behavior. Desired behavior patterns eventually lead to better health. Health education programs encourage the behavior that promote health, prevent illness cures disease, and facilitates rehabilitation.

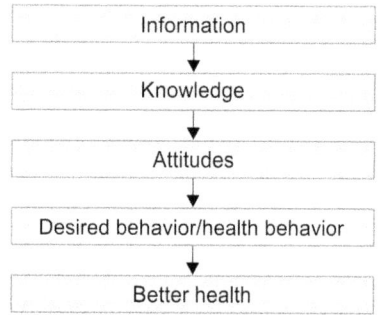

**Fig. 14.5:** Medical model of health education.

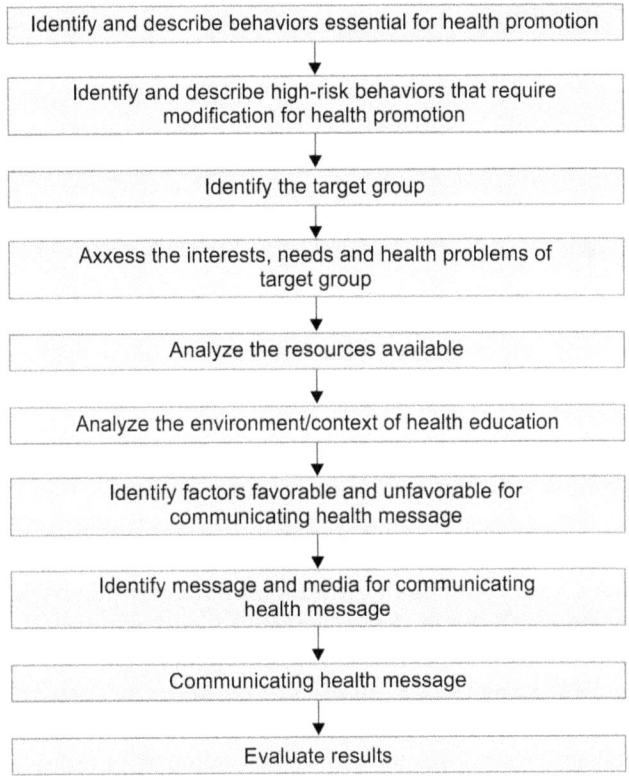

**Fig. 14.6:** Planning for health education.

## Planning for Health Education

As there is no effective treatment for many emerging diseases, and majority of lifestyle diseases and accidents can be prevented by adopting desirable behavior, the role of health education in promoting public health has increased considerably. Since health education depends upon the interests and needs of the target group, behaviors that require modification, resources available, circumstances or context along with other factors, following steps in planning health education need to be modified as desired (**Fig. 14.6**).

## Health Education for Individuals

Health education for individuals usually takes place in hospitals, health centers, or in homes. Depending on the situation, educator may be a medical practitioner, nurse, nursing student, public health nurse, dietician, health inspector or any other member of the health team. Even though individual health education is imparted in the form of personal interview, sometimes it virtually takes the shape of counseling. Practically, counseling is the fullest manifestation of health education at individual level. Since individual health education imparted through one to one interaction, individuals are motivated to adopt healthy lifestyle by adopting desirable behaviors. Time consuming nature of individual health education is its main disadvantage. Only a few individuals can be educated at a given time. The disadvantages will be more if the educator tries to impose his own views and values on the individual.

## Health Education for Groups

Health education for small groups provide an opportunity for two-way communication between the educator and audience. Knowledge of group dynamics and its applications is essential to conduct group health education in a successful manner. In OP Gai's opinion, following are some of the groups commonly organized for health promotion activities: (a) self-help groups, (b) problem-solving groups, (c) task-oriented groups/core groups, (d) disease treatment groups of patients, and (e) special target groups like adolescents, antenatal mothers, etc.

## Health Education with Communities

Health education with communities is carried through mass media of communication. According to Piyush Gupta, there are three widely accepted strategies for mass communication in order to give health education to communities, namely psychodynamic strategy, sociocultural strategy, and meaning construction strategy.

The psychodynamic strategy depends on modifying cognitive factors to influence behaviors. Information provided by the health educator results in new learning. New learning takes place through the modification of internal psychological structure of the individual consisting of needs, fears, attitudes, etc., resulting in the adoption of desired behavior. The disadvantage of psychodynamic strategy is that it does not seem to work consistently. For example, after attending health education on evil effects of smoking, people may avoid smoking only for few days due to the fear of lung cancer. After that they forget the explanation of health educator and starts smoking again.

The sociocultural strategy utilizes the rules of social behavior for individuals and cultural values. In order to bring about desired behavioral changes, health educator highlights the acceptable role behavior, ways to acquire and maintain social status and what social control might operate, if one deviates from the system in addition to the health hazards resulting from unhealthy behavior. Sociocultural strategy is highly useful in giving health education regarding good parenting, alcoholism, drug abuse, etc.

Meaning construction approach aims to remove certain unintended influences developed among the public due to the impact of mass media by way of providing newly constructed or revised meanings for certain objects, events, and issues. For example, in the past, due to the impact of mass media, chubby babies were considered healthier than optimum weight babies. Now, through the same mass media, we are receiving the health message that chubby babies are prone to develop illness during their adulthood when compared to optimum weight babies.

## Concept of Empowerment

In Piyush Gupta's opinion, above discussed strategies are based on persuasion approach. Worldwide, a new concept for communicating health message, namely "concept of empowerment" based on "informed decision-making approach" is gaining acceptance. This relatively new approach empowers individual, family, and community to make their own choice by way of providing proper information and enhancing their problem-solving and decision-making skills. The concept of empowerment is practical, sustainable and more humane in nature. However, in emergency situations like epidemics and disasters or when preventive actions are well defined, it is essential to follow persuasive approach in bringing out desirable behavioral changes.

## Communicating Health Messages

In addition to employing effective communication techniques and selecting appropriate media for communication, educator need to consider the following points while preparing content of health message in order to communicate health messages effectively. (a) content should elicit active participation from the audience, (b) health message should be introduced in an attractive manner, (c) whenever possible explain with the help of appropriate examples and seek examples from the audience, (d) content should be appropriate to the media and method of communication, (e) content should be relevant, condensed in nature and comprehensible, (f) content should respect the belief of all sections of the society, (g) use clear and simple language in preparing content and (h) content should contain enough practical tips related to the topic of health education.

## Methods and Media for Communicating Health Message

K Park suggests following methods and media for communicating health message (**Fig. 14.7**).

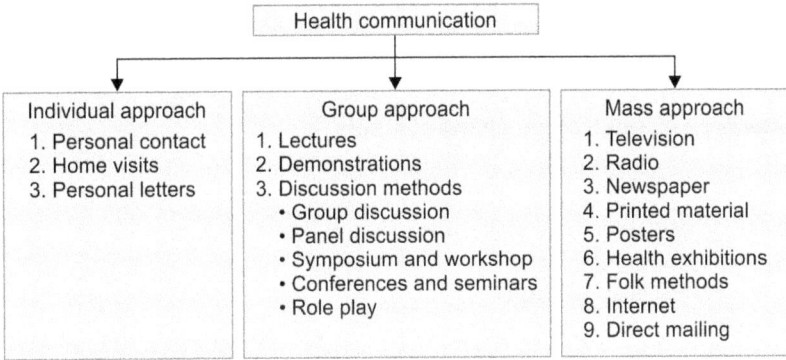

**Fig. 14.7:** Methods and media for communicating health message.
(*Courtesy:* Bhanot Publishers)

## USING MASS MEDIA

Mass media can be used to communicate the right message in a right way at a right time to a large audience. Only "one-way" communication is possible through mass media. Mass media helps in the uniform dissemination of the message, as it reaches to all sections of the society. Mass media usually fails to bring about social and economic changes essential for building a healthy society. K Park believes that mass media alone are generally inadequate in changing human behavior. For effective health communication, they should be used in combination with other suitable methods.

## SUMMARY

Communication is the transfer and understanding of meaning. Communication process consists of seven elements. Effective communication provides numerous benefits. Effective communication techniques help to communicate effectively. Knowledge regarding barriers to communication and methods to overcome barriers is essential for effective communication. An interpersonal relationship is an association or connection between two or more individuals. Knowledge regarding barriers to interpersonal relationship and measures to overcome them is essential to build good interpersonal relationship with patients.

Understanding self is essential for successful nursing practices. The communication and behavioral patterns established the group members is referred to as group dynamics. A team is the group of individuals who functions as a unit for attaining a common goal. Nursing is a conscious practice of human relations. Information, education and communication for health (IEC) is being widely used as a general term for communication activities in health promotion.

## MULTIPLE CHOICE QUESTION

1. **Which one is an example of presentational media:**
   a. Voice
   b. Photograph
   c. Internet
   d. Television

2. **Which one is an example of representational media**
   a. Voice
   b. Good picture
   c. Face
   d. Phone

3. **Which one is an example of mechanical media**
   a. Voice
   b. Face
   c. Internet
   d. Picture

4. **On-line education is an example of:**
   a. Multimedia
   b. Mass media
   c. Audio-video media
   d. Visual media

5. **Filtering is an example of:**
   a. Information related barrier
   b. Physical barrier
   c. Language barrier
   d. Psychological barrier

## ANSWER KEY

| 1. c | 2. b | 3. c | 4. a | 5. a |

# Bibliography

1. Abbot C. ICT: Changing education. London: Routledge; 2001.
2. Ackerman D, Perkins D. Integrating thinking and learning skills across the curriculum. Alexandria: ASCD; 1989.
3. Adam S. EQ intervention: shaping a self-aware generation through social and emotional learning. New York. Greenleaf Book Group; 2020.
4. Aggarwal JC. Development and planning of modern education. New Delhi: Vikas Publications; 1993.
5. Aggarwal JC. Essential of educational technology. New Delhi: Vikas Publications; 1997.
6. Aggarwal JC. Landmark in the history of modern education. New Delhi: Vikas Publications; 1993.
7. Aggarwal JC. Principles methods and techniques of teaching. New Delhi: Vikas Publications; 1993.
8. Aggarwal JC. Teacher education in a developing society. New Delhi: Vikas Publishing; 2017.
9. Aggarwal JC. Theory and principles of education. New Delhi: Vikas Publications; 1993.
10. Ahuja BN. Modern Education and Problems of Indian Education. New Delhi: Surjeet Publications; 1993.
11. Ainsworth L. Curriculum design: How to create curricular units of study that align standards, instruction and assessment? Harcourt: Houghton Mifflin Harcourt Publishing Company; 2014.
12. Akey T. School context and behaviour and academic behaviour. New York, NY: MDRC; 2006.
13. Alan J. Educational technology. London: Routledge; 2001.
14. Alan J. Educational technology. New York: Routledge; 2008.
15. Albert K. Cognitive psychology. London: Larsen and Keller Education; 2018.
16. Alexander PA. Handbook of educational psychology. London: Routledge; 2006.
17. Alexander R. Culture and pedagogy. London: Blackwell Publishers; 2000.
18. Alkharushi H. Effects of classroom assessment practices on students achievement goals. Educational Assessment. 2008; 13(4): 243-66.
19. Allan AG, Floyd B. Curriculum leadership: Strategies for development and implementation. London: Sage Publications; 2018.
20. Allan C, Richard H. Rethinking education in the age of technology: the digital revolution and schooling in America. London. The Teachers College Press; 2010.
21. Allan CO, Daniel U. Foundations of education. New York: Cenage Learning; 2016.
22. Allan CO, Francis PH. Curriculum: foundations, principles and issues. London: Pearson; 2016.
23. Allen M, Brain M. Discipline with dignity. Virginia: ASCD; 2008.
24. Alley LR. What makes a good online course? The administrator's role in quality assurance of online learning. Converge. 2001; 4(11): 50-3.
25. Alvero AM, Austin J. The effects of conducting behavioural observations on the behaviour of the observer. J Appl Behav Anal. 2004; 37:457-68.
26. Alyssa H, Kami T. Design thinking for school leaders. Alexandria: ASCD; 2018.
27. Ananda C. Teacher and education in Indian society. New Delhi: NCERT; 1983.
28. Anderman EM, Corno L. Handbook of educational psychology. New York: Rutledge; 2016.
29. Anderson D. Educational technology. New York: Routledge; 1972.
30. Andrew C. The art of being a brilliant teacher. London: Crown house; 2015.
31. Antony D. Starting to Teach. London: Kogan Page; 1988.
32. Antony E. An Introduction to Applied Cognitive Psychology. London. Psychology Press; 2004.
33. Armeto BT. Research on teaching social studies. London: Macmillan; 1984.
34. Arther J. Principles of guidance. Tokyo: McGraw Hill Book Company; 1985.
35. Ary D, Razavieh A. Introduction to research in education. Belmont: Cengage Learning; 2010.

36. Aschorft K. Teaching and learning in higher education. London: the Falmer Press; 1994.
37. Baddeley AD. The episodic huffer: A new component of working memory? Trends in cognitive science. 2000; 4:417-23.
38. Baddeley AD. Working memory. London: Oxford University Press; 1986.
39. Bailey GD. Improving Classroom Instruction with means-referenced objectives. Educational Technology. 1977: 17(7) 13-5.
40. Bailey R, Barrow R. The sage handbook of philosophy of education. New York: Sage Publications; 2010.
41. Ball DL, Rowan B. Measuring instruction. The Elementary School Journal. 2004; 105(1): 3010.
42. Bambrick P. Driven by data: A practical guide to improve instruction. San Francisco: Jossey-Bass; 2010.
43. Bandura A. A social foundation of thought and action: A social cognitive theory. London: Prentice-Hall; 1986.
44. Bandura A. Influence of models' reinforcement contingencies on the acquisition of imitative responses. Journal of Personality and Social Psychology.1965; 1:589-95.
45. Banks J. Handbook of simulation: Principles, methodology, advances, applications and practice. New York: John Wiley and Sons; 1998.
46. Banks JA. Teaching strategies for ethnic studies. Boston: Allyn and Bacon; 1981.
47. Barrow R. An introduction to philosophy of Education. London: Routledge; 2006.
48. Barun, Barbara J Steven. Nursing theory; analysis, application, evaluation. Philadelphia: JB Lippincott Company; 1994.
49. Bates T. Teaching in the digital age: Guidelines for teaching and learning. London: Center for Open Education; 2015.
50. Baumgartner J. Key factors to successful brainstorming; 2005. http;//www.JPb.com.
51. Beard C, Wilson J. Experiential learning: A best practice handbook for educators and trainers. London: Pearson; 2006.
52. Beard LA, Harper C. Student perception of online versus campus instruction. Education. 2003; 122(4): 658-64.
53. Beijaard D, Meijer PC. Reconsidering research on teachers' professional identities. Teaching and Teacher Education. 2004;20:107-28.
54. Bell B, Cowie B. Formative assessment and science education. Dordrechi: Kluwer; 2001.
55. Bennet JF, Bennet LB. Assessing the quality of distance education programs. The Faculty's perspective. Journal of Computing in Higher Education. 2002; 13(2):71-86.
56. Bennett T, Sealy C. Researched guide to the curriculum: An evidence informed guide for teacher. London: John Catt Educational; 2020.
57. Bently T. Learning Beyond the classroom. London: Routledge; 1998.
58. Berry R. Assessment for learning. Hong Kong: Hong Kong University; 2008.
59. Best JW, Kahn JV. Research in education. New Delhi: Pearson India; 2010.
60. Bevis EM Olivia. Curriculum building in nursing. New York: National League for Nursing; 1989.
61. Bevis EM Olivia. Towards a caring curriculum: A new pedagogy for nursing. New York: National League for Nursing; 1989.
62. Bhatia. Principles of education. New Delhi: Kalyani Publishers; 1987.
63. Bhatia and Bhatia. Principles and methods of teaching. New Delhi: Doaba Publishers; 1984.
64. Bhatia KK. Principles of education. Ludhiana: Prakash Brothers; 1988.
65. Bilon E. Using Bloom's taxonomy to write effective learning objectives: The ABCDs of writing learning objectives: A basic guide. Independly published; 2019.
66. Binance MB. Exploring qualitative methodologies in online learning environments. The Quarterly Review of Distance Education. 2002; 3(3): 251-60.
67. Black P, Wiliam D. Assessment for learning: Putting it into practice. Berkshire: McGraw-Hill Education; 2003.
68. Black P. Formative assessment views through different lenses. The Curriculum Journal. 2008; 16(2):133-5.
69. Bloom B. Taxonomy of educational objectives. London: Longman; 1954.
70. Bondi JC, Wiles JW. Curriculum development: A guide to practice. New Delhi: Pearson; 2019.
71. Bontech B, Petrov M. Playing styles based on experiential learning theory. Computers in Human Behaviour. 2018; 85:321-28.

72. Borich GD. Effective teaching methods: Research based Practice. London: Pearson; 2010.
73. Borredon L, Deffayet S. Enhancing deep learning: Lessons from the introduction of learning teams in management education in France. Journal of Management Education. 2011;35(3):324-50.
74. Bowes D, Johnson J. Experiential learning through classroom experiments. College Teaching Methods & Styles Journal. 2008; 4(4): 7-16.
75. Boyle B, Charles M. Curriculum Development. London: Sage Publications; 2016.
76. Brabacher JS. Model philosophies of education. Mumbai: Tata McGraw-Hill; 1950.
77. Brophy J, Good TL. Teacher behaviour and student achievement. New York: Macmillan; 1986.
78. Broudy. Building a philosophy of education. New Delhi: PH1; 1965.
79. Brown and Pickford. Assessing skills and practice. London: Routledge; 2006.
80. Brown G. Effective teaching in higher education. London: Mauthon Publishers; 1988.
81. Brunner SM, Thomas AS. The effect of instructional facilitation on student college readiness. Journal of Instructional Science. 2017;45: 769-87.
82. Buck J. Assessing quality in distance education. Higher Education in Europe. 2001;26(4):599-602.
83. Burich GA. Effective teaching methods: Research-based practice. Boston: Pearson; 2014.
84. Burkus D. The myths of creativity. San Franciso: Jossey-Bass; 2014.
85. Bush T. The principles of educational management. London: Longman;1994.
86. Butterfields. Educational objectives and National Assessment. Philadelphia: Open University Press; 1995.
87. Byrne B. Qualitative interviewing: Researching society and culture. London: Sage Publications; 2012.
88. Cahn SM. Philosophy of education: The essential Texts. London: Routledge; 2009.
89. Cambell RJ, Robinson W. Assessing teacher effectiveness: Developing a differentiated mode. London: Routledge; 2004.
90. Cameron N, Bogin B. Human growth and development. New York: Elsevier; 2012.
91. Cannan R. A handbook for teachers in universities and colleges. London: Kogan Page; 2000.
92. Canter L. Assertive discipline: positive behaviour management for today's classroom. Bloomington: Solution Tree Press; 2010.
93. Carl A. Teacher empowerment through curriculum development theory into practice. New York: Juta & Company; 2009.
94. Carley JD. School counseling and student outcomes: summary of six statewide studies. Professional School Counseling. 2012; 16:146-53.
95. Carl P. Quality improvement in education. London. David Fulton; 1988.
96. Catherine. Educating able children. London: David Fuston; 1988.
97. Cattin RT, Tiffany W. Blended learning in action: A practical guide toward sustainable change. London: Corwin; 2016.
98. Chandari SS. Monitoring education. London: Cassel;1988.
99. Chander P, Sweller J. Cognitive load theory and the format of instruction cognition and instruction.1991;8: 293-332.
100. Chandra S. Philosophy of education. New Delhi: Atlantic Publishers; 2002.
101. Chandra S. Philosophy of education. New Delhi: Atlantic Publishers; 2006.
102. Chaudhary M. Teaching methodology: Pedagogical principles and effective and effective teaching strategies. Insependly published; 2017.
103. Chauhan S. Innovation in teaching and learning process. New Delhi: Vikas Publications; 1992.
104. Chin P. Using C&IT to support teaching. London: Routledge; 2004.
105. Chizmer JF. Web-based learning environment guided by principles of good teaching practice. Journal of Economic Education. 2000; 298-64.
106. Chkraborthy AK. Principles and practice of education. New Delhi: Lal Book Depot; 2003.
107. Choen L. A guide to teaching practice. London: Routledge; 1996.
108. Choi DG, Vries HJ. Standardization as emerging content in technology education. International Journal of Technology and Design Education. 2011;21(1):111-35.
109. Clare L, Aschbacher PR. Exploring the technical quality of using assignments and student work as indicator of classroom practice. Educational Assessment. 2001;7(1), 39-59.
110. Clark D. Psychological myths in e-learning. Medical Teacher. 2002;24(6): 598-604.

111. Clark JM, Paivio A. Dual coding theory and education. Educational Psychology Review. 1991;3:149-70.
112. Claxton N. Being a teacher. London: Cassell; 1989.
113. Cohen DK, Hill H. Instructional policy and classroom performance. The mathematics reform in California. Teachers College Record. 2000;102(2):294-343.
114. Cohen JL. That's not treating you as a professional; teachers constructing complex professional identities through talk. Teachers and Teaching: Theory and Practice. 2008; 14(2): 79-93.
115. Cohen L. Research methods in Education. London: Routledge; 2001.
116. Coleman HL. Handbook of school counseling. New Jersey/Lawrence: Eribaum; 2009.
117. Conely D. Rethinking the senior year. The National Association of Secondary School Principals. Bulletin. 2001;85:26-41.
118. Conley DT. Rethinking college readiness. New Direction for Higher Education. 2008;144:3-13.
119. Cooper JO. Applied behaviour analysis. London: Pearson; 2007.
120. Cooper PC. Effective teaching and learning. Philadelphia: Open University press; 1996.
121. Corbett M, Dianne G. Rural teacher education: connecting land and people. Singapore: Springer; 2002.
122. Couch J, Towne J. Rewriting education: How technology can unlock every students potential. Texas: Ben Bella Books; 2018.
123. Coxon M. Cognitive psychology. San Fransico: Learning Matters; 2012.
124. Creasia JL, Barbara P. Conceptual foundations of professional nursing practice. London: Mosby; 1991.
125. Creswell JW. Educational research: Planning, conducting and qualitative research. Sydney: Merill Prentice Hall; 2011.
126. Crooks TJ. The impact of classroom evaluation practices on students. Review of Educational Research. 1988; 58:438-81.
127. Curtis D, Carter M. Learning together with young children: A curriculum framework for reflective teachers. London: Redleaf Press; 2017.
128. Curzon. Teaching in further education. London: Cassell; 1990.
129. Daniel J. Foundations of cognitive psychology: core readings. London: Bradford Publishers; 2002.
130. Danielson C. Enhancing professional practice: A framework for teaching. Alexandria: ASCD; 1996.
131. Dash BN. Assessing students: How shall we know them? London: Harper and Row; 1986.
132. David C, Mark S. Human growth and development across the lifespan. New Jersey: Wiley; 2016.
133. Davidson J. Evaluation methodology basics. London: Sage publications; 2005.
134. Davis C, Highton M. Designing learning: From module outline to effective teaching. London: Routledge; 2006.
135. Delers J. The Treasure within: Report of the International commission on education for 21st century; 1996.
136. Delougary NL. Issues and trends in nursing. St. Louis: Mosby; 1995.
137. Denick R, Exley K. Small group teaching: Seminars, tutorials and beyond. London: Routledge; 2004.
138. Denzin NK. The sage handbook of qualitative research. London: Sage publications; 2005.
139. Derrick F. Managing professional development in education. London: Longman; 1996.
140. Dewey J. An introduction to the philosophy of education. New York: McMillan; 1977.
141. Dey C. Teachers matters: Connecting lives, work and effectiveness. Brakshire: Open University Press; 2007.
142. Dhawan L. Philosophy of education. New Delhi: Isha Books; 2005.
143. Dick W, Carey L. The systematic design of instruction. Columbus: Pearson; 2008.
144. Dreyfus H. Mind over machine: The power of human intuition and expertise in the era of computer. Oxford: Blackwell; 1986.
145. Drfden W. Counselling in action. London: Kogan Page; 1988.
146. Duchastel PC, Merrill PF. The effects of behavioural objectives on learning: A review of empirical studies. Review of Educational Research. 1973; 43(1):53-69.
147. DuFour R, DuFour R. Learning by doing: A handbook for professional learning communities at work. Bloomington: Solution Tree Press; 2010.
148. Dunn. The complete guide to learning strategies. Boston: Allyn and Bacon; 1999.
149. Dwyer F. Assessing strategies for developing effective and efficient tests for distance education. International Journal of Instructional Media. 2003; 30(1):11-23.

150. Eaton M. The perfect blend: A practical guide to Designing student-centered Learning Experience. Eugene: International Society for Technology in Education; 2020.
151. Eble EE. Aims of college teaching. London: Jossey-Ban Publishers; 1983.
152. Eccles JS, Fredicks JA. Children's competence and value beliefs from childhood through adolescence. Development Psychology. 2002;38:519-33.
153. Edwards A. Assessing Competencies in Higher Education. London: Kogan Page; 1995.
154. Edward SD. Discourse and cognition: London: Sage Publications; 1997.
155. Ellington H. Handbook of educational technology. London: Kogan Page; 1993.
156. Ellington H. Producing teaching materials. London: Kogan Page; 1993.
157. Ellis J. Essentials of educational psychology. New Delhi: Pearson; 2018.
158. Enthwistle M. Handbook of educational ideas and practices. London: Routledge; 1990.
159. Eric CS, Thomas CM. Learning transformed: 8 keys to designing tomorrow's schools, today. Alexandria. ASCD; 2017.
160. Eric CS. Digital leadership: Changing paradigms for changing times. California: Corwin; 2019.
161. Errant M. Developing professional knowledge and competence. London: Falmer Press; 2002.
162. Etetcher S. Competency based assessment. London: Kogan Page; 1993.
163. Ewan C, While R. Teaching nursing: A self-instructional handbook. London: Croom Helm; 1984.
164. Exley K, Dennick R. Giving a lecture: From presenting to teaching. London: Routledge; 2009.
165. Eyler J. The power of experiential education. Liberal Education. 2009; 95(4):24-31.
166. Eyler JR. How Human Learn: The science and stories behind effective college Teaching. Virginia: West Virginia University Press; 2018.
167. Farringdon D. The nature of expertise: A review. Applied Ergonomics. 2006;37(1):17-32.
168. Ferguson R. Teachers perceptions and expectations and the black-white test score gap. Urban Education. 2003; 38: 460-507.
169. Feryok A. Language teacher cognitions: complex dynamic systems? 2010;38(1): 272-79.
170. Finn CE. Education reforms in the 90s. New York: Macmillan; 1992.
171. Forest N. Qualitative research methods in psychology. Malde head. McGraw-Hill; 2011.
172. Fraenkel JR, Wallen NE. How to design and evaluate research in education? New York: McGraw-Hill; 2003.
173. Frederikson N. Implications of cognitive theory for instruction in problem solving: Review of Educational Research. 1994; 54(3):363-407.
174. Fred G. The nursing curriculum. Theory and Practice. Madras: Chapman and Hall; 1991.
175. Fredicks JA, Paris A. School engagement: Potential of the concept, state of evidence. Review of Educational Research. 2004; 74:59-109.
176. Fuchs LS, Fusch D. Effects of systematic formative evaluation. A meta-analysis. Exceptional children. 1986; 53(3):199-208.
177. Fullman J. Secondary school students' ratings of teacher effectiveness. The High School Journal. 1992;75(3): 168-78.
178. Gagne RM, Briggs LJ. Principles of instructional design. Fort Worth: Harcout Brace. Jovanovich college publishers; 1992.
179. Gallaher HA. Vanston Elementay's innovation teacher evaluation system. Are teacher evaluation scores related to growth in student achievement? Peabody Journal of Education. 2004; 79(4): 79-107.
180. Garrison KL, Fung T. Student role adjustment in online communities of inquiry: Model and Instrument validation. Online Journal of Distance Learning Administration. 2004; 6(1).
181. Gary S, Janice P. Understanding education research: A guide to critical reading. London: Routledge; 2018.
182. George GB. School discipline and self discipline: A practical guide to promoting prosocial student behaviour. New York: Guifors Press; 2010.
183. Gibson, et al. Introduction to counseling and guidance. Michigan: Merrill; 2008.
184. Gibson D, Clark A. Games and simulations in online learning: Research and development frameworks. London. Information Science Publishing; 2007.
185. Gingras S. Best practices in co-teaching & collaboration: The how of co-teaching implementing the models. Manchester: Cognet Catalyst Publications; 2018.

186. Gipps C, Murphy P. A fair test, assessment achievement and equality. Philadelphia:Open University Press; 1994.
187. Glesne C. Becoming qualitative researchers: An introduction. Boston: Pearson; 2011.
188. Glover J, Browning RH. Educational psychology: Its Application and Principles. Tehran. The Academic Publishing; 2007.
189. Goleman D. Emotional intelligence: why it can matter more than IQ. London: Batam; 2006.
190. Good T, Brophy J. Looking in classroom. New York: Harper and Row; 1984.
191. Grace S, Garvestock P. Inclusively and diversity. London: Routledge; 2008.
192. Graham S. 53 interesting things to do in your lecture. London: Technical and Educational Services; 1985.
193. Gronlund NE. Stating behavioural objectives for classroom instruction. New York: Macmillan; 1985.
194. Gronlund NE. Writing instructional objectives for teaching and assessment. New York: Prentice Hall; 2004.
195. Grossman PL. The making of a Teachers: Teacher knowledge and teacher education. New York: Teachers College Press; 1990.
196. Groundlaund NE. Measurement and evaluation in teaching. London: Routledge; 1995.
197. Guba EH. Criteria for assessing the trust worthiness of naturalistic inquires. ECTJ.1981;29(2);75-91.
198. Gyshers NC. Assessing the counselling needs of high school students in Kenya. International Journal for Education and Vocational Guidance. 2006; 8(2): 83-94.
199. Habeshaw EL. Preparing to teach: An introduction to effective teaching in higher education. Bristol: Technical and Educational Services; 1982.
200. Hadavand S. Ten effective commandments in evaluation of training programs monthly management. 2008;15:133-34.
201. Haines C. Assessing students' written work. Making essays and report. London: Routledge; 2006.
202. Hakel MD, Elliet SW. Assessing accomplished teaching: Advanced-level certification programs. Washington DC: National Academies Press; 2008.
203. Halstead J, Billings D. Teaching and nursing: A guide for faculty. St. Louis: Elsevier; 2005.
204. Halverson R, Collins A. Rethinking education in the age of technology. New York: Teachers College Press; 2018.
205. Hamilton B. Integrating technology in the classroom: Tools to meet the needs of every student. Virginia. International Society for Technology in Education; 2015.
206. Hancock A. The evolving terrain of distance learning. Satellite Communication. 1999; 23(3):24-8.
207. Handler B. Teacher as curriculum leader: A consideration of the appropriateness of that role assignment to classroom-based practitioners. International Journal of Teacher Leadership. 2010; 3.
208. Hanstedt P. General education Essentials: A guide for college faculty. San Francisco: Jossey-Bass; 2012.
209. Harrison C. Teachers developing assessment for learning: mapping teacher change. Teacher Development. 2005; 9:255-64.
210. Hartiey J, Davies IK. Preinstructional strategies: The role of pretest, behavioural objectives, overviews and advance organizers. Review of Educational Research. 1976; 46(2): 239-63.
211. Hass G. Curriculum planning: A contemporary approach. London: Pearson; 2008.
212. Hattie J. The power of feedback. Review of Educational Research. 2007;77(1): 81-112.
213. Hattie J. Visible learning. New York: Routledge; 2008.
214. Hattie J. Visible learning for teacher. London: Corwin; 2013.
215. Hayes H. Curriculum: 21 essential education for a changing world. Alexandria: ASCD; 2010.
216. Heather D, Patrick G. Classroom management in the digital age: effective practices for technology-rich learning spaces. Edtech Team; 2016.
217. Heidgerken EL. Teaching and learning in schools of nursing. Philadelphia: London; 1982.
218. Herne S. Study to teach: A guide to studying in Teacher education. London: Routledge; 2000.
219. Heubert JP, Hause RM. High stakes testing for tracking promotion and graduation. Washington DC: National Academy Press; 1999.
220. Heyden SM. Counselling children and adolescents. Belmont: Brooks; 2011.
221. Hinchiliff S. The practitioner as a teacher. Tokyo: WBC Publishers; 1996.
222. Hoberman M. Highly effective teaching strategies: winning in the classroom. London: Grade Success; 2017.

223. Holt J. How children learn. Cambridge: Perseus Books; 1983.
224. Hopkins D. Educational and development psychology. London: Clanryne International; 2018.
225. Hosp MK, Howell KW. The ABCs of CBM: A practical guide to curriculum based measurement. London: The Guiford Press; 2016.
226. Howard MK. School discipline, classroom management, and student self management. California: Corwin; 2012.
227. Howes C, Clifford R. Ready to Learn? Children's pre-academic achievement in pre-kindergarten programs. Early Childhood Research Quarterly; 2008.
228. Howland JL, Moore JL. Student perceptions as distance learners in internet based courses. Journal of Distance Education. 2002,23(2): 183-96
229. Hubbard R. Learning how to learn. London: Effective Education Publishing, 2000.
230. Huse I, McDavid JC. Program evaluation and performance measurement. An introduction to practice. London: Sage Publications; 2004.
231. Ian F. Delivering a course. London: Kogan Page; 1995.
232. Ian F. Evaluating a course. London: Kogan Page; 1995.
233. Ian F. Planning a course. London: Kogan Page; 1995.
234. Ian F. Preparing a course. London: Kogan page; 1995.
235. Irons A. Enhancing learning through formative assessment and feedback. London: Routledge; 2007.
236. Jacob BA, Lefgren L. Can principals identify effective teachers? Evidence on subjective performance evaluation in education. Journal of Labor Economics. 2008; 26(1): 101-36.
237. Jacobs J. Experiential education: The main dish, not just a side course. Colorado: Association for Experiential Education;1999.
238. James FM. Teaching the teacher: Lesson learned from teaching. London: IUNIVERSE; 2007.
239. James M. Using assessment for school improvement. London: Heinemann;1998.
240. Janet C. Teaching and learning with multimedia. London: Routledge;1997.
241. Jarmon L, Trivedi A. Virtual world teaching, experiential learning and assessment: An interdisciplinary communication course in second life. Computers and Education. 2009;53(1):168-82.
242. Jennifer J, Pam H. Transformational 21st century education: Essential tools for the development of social, emotional and academic excellence. London: Roots N Wings; 2020.
243. Joannason. Improving education. London: Cassell; 1999.
244. Joanne S, Mark L. Pirot: A vision for the New University. Charleston: Advantage Media Group; 2019.
245. John L, John M. Setting the standard for project based learning. Alexandria: ASCD; 2015.
246. John S, Andrew E. Human growth and development: An Introduction for social works. London: Routledge; 2013.
247. Johnson L. Teaching outside the box: How to Grab your students by their brains. New York: Jossey-Bass; 2009.
248. John TA, Kara LV. Clarity for learning: Five essential practices that empower students and teachers. London: Corwin;2018.
249. Jonatha F, Mark S. Psychology in the classroom: A teacher's guide to what works. New York: Routledge; 2018.
250. Jones N. Practical counselling skills. London: Rinehart and Winston; 1988.
251. Kahn P, Walsh L. Developing your Teaching: Ideas, Insights and Action; London: Routledge; 2006.
252. Kane MT. Educational measurement. New York. Prayer Publishers; 2006.
253. Karchmer R. Improving online teacher education: Digital tools and E practices. London: Teachers College Press; 2020.
254. Kate A. Improving teaching and learning in core curriculum. London: Falmer Press; 2000.
255. Kearsley G. Online education: Learning and teaching in cyberspace. Belmant: Wadsworth; 2000.
256. Kelley K, Kim R. Bring the world to your classroom: Using Google Geo tools London. Edtech Team; 2018.
257. Kellogg R. Fundamentals of cognitive psychology. New York: Sage Publishers; 2015.
258. Khnyfr H. The higher education system in the world with strategy. Journal of Cultural Management. 2005;3(9):10.
259. Kinra AK. Guidance and counseling. Noida: Pearson India; 2008.

260. Kline P. An easy guide to factor analysis. London: Routledge; 1994.
261. Knight J. High impact instruction: A framework for great teachers. London: Corwin; 2012.
262. Kochar SK. Guidance and counselling in colleges and Universities. New Delhi: Sterling Publishers; 2001.
263. Kochar SK. Guidance in Indian Education. New Delhi: Sterling Publishers; 1998.
264. Kochar SK. Secondary school administration. New Delhi: Sterling Publishers; 2000.
265. Kolb AY, Kolb DA. Experiential learning theory: Encyclopedia of the sciences of Learning. Boston: Springer; 2012.
266. Kolb DA. Experiential Learning. New Jersey: Prentice Hall; 1984.
267. Kolb L. Learning first, technology second: The educators guide to designing authentic lessons. London: International society for Technology in Education; 2017.
268. Konga P, Lam C. Student engagement in mathematics: Development of instrument and validation of construct. Mathematics Education Research Journal. 2003;15:4-21.
269. Kosslyn S. Active learning online: Five principles that make online courses come alive. London: Alinea Knowledge; 2020.
270. Kossyln S. The science of learning: Mechanisms and principles. London: Universities Press; 2017.
271. Kothleem MG. Cognitive psychology. New York: Sage Publications; 2013.
272. Krawczyk D. Reasoning; the neuroscience of how we think. London: Academic Press; 2017.
273. Krebs D, Zvi G. The genius hour guidebook: Fostering passion, wonder, and inquiry in the classroom. London: Routledge; 2015.
274. Krtriacov C. Essential teaching skills. Cheltenham: Nelson Thomas Ltd; 2001.
275. Kumar KL. Educational Technology. New Delhi: New Age International; 1996.
276. Lamberts K, Shanks D. Knowledge concepts and categories. London: Psychology Press; 2016.
277. Lang J. Small teaching: Everyday lessons from the science of learning. SanFrancisco: Jossey-Bass; 2016.
278. Laurillard DM. Rethinking university teaching: A framework for the effective use of educational technology. London: Routledge; 1993.
279. Leader W. Lecturing at your Best. London: TC1;1983.
280. Leigh HN, Tracey MW. A review and new framework for instructional, design practice variation research: performance improvement. Quarterly. 2010; 23(2): 33-46.
281. Lemor D. Teaching in the online classroom: Surviving and thriving in the new normal. London: Wiley Publishing; 2020.
282. Lemor D. Teach like a champion. London: Wiley Publishing; 2014.
283. Linda BN. Teaching at its best: A research based resource for college instructors. London: John Wiley & Sons; 2016.
284. Lok JCH. Educational psychology. Independently Published; 2019.
285. Loughram J. International handbook of teacher education. Singapore: Springer; 2016.
286. Loughran J, Russell T. Teaching about teaching: Purpose, passion and pedagogy in teacher education. London: The Falmer Press;1997.
287. Louischan A. A guide to teaching practice. London: Routldege; 1996.
288. Low WC. Changes in instructional development: The aftermath of an information processing take over in psychology. Journal of Instructional Development. 1980; 4(2):10-8.
289. Lugher M. Teaching and learning in changing times. London: Black Well; 1996.
290. Lynch DJ. Confronting challenges: motivational beliefs and learning strategies in difficult college courses. College Student Journal. 2008; 42: 416-21.
291. Macloskey. Current issues in nursing. London: St. Louis Company; 1994.
292. Mager R. Preparing instructional objectives. San Francisco: Fearon; 1962.
293. Mangal SK. Advanced educational psychology. New Delhi: PHI Learning Pvt. Ltd; 2002.
294. Mangal SK. Essential of educational technology. New Delhi: PHI Learning Pvt. Ltd; 2009.
295. Mangal SK. Essentials of educational psychology. New Delhi: PHI Learning Pvt. Ltd; 2007.
296. Marcelino MJ. ICT in education: Multiple and inclusive perspectives. Singapore: Springer; 2015.
297. Margaret S. Theory of education. London: Longman; 1988.
298. Maria W. Counselling in further education and higher education. Philadelphia: Open University Press; 1996.

299. Marks H. Student engagement in instructional activity: patterns in the elementary, middle and high school years. American Educational Research Journal. 2002; 37:153-4.
300. Marks H. Student engagement in the classroom of restructuring school. Washington: Office of Educational Research and Improvement;1995.
301. Martin H. Teaching and learning in changing times. London: Blackwell; 1996.
302. Martin M. The curriculum a comparative perspective. London: Unwin;1989.
303. Marzano RJ, Kendall JS. Designing and assessing educational objectives: Applying the new taxonomy. London: Corwin Press; 2008.
304. Matsumra LC, Pascal J. Measuring instructional quality in accountability systems; classroom assignments and student achievement. Educational. Assessment. 2002;8(3):207-29.
305. Mayer RE, Bove W, Mars R, Tapangco L. When less is more: meaningful learning from visual and verbal summaries of science textbook lessons. Journal of Educational Psychology.1996;88:64-73.
306. Mayesky M. Creative actives and curriculum for young children. New Delhi: Cenage Learning; 2014.
307. Mckenney S, Reeves TC. Conducting educational design research. London: Routledge; 2012.
308. McKernan J. Curriculum action research. London:Kogan Page;1996.
309. McMillan JH. Classroom assessment: principles and practice for effective standards based instruction. London: Pearson; 2014.
310. McTighe J, Silver HF. Teaching for deeper learning: Tools to engage students in meaning making. Alexandria: ASCD; 2020.
311. Medley DM, Coker H. The accuracy of principal's judgment of teacher performance. Journal of Educational Research.1987;80:242-7.
312. Merriam SB. Qualitative research and case study application in education. San Francisco: Jossey-Bass; 1998.
313. Messik S. Individuality in Learning .San Francisco: Jossey-Bass; 1979.
314. Michael S. Foundations of educational technology. New York: Routledge; 2012.
315. Michael WE. Cognitive psychology: A student Handbook. London: Psychology Press; 2015.
316. Michalko M. Cracking creativity: The secrets of creative genius. London: Ten Speed Press; 2001.
317. Michelle DM. Minds online: Teaching effective with technology. London: Harvard University Press; 2016.
318. Michelle LR, Marjorie J. Developmentally appropriate curriculum: Best practices in early childhood education. London: Pearson; 2018.
319. Miller M. Do more with Google classroom. London: Dave Burgers Consulting; 2020.
320. Mohan R. Measurement, evaluation and assessment in Education New Delhi: PHI; 2006.
321. Moreno R, Mayer RE. A split-attention effect in multimedia learning: Evidence for dual processing systems in working memory. Journal of Educational Psychology; 1998.
322. Morrison GR, Ross SM. Designing effective instruction. New Jersey: Wiley & Sons; 2013.
323. Morrison GS. Early childhood education today. London: Pearson; 2012.
324. Morryvan M. The effective use of role play. London: Kogan Page; 1994.
325. Moss CM, Brookhart SM. Advancing Formative Assessment in every classroom: A Guide for Instructional Leader. Alexandria: ASCD; 2009.
326. Mukhopadhyay B. Guidance and counselling manual. New Delhi: Sterling Publications; 2001.
327. Muro E, Mathei R. Counselling: A skill approach. Bristol: Merheven; 1983.
328. Murry P. Curriculum development and design. London: Routledge; 1998.
329. Murthy SK. Teacher and education in Indian society. Ludhiana: Prakash Brothers;1992.
330. Namitha R, Toolika W. Guidance and counselling for children and adolescents in schools. London: Sage Publications; 2011.
331. Narayana SR, Prem S. Counselling and guidance. New Delhi: Tata McGraw Hill; 2009.
332. National Research Council. Engaging schools: Fostering high school students motivation to learn. Washington, DC: National Academic Press; 2003.
333. Naude L, Kruger IS. Learning to like learning: An appreciative inquiry into emotions in education. Social Psychology of Education. 2014; 17(2): 211-28.
334. Neisser U. Cognitive psychology. London: Psychology Press; 2014.
335. Nelson J, Lott L. Positive discipline in the classroom. London: Harmony; 2013.

336. Newble D. A handbook for teachers: A guide to improving teaching methods. London: Kogan Page; 1989.
337. Newmann FM. Student engagement and achievement in American Secondary schools. New York: Teachers College Press; 1992.
338. Nicholis H. Creative teaching. An approach to the achievement of educational objectives. London: Routledge; 1985.
339. Nicholson DW. Philosophy of education in action. Oxyon: Routledge; 2016.
340. Noddings N. Philosophy of education. Boulder: Westview Press; 2016.
341. Nosich GM. Learning to think things through: A guide to critical thinking across the curriculum. London: Pearson; 2011.
342. Novakowski J. Classifying classification science and children. 2009; 46(7):25-9.
343. Nussbaum S. The connected educator. Bloomington: Solution Tree Press; 2011.
344. Nuttall J, Jones M. Teacher education policy and practice: Evidence of impact, impact of evidence. Singapore: Springer; 2011.
345. Onwllegbuzie AJ, Leech NL. Linking research questions to mixed methods data analysis procedure. The Qualitative Report. 2006; 11:479-98.
346. Ormred J. Educational psychology: Developing learners. Boston: Pearson; 2011.
347. Ormrod JE. Educational psychology: Developing learners; 2006.
348. Ormrod JE. Essentials of educational psychology: Big ideas to guide effective teaching. London: Pearson; 2018.
349. Pallant J. SPSS survival manual: A step by step guide to data analysis using the SPSS. Maidenheed: Open University; 2013.
350. Pal Y. Report of the committee to advice on renovation and rejuvenation of higher education. National seminar on Quality, Expansion and Inclusion in India Higher Education. Calicut, India.2009;1-8.
351. Pandy RS. Principles of education. Agra: Pustak Mandir; 1991.
352. Papham WJ. educational assessment: what school leaders need to know? London: Corwin; 2010.
353. Parker J, Crabtree SA. Human growth and development in adults: Theoretical and practice perspectives. Bristol: Policy Press; 2020.
354. Parsons RD. Thinking and acting like a cognitive school counselor. London: Corwin; 2009.
355. Patterson CH. An introduction to counseling on the school. New York: Harper and Row Publishers; 1971.
356. Patton MQ. Qualitative research and evaluation methods. London: Sage Publications; 2002.
357. Paul G. The student centered school. London: Blackwell; 1990.
358. Pavio A. Mental representation: A dual coding approach. New York: Oxford University Press; 1986.
359. Penny CG. Modality effects and the structure of short-term verbal memory. Memory and Cognition. 1989;17:398-442.
360. Perpalin. How schools improve. London: Cassell; 1994.
361. Peter RS. The philosophy of education. London: Oxford University Press; 1975.
362. Peterson ADC. Schools across frontiers. La Salle: Open Press; 1987.
363. Peterson E, Siadat MV. Combination of formative and summative assessment instruments in elementary algebra classes: A prescription for success. Journal of Applied Research in the Community College. 2009; 16(2): 92-102.
364. Petride LA. Web-based technologies for distributed distance learning creating learner-centered educational experiences in the higher education classroom. International Journal of Instructional Media. 2007; 29(1):69-77.
365. Petrina S. Advanced teaching methods for the technology classroom. London: Information Science Publishing; 2007.
366. Pianta RC, Hamre BK. Classroom Assessment scoring system: Preschool version Baltimore: Brookes Publishing; 2006.
367. Pinker S. How the mind works. London: WW Norton and Company; 2009.
368. Poole DM. Students participation in a discussion oriented online course. A case study. Journal of Research on Computing in Education; 2000.
369. Posner GJ, Strike KA. Ideology versus technology: The bias of behavioural objectives. Educational Technology.1975:15(5): 28-33.

370. Posner JU. Course design. London: Longman; 1986.
371. Pratt D. Curriculum planning: A handbook for professionals. London: Warsworth Publishing Company; 1994.
372. Quinn FM. The principles and practice of nursing education. Madras: Chapman and Hall; 1995.
373. Rahman Z. Modern teaching methods and techniques. Bengaluru: Anmol Publishers; 2004.
374. Rai BC. Principles of Education Lucknow: Prakash Kendra;1986.
375. Rai BC. Techniques of teaching. Lucknow: Prakash Kendra; 1993.
376. Rai BC. Theory of education. Lucknow. Prakash Kendra; 1990.
377. Ramparsed R. A strategy for teacher involvement in curriculum development. South African Journal of Education; 2000.
378. Raudenbush SW. Magnitude of teacher expectancy effects on Pupil IQ as a function of the credibility of expectancy induction: A synthesis of findings from 18 experiments. Journal of Educational Psychology. 1998;76: 85-97.
379. Razanoonis. Educational planning: A long term perspective. New Delhi: Concept Publishing Company; 1989.
380. Reisberg D. Cognition: Exploring the science of the mind. London: WW. Norton and Company; 2018.
381. Reiser RA, Dempsey JV. Trends and issues in instructional design and technology. New Delhi: Pearson India; 2017.
382. Reti PG. Some guidelines on the classroom use of performance objectives. Programmed Learning and Educational Technology.1975;12(1):29-33.
383. Richard P. Cognitive neuroscience: A very short introduction. New York: Oxford University Press; 2016.
384. Robert C. A handbook for teachers in colleges and Universities. London: Kogan Page; 2000.
385. Robert JM. Designing and assessing educational objectives. New York: Sage Publications; 2008.
386. Roblyer MD, Huges JE. Integrating educational technology into teaching. New Delhi: Pearson India; 2018.
387. Ronghuai H. Educational technology: A primer for 21st century. Singapore: Springer; 2019.
388. Ross SM. Simulation. New York: Elsevier; 2005.
389. Rowntree D. Assessing students: How shall we know them? London: Harper and Row; 1987.
390. Rowntree D. Teaching with audio in open and distance learning. London: Blackwell; 1994.
391. Roy S. Theories and philosophies of education. New Delhi: Soma Book Agency; 1989.
392. Ryan S. The virtual university. London: Kogan Page; 2000.
393. Safaya RN, Shahida BD. Development of educational theory and practice. New Delhi: Dhanapat Rai and Sons; 1994.
394. Sampath K. Introduction to educational technology. New Delhi: Sterling Publishers; 2001.
395. Sandra D. Teaching nursing. Canada: Addison-Wesley Nursing; 1990.
396. Santrock JW. Life span development. New Delhi: McGraw-Hill Education; 2017.
397. Saudra C. Psychology. New Delhi: Pearson India; 2017.
398. Saxena NR. Teachers education. New Delhi: Recall Book Depot; 2020.
399. Schrum L. Oh what wonder you will see. Distance education past, present and future. Learning and Leading with Technology. 2002;30(3): 6-9, 21-21.
400. Semeyers P. International handbook of philosophy of education. Singapore: Springer; 2010.
401. Senge P. The fifth discipline: The art and practice of the learning organisation. London: Random House; 2008.
402. Sewtt J. Methods of teaching: A handbook of principles. London: Book on Demand Ltd; 2013.
403. Shalini P. Child development and pedagogy for CTET & STET. New Delhi: Disha Publication; 2015.
404. Sharma AR. Educational technology. Agra: Vinod Pustak; 1992.
405. Sharma RH. Technology of teaching. Meerut: International Publishing House;1993.
406. Sharma RM. Advanced educational technology. Meerut: Eagle Books; 1989.
407. Sharma RN. Guidance and counselling in India. New Delhi: Atlantic Publishers; 2004.
408. Sharma S. School administration and health education. Agra: Vinod Pustak Mandir;1993.
409. Shepard CA. The role of assessment in a learning culture. Educational Researcher. 2000;29(7):4-14.
410. Shernoff D, Shernoff E. Student engagement in high school classroom from the perspective of flow theory –school psychology quarterly. 2003;18:158-76.

411. Shimsh A. Philosophical investigation of the role of teacher: A synthesis of Plato, Confucius, Blubber and Freire. Teaching and Teacher Education. 2008;24(3):515-35.
412. Shivarudrappa. Philosophical approach to education. New Delhi: Himalaya Publishers; 1985.
413. Shute VJ. Focus on formative feedback. Review of Educational Effects. 2008; 78(1): 153-89.
414. Siegel H. The Oxford handbook of philosophy of education. New York: Oxford University Press; 2009.
415. Siegel H. The Oxford handbook of philosophy of education. New York: Oxford University Press; 2012.
416. Singh A. Higher education in India. New Delhi: Konark Publishers; 1996.
417. Singh AK. Tests, measurements and research methods in behavioural sciences. New Delhi: Bharti Bhavan; 2019.
418. Singh JA. Philosophical foundation of education. New Delhi: APH Publishing Corporation; 2007.
419. Singh S. Philosophy and ideology of western political thinkers. New Delhi: Kanishka Publishers; 1990.
420. Slavin RE. Educational psychology. London: Pearson; 2013.
421. Smith E. Cognitive psychology. Chennai: Pearson India; 2006.
422. Smith P. Free range learning in the digital age: The emerging revolution in college career and education. New York: Select Books; 2018.
423. Snider SJ. Cognitive and affective learning outcomes resulting from the use of behavioural objectives in teaching poetry. Journal of Educational Research. 1975;68(9):333-8.
424. Soman EK. Educational measurement and evaluation. Calicut: Goutham Publications; 1998.
425. Sousa DA. How the brain learns. London: Crowin; 2016.
426. Spector JM. Foundations of educational technology. Integrative approaches and interdisciplinary perspectives. London: Routledge; 2011.
427. Srinivasan MV. Education in contemporary India. New Delhi: Pearson India;2019.
428. Srivastava DS, Kumari S. Education instruction methods. New Delhi: Isha Books; 2009.
429. Sternberg RJ. Thinking styles. Boston: Cambridge Universities Press; 1997.
430. Stewart W. An A to Z of counselling Theory and practice. London: Stanley Thrones; 1992.
431. Strong R, Silver HF. Teaching what matters most: standards and strategies for raising student achievement. California: ASCD; 2001.
432. Sukia SD. Educational administration. Agra: Vinod Pustak Mandir;1986.
433. Susan A. How learning works: Seven research based principles for smart teaching.
434. Sutherland M. Theory of education. London: Longman; 1988.
435. Sweller J, Pass F. Cognitive architecture and instructional design. Educational Psychology Review.1998;10:251-96.
436. Sylvia D. Sketch notes for educators: 100 Inspiring illustrations for lifelong learners. London: Elevate Books; 2019.
437. Taneja VR. Educational thought and practice. New Delhi: Sterling Publishers; 1993.
438. Taylor C. Monitoring education. London: Cassell; 1998.
439. Terry D, Zakrajsek T. The new science of learning: How to learn in harmony with your brain. Sterling, VA, United States: Stylus Publishing; 2018.
440. Tesser M. Planning and conducting formative evaluation: Improving the quality of education and training. London: Kogan Page; 1995.
441. Tessmer M, Wedman WB. A layer of necessity instructional development model. Educational Technology Research and Development.1994; 38(2):77-85.
442. Thomas A, Patricia C. Classroom assessment techniques. Bloomington: Jossey-Bass; 1993.
443. Thomson S. Creativity is everything: rethinking technology, schools, humanity. Independently published; 2020.
444. Tomei LA. Online courses and ICT in education. New York: Information Science Reference; 2011.
445. Tom R. Teacher who Teach Teachers. London: The Falmer Press;1995.
446. Townsend T. Handbook of teacher education. Singapore: Springer; 2007.
447. Tuckman B, Moneth D. Educational psychology. London: Cenage Learning; 2010.
448. Tyler RW. Basic principles of curriculum and instruction. Chicago: University of Chicago Press; 1972.
449. Venkittaswaran S. Principles of education. New Delhi: Vikas Publishers;1993.
450. Vishala M. Guidance and counselling: for teachers, parents and students. New Delhi: S Chand and Company; 2006.

451. Waitzkin J. The art of learning:An inner journey to optimal performance. New York: Free Press; 2007.
452. Warner D. Higher education management. London: Open University Press;1996.
453. Watson E, Bush B. The science of learning: 77 studies every teacher needs to know. London: Routledge; 2019.
454. Weisberg RW. Creativity: Understanding innovation in problem solving, science, invention and the Arts. London: Wiley; 2006.
455. Wenger E. Communities of practice: Learning meaning and identity. Cambridge: Cambridge University Press;1998.
456. Westwood P. What teachers need to know about teaching methods? Victoria: ACER Press; 2008.
457. Wheeler S. Students perception of learning support in distance education. Quarterly Review of Distance Education. 2002;3(4):419-30.
458. White RV. The ECT curriculum: Design, innovation and management. Oxford: Blackwell; 1988.
459. Whitney HR. Universal design for learning in action: 100 ways to teach all learners. Baltimore: Brooks Publishing; 2014.
460. Wight AR. Beyond behavioural objectives. Educational Technology. 1972; 12(7):9-14.
461. Wiles J. Leading curriculum development. London: Crowin; 2009.
462. Wilkinson B, Vanghan A. Educational psychology for learner: Connecting theory, research and application. London: Kendall Hunt Publishing; 2019.
463. William D. Embedded formative assessment. Bloomington: Solution Tree Press; 2011.
464. Willms JD. Student engagement at school: A sense of belonging and participation Paris. OECD;2003.
465. Winch C. Key concepts in the philosophy of education. London: Routledge; 1996.
466. Wisker G, Exley K. Working one- to-one with students. London: Routledge; 2008.
467. Witkin HA. Cognitive Styles. Boston: Cambridge Press;1981.
468. Woods N. Formative assessment and self-regulated learning. The Journal of Education. 2015; 13(1): 15-20.
469. Woolfolk A. Educational psychology. London: Pearson; 2012.
470. Woollard J. Learning and teaching using ICT in secondary schools. Southernbay East: Learning Matters Ltd; 2007.
471. Wright C. Issues in Education and Technology. London: CWS; 2000.
472. Wynd WR, Bozman CS. Student learning style: A segmentation strategy for higher education. Journal of Education for Business. 1996; 71(4): 232-5.
473. Yin RK. Case study research: Design and methods. London: Sage Publications;1994.
474. Yon M, Kohut G. Evidence of effective teaching perception of peer reviewers. College Teaching. 2002; 50(3):104-10.
475. Zerwekh J, Claborn JC. Nursing today, transition and trends. Philadelphia: WB Saunders Company; 1994.

# INDEX

**Note:** Page numbers followed by '*b*' box; '*f*' figure; and '*t*' indicate table respectively.

## A

Ability-based learning 22
Accelerates learning 123
Access to information 20
Achieve learning objectives 196
Achievement tests 292
 construction and administration of 307
Action-oriented 65
Activated demonstration 223
Active
 learning strategies 126
 listening 236
 participation, increases 124
Activity, principle of 84, 146
Adaptation 62
Addie model 219
Addressing learner's needs 138
Adequate nurse educators 30
Adequate pacing 171
Adequate student support 116
Adequate teacher and parental support 116
Adjustmental 320
Admission service 330
Advanced beginner 224
All tech-all human 4
 21st century concept of education 5*f*
Analysis 60, 64
Anecdotal records 288
 uses of 288
Application 60
Applying 64
Appointment and establishing relationship 337
Appraisal, methods of 23
Appropriate channel, principle of 367
Appropriate feedback, principle of 367
Appropriate student behavior 233
Appropriate test item, selection of 292
Arouse interest 82
Arouse students' interest 177
Artificial intelligence 253
Asking questions, purposes in 157
Assertive communication 375
Assertive discipline 350
Assessment 136, 276
 and evaluation 277
 components of 276
 proper 139
Assignment 202, 217
 guidelines for preparing 202
 principles of planning 202
 types of 203
Assist in good course design 57
Assist to build promising career 25
Asynchronous online teaching 211
Attention 122, 236
Attitude 63*b*
 reformation of 12
Audience, experience of 369
Audio media 369
Audio-video media 369
Audiovisual aids 253, 257*t*
 advantages of 259
 classification of 256
 description of 260
 judicious use of 171
 principles in use of 256
 purposes of 256
 use of 258
Auditory 129
 learners 129
Authentic assessment, foundation for 57
Autonomous development 15
Autonomous institutions 28
Autonomy 362
 in learning 135
Avocational guidance 329
 in nursing education 329
Awareness, lack of 322
Awareness of
 learner 163
 self teacher 163
 teacher-student interactions 163
 teaching practice 164
Awareness regarding needs, lack of 379
Axiology 34

## B

Background barriers 372
Barriers to
 communication 372
 interpersonal relationship 379
 learning 116
Beattie's fourfold model 72
Bedside clinic 199
Behavior modification 139
Behavioral learning theories, types of 114
Behavioral objective
 based on well-defined 7
 components of 66
 criteria of 65
 model 71
 strengths of 67
 weaknesses of 68
Behavioral support 231
Behavior-centered objective 65
Behaviorism 113
 and learning, key features of 114

Bellon's opinion 164
Benchmarks 97
Better classroom
 communication 233
 management 138
Biological pragmatism 44
Blended
 curriculum 78
 learning 121, 251
 teaching 212
Bloom's taxonomy 62, 63
 and nursing education 63b
 of educational objectives 58
 revised 63
Blueprint for test, preparation for 308
Bluffing, special scoring problem 304
Body, all-round development of 85
Body language, proper 171
Budgetary provisions 343

### C

Capability 362
Cartoons 269
Central objective 62
Central tendency error 290
Centralized and decentralized services, combination of 341
Chalkboard 260
 demerits of 262
 effective use of 261
 use of 261
Challenges 98
 before nursing education 29
 from new educational programs 28
Character building, principle of 85
Character development 14
Characterization 61
Charting and patient progress notes 311
Charts 264
 effective use of 266
 preparation of 265
 purposes of 264
 types of 264
  chain chart 265
  evolution chart 265
  narrative chart 265
  tabulation chart 265
Child, abilities of 7
Child-centered curriculum 84
Child-centered education 41
Child-centeredness 343
Chunk lessons 214
Citizenship 14, 25
Clarify
 and condense information 370
 information and concepts 177
 and mastery over content, principle of 229
Class and curriculum structure 136
Class teachers counselors 335
Classes using lecture capture 219
Classroom climate for proper communication 238

Classroom communication 234, 237
 barriers of 239
 competencies of teacher 238
 competencies, improving 237
 importance of 235
 types of 235
Classroom discipline 351
Classroom discussion techniques 178
Classroom environment 233
Classroom management 227
 approach for effective 230
 components of 232
 factors influencing 233
 goals of 228
 importance of 231
 principles of 229
Classroom rules, effective use of 231
Clear direction, signposting for 173
Client-centered counseling 337
Clinical evaluation
 methods and tools 310
 purposes of 310
Clinical experience, organization of 94, 95
Clinical questioning 223
Clinical rotation plan, factors influencing 95
Clinical teaching 193
 challenges in 195
 methods 197
  classification of 197
 objectives of 194
 outcomes of 195
 principles of 194
 selection of clinical area 196
Cognitive domain 59
Cognitive impact 134
Cognitive neuroscience
 appreciating developments in 30
 development in 19
 recent developments in 97
Cognitivism 114
 and learning, key features of 115
Coherent curriculum 79
Collaboration 4
Communicate ethically 370
Communicating health message 387
 methods and media for 387, 387f
Communicating teacher expectations, principle of 229
Communication 4, 380
 and human relations 365
 behaviors, objective evaluation of 237
 competencies 237
  in teaching 236
  three basic skills for 236
 different media and channel of 369
 in classroom 238
 in nursing 370f
  significance of 366
 ineffective 379
 principles of 366
 problems in clinical area 375
 process 365, 367f
  and elements 367

# Index

situations, principle of 367
skills, developing 239
technologies in education 361
technologies, use 370
theory 373
    in nursing 373
types of 368f, 368
Community living, promotion of 377
Community participation 22
Competence 135
    and worth, principle of 300
Competency-based education 17
Competency-based learning 220
Competent nurse educators, shortage of 28
Competent professional nurse 192
Complex competencies, measure 250
Comprehensive 83
Comprehensiveness and balance, principle of 85
Computer instruction
    advantages of 271
    disadvantages of 272
Computer-assisted instruction 270
Computer-managed instruction 271
Computers in nursing education 269
Computers tool, using 271
Concentration, lack of 322
Concepts, difficult 170
Conducive environment, absence of 379
Conduct management 232
Conflict resolution 380
Connecting
    to community needs, principle of 85
    to life, principle of 84, 147
    with social life, principle of 85, 147
Connectivism 116
Conservation 40
Conservative principle 84
Construct validity 306
Constructing essay questions, suggestions for 301
Constructivism 115
Content 376
    better understanding of 221
    management 232
    standards 97
    validity 305
Context specific 154
Continuity 83, 156, 343
Continuous comprehensive evaluation 285f
Continuous evaluation, importance of 285f
Continuous experience 46
Continuous process 316
Control annoying mannerisms 171
Control over students by faculty 196
Cooperation 343
Core curriculum 97
Corrective discipline 351
Correlating theory and practice 29
Correlation chart, preparation of 94
Correlation, principle of 147
Cost effective 221

Counseling 196, 335, 336
    approaches to 337
    characteristics of 318
    classification of 336
    concept of 317
    do's and don'ts in 341t
    interview 338
    meaning 317
    phases of 337
    service 332, 342
    techniques 337
Course planning
    elements of 100
    principles of 100
Courses in curriculum, proper placement of 57
Covenant management 232
Covert statements 376
Creating 64
    learner-centered classroom 57
    quality course content 362
    safe and positive learning environment 137
Creative
    curriculum 78
    discipline, positive environment for 260
    education 21
    principle 84
    types of 203
Creativity 362
    principle of 146
Criterion-referenced evaluation 284
Criterion-related validity 305
Critical thinking 4, 36, 170
    skills, develop 362
    promotion of 21
Cultural
    barriers 241
    development 14
    environment, enrichment of 40
Cultural heritage 12
    promotion and transmission of 40
Cumulative record 292
Current trends in education 20
Curriculum 70, 111
    agenda of important cultural issues 72
    changes 26
    components of 72
        nursing 73
    development 81
        aspects of 88
        factors influencing 86
        principles of 84
        responsibility of 79
        steps in 88, 88f
        team 81
    evaluation of 84, 96
        principles of 96
    evolving 78
    for excellence 79
        in nursing education 97
    implementing 84

map of key subjects 72
models of 71
modern concept of 71
nature of 74
objectives 74
opportunities for students 74
organization of 81
planning 196 80
related barriers 241
related issues 29
revision
    approaches to 99
    changing curriculum 98
    stages of 99
schedule of basic skills 72
student experience 74
subject matter 74
types of 75
    essential 76
    explicit 75
    hidden 75, 77
    illegitimate 77
    legitimate 77
    null 75, 77
    official 76
    received 76
    societal 76
Cybernetic machines 249
Cybernetics 248

## D

Data, collection and analysis of 343
Decentralized services 341
Degree program, preference to 27
Democracy, principle of 85
Democratic behavior 229
Demonstration 174
    advantages of 175
    disadvantages of 176
    phases of 174
Descriptive ethics 356
Descriptive graphic rating scale 289
Desirable curriculum, criteria for 74
Desirable personal traits 160
Developing clinical rotation plan, principles of 95
Developing life skills, WHO 13
Developing official curriculum, steps in 81
Development, level of 371
Developmental 320
    needs of adolescents 322
Diagnostic function 281
Digital course materials 253
Digital teaching 206
    approaches to teaching 208
    design of teaching methods in 209
    principles of 207
    role of teacher in 209
    teaching skills in 208
Dignity of labor, principle of 85
Diminishing government role 27
Directing and distributing 159

Discipline 54, 347
    aims of 349
    eclectic approach to 351
    functions of 348
    modern concept of 348
    need for 348
    principles of 349
    strategies/approaches 351
    types of 349
    with dignity, implementing 30
Discussion method
    advantages of 179
    disadvantages of 180
Discussion, preparing students for 170
Division, principle of 147
Draft curriculum, preparation of 84
Dynamic process 191

## E

Eclectic counseling 337
Eclecticism 50
    meaning of 52
    need for eclecticism in education 50
    need of 53
    philosophy of nursing education 52, 53$f$
    salient features of 51
Edgar Dale's cone of experience 255, 256$f$
Education
    according to nature 43
    act integrative force 12
    agencies of 19
    aims of 13
    and life 19
    based on child's psychology 42
    bipolar process 9
    commercialization of 23
    concept of 2, 2$f$, 4
    deliberate process 11
    earlier concept of 2
    for leisure 14
    for occupational placement 12
    functions of 11
    imparts values 12
    lifelong process 9
    meaning of 1
    modern concept of 3
    multipolar process 9
    natural development of child's power 42
    nonformal type of 22
    philosophy, importance of 36
    planned activity based on objectives 11
    principles of 6, 7$f$
    process of 8, 282
    purposeful activity 11
    system 244
    technology of 244
    transformational 16
    tripolar process 9
    types of 17
Educational guidance 325
    in nursing education 325
    principles of 325

Educational hardware and corresponding software 254t
Educational implications of
   existentialism 50
   idealism 38, 39f, 42f, 45f
   naturalism 42
   pragmatism 45
   realism 48
   theistic realism 49
Educational information 331
Educational objective
   central 58
   classification of 57
   contributory 58
   formulation of 89
   indirect 58
   institutional or general 57
   instructional 58
   intermediate 57
   purpose of 56
   qualities of 64
   statement of 82
   steps in formulation of 90, 90f
Educational philosophy 34, 35, 37
   functions of 35
Educational psychology 86
Educational quality assurance 23, 26
Educational technology 87
   advantages of 248
   and audiovisual aids 253, 254t
   characteristics of 247
   development of 98, 245
   general objectives of 247
   hardware approach 246
   macro-level objectives of 247
   scope of 248
   significance of 249
   software approach 246
   systems approach 246
   types of 246
Educational webinars 220
Educative process 11
   components and characteristics of 11
   integral part of 8
   revise 8
Effective classroom management, strategies for 230
Effective communication 235, 374
   bilateral 374
   both verbal and nonverbal 374
   in clinical area 375
   in nursing practice, principles of 374
   involves conflict resolution 374
   requires accuracy 374
   requires active listening 374
   requires understanding of 375
   techniques 369
Effective evaluation, principles for 279
Effective feedback
   characteristics of 164
   educative in nature 164
   focuses on future 165
   goal oriented 165

Effective learning initiated by learner 112
Effective questioning, key factors for 159
Effective teaching 233
   characteristics of 153
   learning methods, user of 160
Elicit feedback 371
   from students 171
Embrace boredom, failure to 117
Emergence of
   democratic and student-centered campus 27
   individual teaching unit 23
   new specialities 27
Emergency remote teaching 212
Emotion, components of 133
Emotional
   climate 154
   intelligence and learning 131
Emotions 371
   and learning 132
   characteristics of 133
   in learning, impact of 133
Empathy 380
Empowerment, concept of 386
Enables personalized learning 124
Enabling process 317
Encourage students 165
Encouraging collaboration 217
Encouraging leadership and adaptability 139
Energy and time, saving of 260
Enhanced physical literacy 131
Enhanced student status 27
Entrepreneurship
   aim 26
   curriculum 79
Environment 111
   and learning 137
   issues 116
Epistemology deals 34
Equal opportunity, principle of 229
Essay questions
   advantages and limitations of 301
   forms and uses of 300
Essay tests 300
   suggestions for 301
Establish realistic communication goals 237
Establishing supportive learning culture 138
Esthetics 34
Ethical decision making 356
   factors influencing 357
   steps in 357
Ethical standards for students 358
Ethics
   and evidence-based nursing education 355
   branches of 355
   review 355
Evaluation 60, 275, 276
   academic and nonacademic subjects 279
   and revising of educative process 8f
   assessment 276
   characteristics of 279
   clinical process 312

components of 276
continuous comprehensive 285
functions of 280
general principles of 278
objective-based 280
observation 286
principle of 258
procedure for improving product 279
purpose oriented 279
purposes in nursing education 280
service 333
steps in 286
techniques 278
    and tools of 286
    proper use of 278
tool/characteristics of 305
types of 282
Evidence-based education
advantages of 359
application of 360
Evidence-based teaching in nursing 221
Evolving roles, preparation for 25, 29
Experience, principle of 46
Experiential learning 122
preference to 21
Experiential theory 115
Experimental pragmatism 44
Explanation 156
Explicitness 156
Exploitation phase 374
Extrinsic motivation 134

## F

Facilitates learning 238
Facilitators
and barriers of communication 367
of classroom communication 237
of communication 371
of learning 235
Faculty evaluator, role of 312*b*
Family issues and instability 136
Family problems 116
Feasible and achievable 64
Feedback
appropriate 138
importance of 164
in teaching-learning process 164
providing 191
Final output, assessment of 281
Finalizing curriculum 84
Financial guidance 330
Financial issues 116
Finnish model of education 21
Flash cards 269
Flexibility 221
principle of 229
Flip charts 264
Flipped classroom 219, 223, 251
Focused attention, lack of 116
Focusing behavior 156
Foreign universities, presence of 23

Formal and nonformal education, difference of 18*t*
Formal nursing education 211
Formative and summative evaluation, difference 284*t*
Formative evaluation 282
characteristics of 282
Formulating educational objectives, data required for 89
Fostering motivation 138
Fosters participant democracy 12
Framing question 157
Freedom and responsibility 50
Fruitful learning 7

## G

Gamification 253
Generosity error 290
Geographical consideration 196
Global nurses 25
preparation of 26
Globalization, continuous experience 27
God's gift 14
Good achievement test 305
Good audiovisual aids, characteristics of 260
Good behavioral objective
clear and understandable 65
explain learning outcomes 65
observable 65
stated in a time bound manner 65
student centered 65
Good classroom environment, creator of 160
Good counselor, qualities of 339, 340*t*
Good interpersonal relationship 233
Good learning experience, characteristics of 91
Good nurse educator, qualities of 166
Good observation, requisites of 287
Good quality programs 251
Good relationship with students 137
Good teaching 149, 150
qualities of 148, 159, 160*f*
marks of 148
Good unit, characteristics of 101
Governing rating scales, principle of 291
Grapevine 371
Graphic rating scale 289
Group conference 201
Group dynamics 382
Grouping learning 93
Groups and individuals 382
Guidance 315, 334
aims of 323
Guidance and counseling 315
bases of 319
    pedagogical 320
    philosophical 319
    psychological 319
    sociological 319
differentiation of 318
functions of 320
in nursing education 322
need of 321
personnel 334
purposes of 321

services 330
    basic concepts related to 342
    organization of 341, 343
Guidance areas 325
Guidance, characteristics of 316
Guidance committee 342
Guidance, concept of 315
Guidance, definition of 316
Guidance, functions of teachers 334
Guidance, principles of 323
Guidance program 201
Guidance services, organization of 343
Guided response 62
Guidelines for
    preparing test designs 308
    selection and practice of teaching–learning methods 167
Guiding techniques, discussion 178

## H

Halo effect 290
Handling assignments 154
Handouts, preparation of 267
Happiness curriculum, concept of 98
Harmonious development 15, 24
    of individual 45
Hay McBer model of teacher effectiveness 161, 161f
Health and emotional problems 116
Health behavior and health education 384
Health education 383
    for groups 386
    for individuals 385
    medical model of 384f
    with communities 386
Health guidance 329
    in nursing education 329
Health promotion 384f
Health universities, inadequate representation in 29
Healthcare delivery system, recent trends in 98
Healthcare professions, new generation 29
Healthy society 377
High tech-high touch 193
Higher abilities, development of 260
Higher motivation for learning 132
Higher studies, increased opportunities for 27
Highly structured lesson plan 106f
High-tech high-touch approach 24
    emphasis on 26
    in teaching 139, 239
Honest communication 236
Human instincts, redirection of 43
Human relations 379
    in context of nursing 383
    skill in nursing 380
    understanding self 380
Humanistic existentialism 50
Humanistic pragmatism 44
Humanistic realism 47
Humanistic theory 115
Hunting knowledge 169
Hybrid learning 251

## I

Idealism 37
    and aims of education 39
    and curriculum 40
    and discipline 40
    and methods of teaching 40
    and teacher 41
    principles of 38
Identify 237
Immersive learning 253
Impressions 370
Individual 10, 15
    and groups 382
    background 371
    conference 201
    perfect development of 43
Inductive teaching 156
Informal education 17
Information service 331
Information, related barriers 372
Innate potential 7
Innovative distance education programs 28
Innovative teaching methods in nursing 222
    types of 222
Institutional curriculum 80
Instructional design 22
Integrated lecture 222
Integration 83
    and correlation, principle of 85
    principle of 46, 47
Intellectual aim 14
Interaction
    changing 156
    classification based on 211
Interactive online teaching 211
Interdisciplinary communication, opportunity for 196
Interest 82
    principle of 46
Internal assessment 312
International understanding 15
Interpersonal relationship 376
    in nursing
        importance of 378
        purposes of 378
    meaning 376
    phases of 379
    purposes of 377
    relationship quotient 377
    types of 378
    with students 166
Intervention 338
Intrinsic motivation 134
Inventive and creative powers, development of 39
Issues in guidance program 344
Issues in nursing education 28
Items, construction of 308

## J

Job market, changes in 20
Journaling 126
Judicious use of resources 57

## K

Kinesthetic 129
  learners 129
Knowledge 195
  and skill aim 24
  explosion and scientific advancements 87
  lack of 322
  of terminology 296
  outcomes, measure 296
  structured 169
Kolb's experiential learning model 123f

## L

Language barriers 372
Lawton's cultural analysis model 72
Leadership aim 25
Leadership and coordination 343
Learnability 82
Learner 111, 145, 211
  celebrate achievement of 138
Learner-centered
  education 6
  methods 167
  objectives 65
  principles of teaching 147
Learner, characteristics of 211
Learner, engagement of 124
Learner, enhancing intrinsic motivation of 135
Learner, level of 4, 196
Learner, types of 129
  auditory 130
  kinesthetic 130
  reading and writing 130
  visual 130
Learning 109
  active, democratic and socialization process 7
  activities 112
  adaptation or adjustment 113
  analytics 253
  approaches to 119
  assessment of 8, 250
  both cognitive and emotional 110, 113
  brings behavioral changes 113
  by doing 43
  change in behavior 110
  characteristics of 110
  collaborative 112
  consequence of experience 112
  content 28
  context dependent 110, 113
  continuous 113
  determinants of 127
  dynamic and changes over time 110, 113
  education 112
  environment 136, 362
    safe 123
  evolutionary process 111
  experience 255, 255f
    direct 255
    in total curriculum, placement of 94
    organization of 83, 92
    selection of 91, 92, 92t
    symbolic 255
    vicarious 255
  factors influencing 111, 112f
  fundamental process of life 111
  future of 122
  growth and development 113
  helps in achieving teaching objectives 111
  highly unique and individual 112
  interactive 110, 113
  Kimble's definition 109
  lifelong process 110
  management systems 219
  materials, low quality 241
  nature of 113
  needs 128
  new areas of 169
  nursing
    definition of 139
    principles of 140
  objectives, series of 145
  principle of 47, 111
  proactive role in 24
  process of progress and development 111
  purposeful and goal oriented 111
  relationship between stimulus and response 111
  styles 129
    combination of 130
  systematic organization of experiences 111
  theories 113
  timetable availability 221
  to be 10
  to do 10
  to know 10
  to live together 10
  transferable 111
  types of 117
    chaining 118
    concept 118
    discrimination 118
    problem-based 119
    rule 118
    selection of 119
    signal learning 117
    stimulus-response learning 117
    verbal association 118
  universal process 110
  using learning management systems 219
  with technology 250
Lecture
  concept mapping-based 223
  interactive 173
  purposes of 169
  training for 85
Lecture method 169
  advantages of 172
  disadvantages of 172
Lecturing techniques 170
Lesson planning 103, 105, 106
  criteria of 104
  principles of 104

purposes of 103
steps in 104
Limitations and demerits 287
Liquid crystal display 269
Listening and responding 159
Logical 64
error 291
Loosely structured lesson plan 105f
Loyalties, principle of 85

## M

Man's existence 50
Management skills 154
Managing human resources 227
Managing material resources 228
Managing stress 380
Mass media 369
using 387
Massive open online courses 5
use of 220
Master plan for curriculum, preparation of 93
Mastery
develop 148
of competencies 160
Matching item 299
Materialistic world 38
Maximum performance evaluation 284
Measurement 276
function 281
Mechanism 62
Meeting individual differences 260
Mental and emotional development 15
Merits of
chalkboard 262
direct observation 286
objective type tests 299
Meta ethics 356
Meta learning 125
Metaphysics 34
Methods level of students 168
Methods suit to teacher's style 168
Methods to overcome
background barriers 373
barriers to communication 372
information related barriers 372
language barriers 373
physical barriers 372
psychological barriers 373
Methods used creatively 168
Microteaching 188
demerits of 191
merits of 191
phases, activities and components of 189
setting, creation of 190
simple outline of 189
Middle level faculty members, shortage of 29
Mind and spirit 85
Mind, real knowledge in 38
Minutes preceptor model 224
Mistrust 379
Mobile technology 253

Model lesson
criticism of 190
observation of 190
Models 268
Modern education 87
concept of 3f
Modern learning, key concepts of 110
Moral development 14
Moral sense, development of 40
Motivating function 281
Motivation 122
and learning 134
components of 134
principle of 146
types of 134
Motivational impact 133
Multimedia 369
Multiple choice item, characteristics of 294
Multiple choice items, uses of 296
Multiple level entries to profession 28
Multiple-response item 298
Multisensory media 369
Mutual respect, lack of 379

## N

National Accreditation Board for Hospitals and Healthcare 28
National Assessment and Accreditation Council Accreditation 28
Naturalism 41
and aims of education 43
and curriculum 43
and discipline 44
and methods of teaching 43
and teacher 44
different forms of 41
principles of 41
Negative education in early childhood 42
Neorealism 48
Nonverbal
communication 235
cues 376
Normative ethics 355
Norm-referenced evaluation 284
Novice 224
Nurse educator 180b
Nurses learners, huge number of 211
Nursing care 139
conference 200
plan 197, 311
study 198
Nursing curriculum, nature of 74
principles related to development of 85
Nursing education 23, 26, 63, 63b, 98, 326, 360
aims of 24, 24f, 53
basis of 1
classification of achievement tests 293fc
maintaining autonomy of 30
nonformal 17, 211
promote democratic approaches in 26
Nursing etiquette, contemporary expectations of 370

## 412  Index

Nursing in health care, safeguard role of 25
Nursing rounds 200
Nursing universities, establishment of 28

## O

Objective test 292
Objective type tests, limitations of 299
Objectives, meaningful statement of 65
Observable 64
Observation
   and experimentation 43
   proper execution of 287
   proper planning of 287
   recording of 287
Observational learning 122
   processes of 122
Occupational information 332
Online collaborative learning 220
Online content, classification based on 211
Online education 206
   fully 251
Online learning 218
   and teaching methods 219
   increasing student engagement in 218
Online teaching 211
   advantages of 215
   assessment in 216
   challenges of 216
   classification of 211
   disadvantages of 215
   evaluation of 214
   implementation of 213
   in nursing education 211
   linear 212
   principles of 212
   steps in conducting 213
Open educational resources 251
Opportunities for students 221
Optimum learning 124
Oral examination, forms of 304
Oral examinations 304
Organization 61
   forms of 341
Organizers, role of 181
Organizing learning experiences 93
   elements of 93
Orientation service 330
Orientational 320
Oriented to life 6
Origination 62
Output, maximization of 282
Overhead projector 262
   advantages of 264

## P

Parental habits and involvement 136
Participatory approach 20
Past experiences 371
Pausing and pacing 159
Pedocentric 20
Peer relationships 136

Peplau's interpersonal relations theory 373
Perception 62
Perception barriers 241
Performance criteria 66
Personal attributes, principle of 229
Personal bias errors 290
Personal communication strengths 237
Personal guidance 327
   in nursing education 327
Personal qualities 166
Personality 136
Personal-social development, evaluating 290
Personal-social information 332
Philosophy 33
   and aims of education 36
   and curriculum 36
   and education 33
   and methods of teaching 36
   branches of 34
   of nursing education 51, 86
   of nursing education, factors influencing 52
   of teacher 37
Physical barriers 240, 372
Physical control, principle of 258
Physical factors 196
Physical health 14
Physical literacy 15
Pitching and putting clearly 159
Placement service 332
Planning achievement test 307
Planning assignments 203
Planning curriculum, elements in 80, 80f
Planning for health education 385, 385f
Planning online teaching 213
Play-way method 43
Polite language, use 231
Positive learning environment, characteristics of 137
Positive student-teacher interaction 8
Positive thinking, promotion of 377
Posters 269
Practical examinations 305
Practical guidelines for
   classroom management 234
   conducting online teaching 214
   discipline 353
Practical information 370
Practice, communities of 220
Pragmatism 44
   and aims of education 45
   and curriculum 46
   and discipline 47
   and methods of teaching 46
   and teacher 47
   definition of 44
   forms of 44
   principles of 44
Prediction 281
Predictive validity 305
Preparation for life, principle of 84
Preparatory assignments 203

Present-day learners, characteristics of 130
Preventive discipline 350, 351
Proactive apex bodies 27
Problem-solving 127
    skills, develop 177
Procedure evaluation 290
Process 376
Product evaluation 290
Profession 378
Professional attitudes 195
Professional competence 166
Professional decision maker 160
Professional development 25
Professional incompetence 379
Professionalism 380
Proficient 224
Proforma for lesson plan 105
Prognosis 281
Program, appraisal of 342
Progressive learning, principle of 47
Promising career 27
Promote collaborative learning 362
Promoting collaboration 137
Psychological barriers 372
Psychological factors 239
Psychological impact 133
Psychomotor domain 61
Publishing curriculum 84
Pupils, types of 190

## Q

Quality conscious institutions 28
Questioning
    common errors in 159
    functions of 157

## R

Rating scales 288
    numerical 288
    types of 288
    uses of 290
Readiness
    and motivation, principle of 366
    to learn 128
Reading 129
Realism 47
    and aims of education 48
    and curriculum 48
    and discipline 49
    and methods of teaching 49
    and teacher 49
    forms of 47
    principles of 48
Realistic high-tech procedural simulators 184
Refeedback session 191
Reflection in learning, importance of 124
Reflective learning 124
Reflective student, learning how to learn 125
Reflective teacher 162
    characteristics of 162

Reinforcement 113
    of behavior 145
Relatedness 135
Relationship and roles 371
Relationship-based education 16, 17
Relationship management 132
Relationship philosophy and education 34
Relevance 98
    to life 83
Relevant 64
    knowledge, skills and attitude 139
Reliability 306
Reliance on technology 26
Remedial
    assignments 203
    service 333
Remembering 63
Remembering and forgetting 140
Replanning session 191
Reproduction 122
Research orientation 98
Research, promoting 25
Research service 333
Resolution phase 374
Resource unit 102
Resources
    for learning, combination of 130
    sharing of 30
Responding 61
Response, principle of 258
Responsibility and authority, allocation of 342
Restricted response questions 300
Restructuring traditional programs 23
Reteaching session 191
Retention 122
Revelation technique 263
Revision and practice, principle of 147
Revisional assignments 203
Role model 161
    for students 196
    principle of 229
Role playing 184, 188
Rotation plan, types of 96

## S

Safe and effective learning environment 228
Safeguarding nursing 29
    profession 29
Sample evaluation strategies 311*t*
Scenario-based learning 120
Scheme for evaluation, preparation of 309
Scoring essay questions, suggestions for 303
Secularism and socialism, principle of 85
Selecting appropriate media 252
Selecting course content, principle of 100
Selection 281
    and statement of objectives 89
    of appropriate technology and media 8
    of assessment strategies 83
    of content 82
    of learning experiences 82, 90

of particular teaching skill 190
of subject matter 82
principle of 147, 256
Self-actualization 54
Self-assessment techniques 313
Self-awareness 132
types of 380
Self-control, principle of 229
Self-directed learning 139, 362
Self-discipline 350
Self-education 44
aim 15
Self-effort 44
Self-esteem of students, improve 235
Self-evaluation 161
Self-expression 43
Self-knowledge 50
and self-directive 343
Self-management 132
Self-preservation 43
Self-realization 14, 39
Self-reporting techniques 313
Self-sufficiency 82
Semantic barriers 240
Seminar 180, 181
and symposium, difference 183t
meaning 181
Seminar, role of
chairperson 182
different personnel 181
participants 182
speakers 182
Seminar technique 182
Sense realism 48
Sequence 83, 159
of stimulus-response situations 145
Service sector 29
Set 62
high expectations 139
Setting and implementing rules 233
Setting goals 338
Setting learner-friendly objectives 67
Severity error 290
Sharing and interaction, principle of 366
Shifting sensory channels 156
Short-answer item, uses of 293
Simplicity 156, 343
Simulations
advantages of 187
based learning 120
disadvantages of 187
exercise 184
game 184
meaning 184
preferred method of teaching 27
purposes of 185
role of teacher 186
types of 184
value of 185
Skills 195
acquisition phase 190

acquisition, Dreyfus model of 224
aim over knowledge aim, dominance of 27
discussion 179
of explanation 155
of promoting student participation 155
of reinforcement 155
of stimulus variation 155
of using examples 155
practice of 191
questioning 155
Slides 267
Small group methods 167
Smart attributes 67
Smart learning environment 253
Social aim 13, 25
Social awareness 132
Social behavior and nursing practice 381
Social discipline 47
Social efficiency 46
Social guidance 328
in nursing education 329
Social harmony 378
Social impact 134
Social media
overuse of 117
promoting judicious use of 30
Social personality, formation of 12
Social realism 48
Social realities, consistent with 82
Social sensitivity 236
Societal curriculum 80
Society 86
Soft skills
consideration to 28
development of 26
Solving technical difficulties 217
Sound psychological principles 168
Space and territory 371
Specialization 343
Speech patterns, changes in 156
Spiritual values, cultivation of 40
Staff nurses 29
Standard 66
Standardized communication tools 375
Standardized patient examination 311
State precise responsibility 371
Status, conferring of 12
Stenhouse's process model 72
Stimulus variation 155
Stress management 132
Structuring 159
Struggle for existence 43
Student
academic progress of 235
assessment of 161
behavior 66
modification of 235
centric teaching-learning process 25
counseling
problems in 339
purposes of 335

Index  415

faculty relationship 361
    elements of 361
    information service 331
    motivation generates 148
    motivation, factors affect 135
    prior knowledge 147
    student relationship 239
    support 231
    teachers, orientation of 190
Study assignments 203
Subject-centered objectives 65
Subject matter, in-depth knowledge of 160
Suitability 83
    of message, principle of 366
Summative evaluation 283
    characteristics of 283
Supernaturalism 49
Support student-centered 362
Supportive discipline 351
Syllabus and curriculum 97
Symposium 183
    disadvantages of 184
    role of different personnel 183
    technique 183
Synchronous online teaching 211
Synthesis 60

**T**

Tactile learners 129
Teachable moments 165
Teacher 54, 145
    and students 237
        inappropriate behavior of 239
    awareness 161, 163, 237
    behavior 136
        principle of 229
    centered classroom environment 239
    centered objectives 65
    clarity 154
    ensure accessibility to 236
    enthusiasm 153
    expectations 153, 161, 162
    feedback 154
    movements 156
    observational skill 154
    performance, assessment of 251
    preparation 238
    professional growth of 236
    role of 20, 42
    student interaction 162
Teaching and learning 221, 360
    innovation in 23, 26
    nursing in digital age 206
    quality, improve 362
Teaching brain's 163
Teaching community settings 224
Teaching, context of 164
Teaching, different modes of 131
Teaching effectiveness 222, 360
Teaching in systematic manner 57
Teaching ineffectives 241

Teaching learning process 20, 143, 144, 145, 166, 167, 216, 229, 235, 238
Teaching, maxims of 150
Teaching, meaning of 143
Teaching, methods of 54, 136
    classification of 167, 197$t$
    combination of 131
    formulation of 47
Teaching nursing 67, 143, 191
    principles of 192
Teaching, principles of 145
Teaching psychomotor skills 193
Teaching resources, quality of 217
Teaching session 191
Teaching skills 154
    component of 155$t$
    discussion of 190
    integration of 191
Teaching strategies 167
    and interventions 222, 360
Teaching styles 152
    delegating 153
    direction 152
    discussion 153
Teaching system 94
Teaching unit 102
Teaching with models 268
Teaching with technology 250
Team-based learning 126
    key components of 126
Teamwork 382
    promote 236
Technological advancements 87
Technology
    and media 252
    driven teaching process 28
    exerts 22
    in teaching, impact of 251
Termination and follow-up 338
Test
    administration 309
    blueprint for unit on oxygenation 309$t$
    design, developing 307
    organization of 309
Testing 276
Theistic realism 49
    and aims of education 49
    and curriculum 49
    and discipline 49
    and methods of teaching 49
    and teacher 49
Theory and practice 29
Thinking and learning, principles 117, 130
Time management 172
    lack of 117
Time-bound 65
Timely manner, proper intervention in 233
Total education system 281
Transnational acceptance 27
Transparencies, effective use of 263
Treat students fairly 161

Trends in education, factors influencing 19
Trends in educational technology 253
Trends in nursing education 26
True-false item, uses of 294

## U

Understanding 63
    role of teacher 238
    self and nursing practice 381
    self, importance of 381
Unequivocal 64
Uniformity and standardization 27
Unique status for nursing education 28
Unit planning
    elements of 101
    principles of 102
    steps in 102
Unit test, design for 307
Units, types of 101
Universal education 39
Universal mind, presence of 38
Up-skilling through online courses 131
Usability 306
Utilitarian aim 13
Utility 82
    principle of 46

## V

Validity 82
    improve 306
    types of 305
Value based education in nursing 358
Value development 358
    strategies 358
Value education 16
    promotion of 21
Valuing 61
Variety 82
    and flexibility, principle of 85
Verbal communication 235
Virtual reality in education 253
Visual 129
    learners 129
    materials and audiovisual materials 258$t$
    media 369
Vocational aim 13
Vocational guidance 326
Voice gradation 170
Voice quality 170

## W

Webinars by experts 223
Weightage to
    content areas 307
    difficulty level 308
    form of questions 308
    instructional objectives 307
Wholeness 343
Working phase 374
Writing behavioral objectives, advantages of 66
Writing good objectives 66
Writing learners 129
Writing objectives in
    affective domain 61$t$
    cognitive domain 59$t$
Written communication 235

EU GSPR Authorised Reprsentative
Logos Europe, 9 rue Nicolas Poussin
1700, La Rochelle, France
Phone: +33 (0) 6 67 93 73 78
E-mail: contact@logoseurope.eu

www.ingramcontent.com/pod-product-compliance
Ingram Content Group UK Ltd.
Pitfield, Milton Keynes, MK11 3LW, UK
UKHW050456150426

5217IPUK00025B/1707